Universal Access and Assistive Technology

Springer-Verlag London Ltd.

Simeon Keates, Patrick Langdon,
P. John Clarkson and Peter Robinson (Eds.)

Universal Access and Assistive Technology

Proceedings of the Cambridge Workshop on UA and AT '02

With 126 Figures

Springer

Simeon Keates, MA, PhD
Patrick Langdon, BSc, PhD
P. John Clarkson, MA, PhD, MIEE, CEng
University of Cambridge, Department of Engineering, Trumpington Street, Cambridge, CB2 1PZ, UK

Peter Robinson, MA, PhD, FBCS, CEng
University of Cambridge, Computer Laboratory, William Gates Building, JJ Thomson Avenue, Cambridge, CB3 0FD, UK

British Library Cataloguing in Publication Data
Universal access and assistive technology : proceedings of
the Cambridge Workshop on UA and AT '02
1.Self-help devices for the disabled 2.Physically
handicapped - Rehabilitation - Technological innovations
3.User interfaces (Computer systems)
I.Keates, Simeon
617' .03

Library of Congress Cataloging-in-Publication Data
A catalog record for this book is available from the Library of Congress.

ISBN 978-1-4471-3721-4 ISBN 978-1-4471-3719-1 (eBook)
DOI 10.1007/978-1-4471-3719-1

http://www.springer.co.uk

Originally published by Springer-Verlag London Limited in 2002.

Typesetting: Electronic text files prepared by editors

69/3830-543210 Printed on acid-free paper SPIN 10867632

Preface

The first Cambridge Workshop on Universal Access and Assistive Technology (CWUAAT) was held at Trinity Hall, Cambridge, in March 2002. It was inspired by the earlier, highly successful Cambridge Workshops on Rehabilitation Robotics organised by the late Robin Jackson. Robin was the founder of Rehabilitation Research at Cambridge which now continues in the Engineering Design Centre within the Department of Engineering, led by John Clarkson and Simeon Keates, and in the Rainbow Group within the Computer Laboratory led by Peter Robinson.

CWUAAT represents the first in a new series of workshops that we are aiming to hold every two years which, reflecting the spirit of recent moves to extend the rights for universal accessibility, will encourage discussion of a broad range of interests. There will be a general focus on product/solution development. Hence it is intended that the principal requirements for the successful design of assistive technology shall be addressed, where these range from the identification and capture of the needs of the users, through to the development and evaluation of truly usable and accessible systems for users with special needs.

The best submissions received for the first CWUAAT are contained in this book, where the contributors are all leading researchers in the fields of Universal Access and Assistive Technology and represent a large part of the international research community. They include, though not exclusively, computer scientists, designers, engineers, industrial representatives, ergonomists and sociologists.

Universal Access and Assistive Technology have increasingly important roles to play in the future as the global population grows older and many more people exhibit some degree of functional impairment. Hence, there is a need to encourage wide-ranging discussion, co-operation and collaboration within and between the Universal Access and Assistive Technology research communities. Thus one of the principal aims of the first CWUAAT and this book is to promote such discussion.

The book begins with the keynote (Chapter 1) which provides an important commercial perspective on the issues that follow. It is clearly argued that any organisation can aspire to provide substantially better service and employment prospects to the widest possible range of people.

Part I – Design Issues for Universal Access and Assistive Technology – focuses on defining design exclusion (Chapter 2), design evaluation (Chapter 3), approaches to user-centred design (Chapters 4, 5 and 7) and user assessment (Chapter 6).

Part II – Enabling Computer Access and New Technologies – addresses novel input systems (Chapters 8 and 9), access solutions to software and information (Chapters 10 through 14) and the application of new technologies (Chapters 15 through 18).

Part III – Assistive Technology and Rehabilitation Robotics – looks at the specification (Chapter 23) and design (Chapters 24 through 29) of Assistive Technology and a number of examples of Rehabilitation Robotics (Chapters 19 through 22).

In summary, the book provides a snapshot of the best current thinking on Universal Access and Assistive Technology, with 84 contributors from academic, public and commercial institutions spread across four continents.

Finally, our thanks must go to all those who contributed to the success of CWUAAT and to the compilation of this book. Many thanks are due to all the contributors who, with the assistance of the Programme Committee, were responsible for setting the high standards of reporting seen in this book. Particular thanks are also due to Christa Croghan who, with the staff at Trinity Hall, so enthusiastically helped to organise and host the workshop. Finally, our special thanks go to Professor Joanne Coy for an inspiring and thought-provoking keynote and to Consignia for sponsorship of the workshop and the production of this book.

John Clarkson and Simeon Keates
Cambridge Engineering Design Centre
University of Cambridge
March 2002

Contents

List of Contributors xi

Keynote

1. **Commercial Perspectives on Universal Access and Assistive Technology**
   J. Coy 3

Part I Design Issues for Universal Access and Assistive Technology

2. **Defining Design Exclusion**
   S. Keates and P.J. Clarkson 13

3. **Quantifying Design Exclusion**
   P.J. Clarkson and S. Keates 23

4. **Countering Design Exclusion**
   S. Keates and P.J. Clarkson 33

5. **Inclusive Design – Developing Theory Through Practice**
   R.R. Gheerawo and C.S. Lebbon 43

6. **A Systematic Basis for Developing Cognitive Assessment Methods for Assistive Technology**
   R. Adams, P. Langdon and P.J. Clarkson 53

7. **Control of Virtual Environments for People with Intellectual Disabilities**
   P.J. Standen, T.L. Lannen and D.J. Brown 63

Part II Enabling Computer Access and New Technologies

8. Why Are Eye Mice Unpopular? – A Detailed Comparison of Head and Eye Controlled Assistive Technology Pointing Devices
R. Bates and H.O. Istance 75

9. Cursor Characterisation and Haptic Interfaces for Motion-impaired Users
F. Hwang, P. Langdon, S. Keates, P.J. Clarkson and P. Robinson 87

10. Web-based Multimodal Graphs for Visually Impaired People
W. Yu, D. Reid and S. Brewster 97

11. Automatically Rearranging Structured Data for Customised Special-needs Presentations
S.S. Brown and P. Robinson 109

12. Bridging the Education Divide
M. Pieper, H. Morasch and G. Piéla 119

13. Contextual On-line Help: A Contribution to the Implementation of Universal Access
A. Capobianco and N. Carbonell 131

14. 3rd Age Interfaces: A Usability Evaluation of the 'Your Guide' Kiosk Prototype from an Older User's Perspective
R.T.P. Young 141

15. Virtual Environments for the Training of the Visually Impaired
D. Tzovaras, G. Nikolakis, G. Fergadis, S. Malassiotis and M. Stavrakis ... 151

16. User Involvement in the Design of a New Multimedia Communication Service
N. Hine, J.L. Arnott, W. Beattie and P. Sergeant 161

17. Issues Surrounding the User-centred Development of a New Interactive Memory Aid
E. Inglis, A. Szymkowiak, P. Gregor, A.F. Newell, N. Hine, B.A. Wilson and J. Evans 171

18. Games Children with Autism Can Play With Robota, a Humanoid Robotic Doll
K. Dautenhahn and A. Billard 179

Part III Assistive Technology and Rehabilitation Robotics

19. Progress of a Modular Prosthetic Arm
A.S. Poulton, P.J. Kyberd and D. Gow 193

20. Development of a Novel Type Rehabilitation Robotic System KARES II
Z. Bien, D-J. Kim, D.H. Stefanov, J-S. Han, H-S. Park and P-H. Chang 201

21. Improving the Flexibility of an Assistive Robot
M.R. Hillman, N.M. Evans and R.D. Orpwood 213

22. Commercialising Assistive and Therapy Robotics
M.S. Colello and R.M. Mahoney 223

23. Improved Assistive Technology Prescription via Usage Log Analysis
C. Roast, P. O'Neill and M. Hawley 235

24. Virtual Interface Development and Sensor-based Door Navigation for Nonholonomic Vehicles
R.S. Rao, K. Conn, S.H. Jung, J. Katupitiya, T. Kientz, V. Kumar, J. Ostrowski, S. Patel, C.J. Taylor 245

25. An Ergonomic One-handed Wheelchair
L.A. Porter and S. Lesley 257

26. Gathering User Needs in the Development of the POWER-HAND Opening Aid – A Successful Consumer Product for the Wider Market
J. Smith, R. Huxley, M. Topping, S. Alcock and P. Hawkins 267

27. Locomotion Assistance for the Blind
R. Farcy and Y. Bellik 277

28. 'Keep Taking the Medication': Assistive Technology for Medication Regimes in Care Settings
S. Kember, K. Cheverst, K. Clarke, G. Dewsbury, T. Hemmings, T. Rodden and M. Rouncefield 285

29. "I can't talk now" and Other Design Stories: Four Assistive Technologies for People With and Without Disabilities
G. Pullin 295

Index of Contributors 305

List of Contributors

Adams R., The Papworth Trust, Papworth Everard, Cambridge, UK, ray_adams@papworth.org.uk
Alcock S., Centre for Rehabilitation Robotics, Staffordshire University, School of Art and Design, College Road, Stoke-on-Trent, UK, S.A.Alcock@staffs.ac.uk
Arnott J.L., University of Dundee, Department of Applied Computing, Dundee, Scotland, UK, jarnott@computing.dundee.ac.uk
Bates R., Department of Computing Science, De Montfort University, Leicester, UK, rbates@dmu.ac.uk
Beattie W., NCR Financial Solutions Group Ltd., Kingsway West, Dundee, Scotland, UK, beattw@exchange.scotland.ncr.com
Bellik Y., LIMSI-CNRS, B.P. 133, Bât 508, Orsay Cedex, France, bellik@limsi.fr
Bien Z., Department of EECS, KAIST, 373-1 Guseong-Dong, Yuseong-Gu, Daejeon, Republic of Korea, zbien@ee.kaist.ac.kr
Billard A., Computer Science Department, University of Southern California, Hedco Neuroscience Building, 3641 Watt Way, Los Angeles, CA, USA, billard@usc.edu
Brewster S., Department of Computing Science, University of Glasgow, Glasgow Scotland, UK, stephen@dcs.gla.ac.uk
Brown D.J., Department of Computing, Nottingham Trent University, Newton Building, Burton Street, Nottingham, UK, david.brown@ntu.ac.uk
Brown S.S., University of Cambridge Computer Laboratory, William Gates Building, JJ Thomson Avenue, Madingley Road, Cambridge, UK, Silas.Brown@cl.cam.ac.uk
Capobianco A., LORIA, CNRS & INRIA, BP 239, Vandoeuvre-lès-Nancy Cedex, France, Antonio.Capobianco@loria.fr
Carbonell N., LORIA, CNRS & INRIA, BP 239, Vandoeuvre-lès-Nancy Cedex, France, Noelle.Carbonell@loria.fr
Chang P-H., Department of ME, KAIST, 373-1 Guseong-Dong, Yuseong-Gu, Daejeon, Republic of Korea, phchang@mecha.kaist.ac.kr
Cheverst K., Department of Computing, SECAMS Building, Lancaster University, Lancaster, UK, kc@comp.lancs.ac.uk

Clarke K., Department of Computing, SECAMS Building, Lancaster University, Lancaster, UK, k.m.clarke@lancaster.ac.uk

Clarkson P.J., Engineering Design Centre, Department of Engineering, University of Cambridge, Trumpington Street, Cambridge, UK, pjc10@eng.cam.ac.uk

Colello M.S., Applied Resources Corp., 1275 Bloomfield Avenue, Fairfield, NJ, USA, mattsr@appliedresource.com

Conn K., University of Kentucky, Electrical and Computer Engineering, 453 Anderson Hall, Lexington, Ky. 40506-0046, e-mail: krala4444@hotmail.com

Coy J., Consignia, Wheatstone Road, Dorcan, Swindon, UK, joanne.coy@consignia.com

Dautenhahn K., Adaptive Systems Research Group, Department of Computer Science, The University of Hertfordshire, College Lane, Hatfield, UK, K.Dautenhahn@herts.ac.uk

Dewsbury G., Department of Computing, SECAMS Building, Lancaster University, Lancaster, UK, g.dewsbury@lancaster.ac.uk

Evans J., MRC Cognition and Brain Sciences Unit, Box 58, Addenbrooke's Hospital, Cambridge, UK, Jonathan.Evans@POW.lifespan-tr.anglox.nhs.uk

Evans N.M., Bath Institute of Medical Engineering, Wolfson Centre, Royal United Hospital, Bath, UK, N.M.Evans@bath.ac.uk

Farcy R., Laboratoire Aimé Cotton, CNRS, Bat 505, Orsay Cedex, France, rene.farcy@lac.u-psud.fr

Fergadis G., Informatics and Telematics Institute, Center for Research and Technology Hellas, 1st Km Thermi-Panorama Road 57001, Thermi – Thessaloniki, Greece, fergadis@iti.gr

Gheerawo R.R., The Helen Hamlyn Research Centre, Royal College of Art, Kensington Gore, London, UK, rama.gheerawo@rca.ac.uk

Gow D., Bioengineering Unit, Princess Margaret Rose Hospital, Edinburgh, Scotland, UK, gowd@rehabtech.org.uk

Gregor P., Department of Applied Computing, Dundee University, Park Wynd, Dundee, UK, pgregor@computing.dundee.ac.uk

Han J-S., Department of EECS, KAIST, 373-1 Guseong-Dong, Yuseong-Gu, Daejeon, Republic of Korea, pyodori@ctrsys.kaist.ac.kr

Hawkins P., Centre for Rehabilitation Robotics, Staffordshire University, School of Art and Design, College Road, Stoke-on-Trent, UK, RehabRobotics@compuserve.com

Hawley M., Barnsley District General Hospital NHS Trust, Gawber Road, Barnsley, UK, Mark.Hawley@bdgh-tr.trent.nhs.uk

Hemmings T., School of Computer Science & Information Technology, Jubilee Campus, Nottingham, UK, tah@cs.nott.ac.uk

Hillman M.R., Bath Institute of Medical Engineering, Wolfson Centre, Royal United Hospital, Bath, UK, M.R.Hillman@bath.ac.uk

Hine N., University of Dundee, Department of Applied Computing, Dundee, Scotland, UK, nhine@computing.dundee.ac.uk

Huxley R., Rehab Robotics Ltd., Staffordshire University, College Road, Stoke-on-Trent, UK, RehabRobotics@compuserve.com

Hwang F., Engineering Design Centre, Department of Engineering, University of Cambridge, Trumpington Street, Cambridge, UK, fh220@eng.cam.ac.uk

Inglis E., Department of Applied Computing, Dundee University, Park Wynd, Dundee, Scotland, UK, einglis@computing.dundee.ac.uk

Istance H.O., Department of Computing Science, De Montfort University, Leicester, UK, hoi@dmu.ac.uk
Jung S.H., 3401, Walnut Street, Suite 300C, GRASP Laboratory, Philadelphia, PA, USA, sangj@seas.upenn.edu
Katupitiya J., School of Mechanical and Manufacturing Engineering, The University of New South Wales, Sydney, NSW 2052, Australia, j.katupitiya@unsw.edu.au
Keates S., Engineering Design Centre, Department of Engineering, University of Cambridge, Trumpington Street, Cambridge, UK, lsk12@eng.cam.ac.uk
Kember S., Department of Computing, SECAMS Building, Lancaster University, Lancaster, UK, kembers@comp.lancs.ac.uk
Kientz T., 3401, Walnut Street, Suite 300C, GRASP Laboratory, Philadelphia, PA, USA, tkientz@seas.upenn.edu
Kim D-J., Department of EECS, KAIST, 373-1 Guseong-Dong, Yuseong-Gu, Daejeon, Republic of Korea, djkim@mail.kaist.ac.kr
Kumar V., 3401, Walnut Street, Suite 300C, GRASP Laboratory, Philadelphia, PA, USA, kumar@seas.upenn.edu
Kyberd P.J., Cybernetics Department, Reading University, Whiteknights, Reading, UK, p.j.kyberd@reading.ac.uk
Langdon P., Engineering Design Centre, Department of Engineering, University of Cambridge, Trumpington Street, Cambridge, UK, pml24@eng.cam.ac.uk
Lannen T.L., Department of Computing, Nottingham Trent University, Newton Building, Burton Street, Nottingham, UK, tanja.lannen@ntu.ac.uk
Lebbon C.S., The Helen Hamlyn Research Centre, Royal College of Art, Kensington Gore, London, UK, cherie.lebbon@rca.ac.uk
Lesley S., Department of Engineering, University of Cambridge, Trumpington Street, Cambridge, UK, sl2@eng.cam.ac.uk
Mahoney R.M., Rehabilitation Technologies Division, Applied Resources Corp., 1275 Bloomfield Avenue, Fairfield, New Jersey, USA, RMahoney@appliedresource.com
Malassiotis S., Informatics and Telematics Institute, Center for Research and Technology Hellas, 1st Km Thermi-Panorama Road 57001, Thermi – Thessaloniki, Greece, stratos@iti.gr
Morasch H., Fraunhofer Institute FIT, Schloss Birlinghoven, 53754 Sankt Augustin, Germany, morasch@fit.fraunhofer.de
Newell A.F., Department of Applied Computing, Dundee University, Park Wynd, Dundee, Scotland, UK, afn@computing.dundee.ac.uk
Nikolakis G., Informatics and Telematics Institute, Center for Research and Technology Hellas, 1st Km Thermi-Panorama Road 57001, Thermi – Thessaloniki, Greece, gniko@iti.gr
O'Neill P., Barnsley District General Hospital NHS Trust, Gawber Road, Barnsley, UK, Peter.Oneill2@students.shu.ac.uk
Orpwood R.D., Bath Institute of Medical Engineering, Wolfson Centre, Royal United Hospital, Bath, UK, R.D.Orpwood@bath.ac.uk
Ostrowski J., 3401, Walnut Street, Suite 300C, GRASP Laboratory, Philadelphia, PA, USA, jpo@seas.upenn.edu
Park H-S., Department of ME, KAIST, 373-1 Guseong-Dong, Yuseong-Gu, Daejeon, Republic of Korea, james@kaist.ac.kr
Patel S., 3401, Walnut Street, Suite 300C, GRASP Laboratory, Philadelphia, PA, USA, sarangi@seas.upenn.edu

Piéla G., Gutenberg-Schule, Pauluskirchstraße 12, 53757 Sankt Augustin, Germany, gpiela@t-online.de
Pieper M., Fraunhofer Institute FIT, Schloss Birlinghoven, 53754 Sankt Augustin, Germany, michael.pieper@fit.fraunhofer.de
Porter L.A., c/o S. Lesley, Department of Engineering, University of Cambridge, Trumpington Street, Cambridge, UK, lucyabi_porter@hotmail.com
Poulton A.S., Department of Telematics, Faculty of Technology, The Open University, Milton Keynes, UK, a.s.poulton@open.ac.uk
Pullin G., IDEO London, White Bear Yard, 144a Clerkenwell Road, London, UK, gpullin@ideo.com
Rao R.S., 3401, Walnut Street, Suite 300C, GRASP Laboratory, Philadelphia, PA, USA, rahulrao@seas.upenn.edu
Reid D., Department of Computing Science, University of Glasgow, Glasgow, Scotland, UK, reiddh@dcs.gla.ac.uk
Roast C., Sheffield Hallam University, Sheffield, UK, c.r.roast@shu.ac.uk
Robinson P., University of Cambridge Computer Laboratory, William Gates Building, JJ Thomson Avenue, Madingley Road, Cambridge, UK, Peter.Robinson@cl.cam.ac.uk
Rodden T., School of Computer Science & Information Technology, Jubilee Campus, Nottingham, UK, tar@cs.nott.ac.uk
Rouncefield M., Department of Computing, SECAMS Building, Lancaster University, Lancaster, UK, m.rouncefield@lancaster.ac.uk
Sergeant P., University of Dundee, Department of Applied Computing, Dundee, Scotland, UK, psergeant@computing.dundee.ac.uk
Smith J., Centre for Rehabilitation Robotics, Staffordshire University, School of Art and Design, College Road, Stoke-on-Trent, UK, J.K.Smith@staffs.ac.uk
Standen P.J., Learning Disabilities, Division of Rehabilitation and Ageing, ADRU, B Floor Medical School, QMC, Clifton Boulevard, Nottingham, UK, p.standen@nottingham.ac.uk
Stavrakis M., Informatics and Telematics Institute, Center for Research and Technology Hellas, 1st Km Thermi-Panorama Road 57001, Thermi – Thessaloniki, Greece, modestos@iti.gr
Stefanov D.H., Department of EECS, KAIST, 373-1 Guseong-Dong, Yuseong-Gu, Daejeon, Republic of Korea, stefanov@ctrsys.kaist.ac.kr
Szymkowiak A., Department of Applied Computing, Dundee University, Park Wynd, Dundee, Scotland, UK, andrea@computing.dundee.ac.uk
Taylor C.J., 3401, Walnut Street, Suite 300C, GRASP Laboratory, Philadelphia, PA, USA, cjtaylor @seas.upenn.edu
Topping M., Rehab Robotics Ltd., Staffordshire University, College Road, Stoke-on-Trent, UK, RehabRobotics@compuserve.com
Tzovaras D., Informatics and Telematics Institute, Center for Research and Technology Hellas, 1st Km Thermi-Panorama Road 57001, Thermi – Thessaloniki, Greece, Dimitrios.Tzovaras@iti.gr
Wilson B.A., MRC Cognition and Brain Sciences Unit, Box 58, Addenbrooke's Hospital, Cambridge, UK, barbara.wilson@mrc-cbu.cam.ac.uk
Young R.T.P., Consignia, 148 Old Street, London, UK, richard.t.young@consignia.com
Yu W., Department of Computing Science, University of Glasgow, Glasgow, Scotland, UK, rayu@dcs.gla.ac.uk

Keynote

Commercial Perspectives

Chapter 1

Commercial Perspectives on Universal Access and Assistive Technology

J. Coy

1.1 Introduction

Consignia is the largest supplier of UK mail services, the largest retailer in Europe, and employs some 220,000 people. Post Offices offer a wide range of services including pensions, benefit payments, bill payments, government services and an increasing number of financial and banking services. Moreover, in many rural communities, Post Offices provide the only shop within reasonable distance and provide a real point of community exchange and focus. In order for such an organisation to thrive in the coming years, the dynamics of the population it serves and employs must be a prime consideration.

The demographics of Europe indicate that over the next twenty years the population will age considerably: by 2020, half of the working population will be over 50 and the over 80s are the fastest growing population sector (Ballabio, 1998; Coleman, 1993). The implications for all employers and service providers are clear: it makes simple commercial sense to ensure that work, information and services are made more accessible.

Technology and design must be recognised as pivotal in developing a strategy for meeting these needs. Advances in systematic design methodologies, sensors, computing power, computational linguistics etc. are now showing what could be possible: it is a realistic aspiration to provide substantially better service and employment prospects to an older and wider range of people.

This chapter outlines the reasons why Consignia regards accessibility of services and employment as so important. Although Consignia is used as a basis for these arguments, they remain essentially valid for the majority of service providers and employers accordingly.

1.2 Access to Services

1.2.1 Legal Imperatives

The Disability Discrimination Act 1995 (DDA, 1995) is clear in its stipulation, from 2004, service providers will also have to make "reasonable adjustments" to the physical features of their premises to overcome physical barriers to access.

The DDA Code of Practice (DDA COP, 1999) states that reasonable adjustments include an obligation to:

> *'provide an **auxiliary aid or service** if it would enable (or make it easier for) disabled people to make use of services.'*
>
> (Section 4.5, DDA Code of Practice, 1990)

Moreover, it is stated:

> *'It is more likely to be reasonable for a service provider with substantial financial resources to have to make an adjustment with a significant cost than for a service provider with fewer resources. The resources available to the service provider as a whole are likely to be taken into account as well as other calls on those resources. Where the resources of the service provider are spread across more than one business unit or profit centre, the calls on them all are likely to be taken into account in assessing reasonableness.'*
>
> (Section 4.1.2, DDA Code of Practice, 1990)

The COP, defines auxiliary aids; stating that technological solutions are a way forward in facilitating aid:

> *'An auxiliary aid or service might be the provision of a special piece of equipment or simply extra assistance to disabled people from (perhaps specially trained) staff. In some cases a technological solution might be available.'*
>
> (Section 5.17, DDA Code of Practice, 1990)

Further, the COP states that the duty for provision is ongoing; it is necessary to undertake a programme of continuous development, and it is expected that technology will be used in improving provisions (Section 4.9, DDA COP, 1990).

The combined effect of these stipulations implies that a large organisation such as Consignia is expected to exceed the efforts of most organisations. Where facilitating access to a service may involve the application of auxiliary aids; it is expected that larger organisations will commit to a higher level of provision and thus more investment in such aids. The interpretation of 'reasonableness' is also dependent upon prior art; if one Service provider has implemented a solution, the others are, to some extent legally obliged to follow.

1.2.2 Commercial Incentives

The focus has to be achieving the widest possible customer base and therefore upon improving accessibility for people with single major disabilities and people with multiple minor disabilities. The demographic trends in the UK and Europe are worthy of consideration. The population is ageing: studies show that by 2021 half the adult population in the UK will be over 50 (Coleman, 1993). European studies show that by 2020, 25% of the European population will be over 60 years old, compared with 18% in 1990. The largest growing age sector are the over 80s which currently constitute 3% of the population: this figure will double over the next 20 years which means that there will be 18 million over-80s in Europe (Ballabio, 1998). Thus, it is reasonable to anticipate that older people will become an increasingly significant part of the customer base of all service providers. Moreover, it is known that increased age is linked to increasing physical functional limitation, the relationship is illustrated in Figure 1.1 (Vanderheiden, 1990):

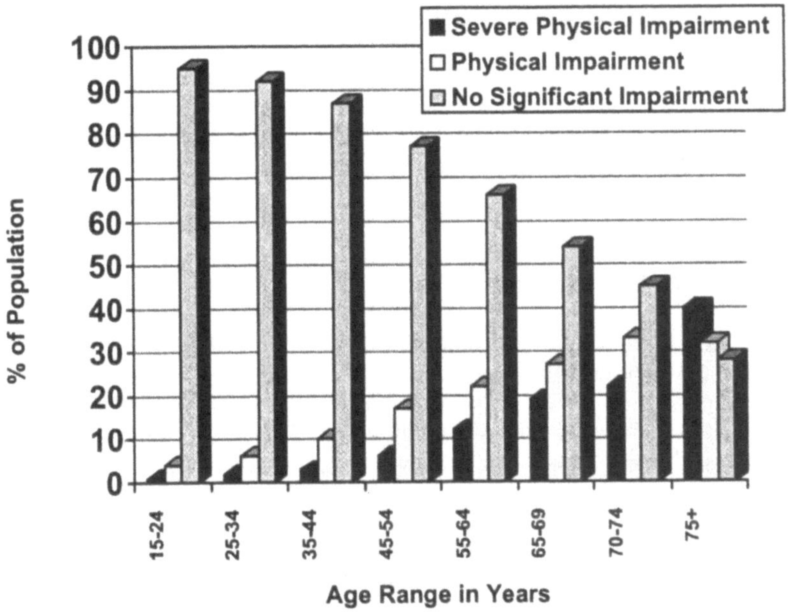

Figure 1.1. Physical impairment as a function of age

In order to thrive as a provider of services, services must be delivered in a way that is cost effective. Moreover, the UK government (a major customer of Consignia) are specifically demanding that their services be accessed electronically. Inevitably, exclusively personal service cannot be viewed as a viable option: it is clear that technology must be employed to deliver the services. These coincident drivers lead to an inevitable conclusion regarding the increasing importance of universal design and assistive technology. In the provision of services, technology provides the opportunity , not merely to maintain quality of service, but to extend and enhance it in a way that has not previously been possible: Consignia is active in developing multimodal interfaces such as the Personal Information Point (Coy *et al.*, 2001), computational linguistics and image generation techniques such as avatars, thus giving opportunities for ensuring that information and transactions can be conveyed in a wide range of accessible formats. Obviously, internet applications such as electronic to physical mail and e-stamps are viewed as a means of bringing more services into people's homes. However, where transactions and information are to be delivered in public spaces (such as Post Offices) the environment imposes further restrictions and requirements for robustness and careful consideration; e.g. speech and aural media can become problematic in a noisy retail space. Further constraints are imposed by floor space return requirements and achieving an integrated functional flow-through in the retail and transaction area (Coy *et al.*, 2001).

1.3 Access to Employment

Caveat: Whilst Consignia has a slightly higher incidence than the general population of post accident trauma and conditions relating to restricted movement (such as arthritis), the statistics quoted within this section of the chapter are unlikely to be at considerable variance with those of other large companies in the UK.

1.3.1 Legal Imperatives

In the U.K., the Disability Discrimination Act (DDA, 1995) and equivalent acts such as the Americans with Disabilities Act (ADA, 1990) place clear requirements upon employers to make adjustments to the workplace in order to create opportunities for people with disabilities. The DDA stipulates that for major employers, the workforce shall include some 3% of employees with physical impairments and that the workplace must not present unnecessary obstacles to employment opportunities. More specifically, the DDA requires that where any physical feature of premises occupied by the employer, or any arrangements made by or on behalf of the employer, cause a substantial disadvantage to a disabled person compared with non-disabled people, an employer has to take such steps as it is reasonable for him to have to take in all the circumstances to prevent that disadvantage - in other words the employer has to make "reasonable adjustments" (DDA COP, 1999).

1.3.2 Commercial Incentives

Simply, failure to recruit people with disabilities and to provide an accessible workplace is to deprive an organisation of a pool of talent and skills which could otherwise be of great benefit. But failure to provide an accessible workplace also results in both a loss of staff who develop physical impairments during the course of their careers and long periods of absence from the workplace during recovery from illness or injury; this is where significant costs are incurred. Figure 1.2 shows how many Consignia employees retire on medical grounds on an annual basis.

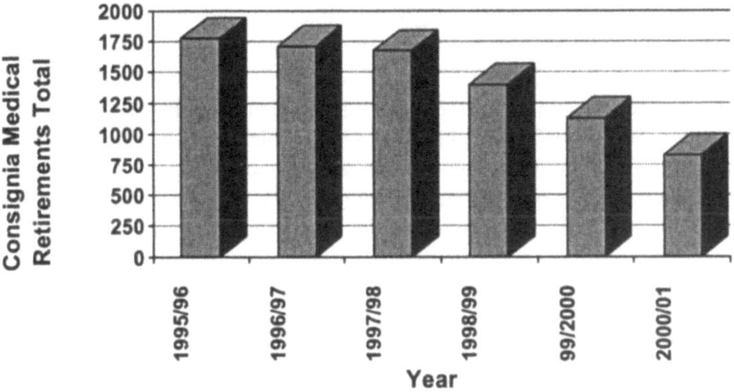

Figure 1.2. Consignia medical retirements total

The costs of pension fund contributions and administration amount to some £80k per person; the annual cost of early retirement on medical grounds has exceeded £120million. This figure does not include the costs of recruitment and training to re-fill the vacant posts. An analysis of these people and their conditions to ascertain the potential for re-deployment is shown in Figure 1.3. It is clear that substantial savings could be made if the workplace was more accessible to the people of categories 1, 2 and 3. However, the costs of early medical retirement are significantly superseded by those of long term absence; the costs to Consignia per annum are currently between £160-£200 million. Technology for rehabilitation and flexible working could clearly provide substantial benefits.

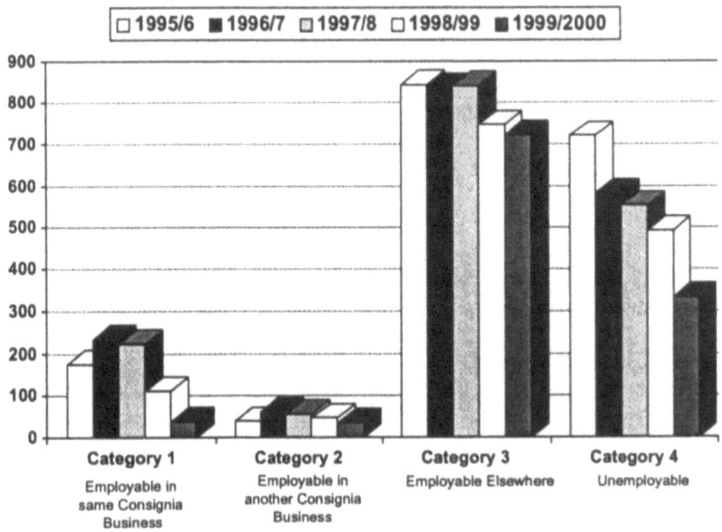

Figure 1.3. Consignia medical retirements by category

Employers may also benefit from considering a direct policy of employing more older and disabled people; it is well established in Consignia that they are make better employees. Consignia statistics consistently show that older employees take less sickness leave than their younger colleagues. Figure 1.4 shows the absences per 1000 staff over the past year, which is not exceptional. These statistics show, that providing appropriate workplace adjustments can be made to accommodate the needs of older people (Figure 1.1), employers could benefit from a significant impact that can be made on the substantial costs of absences.

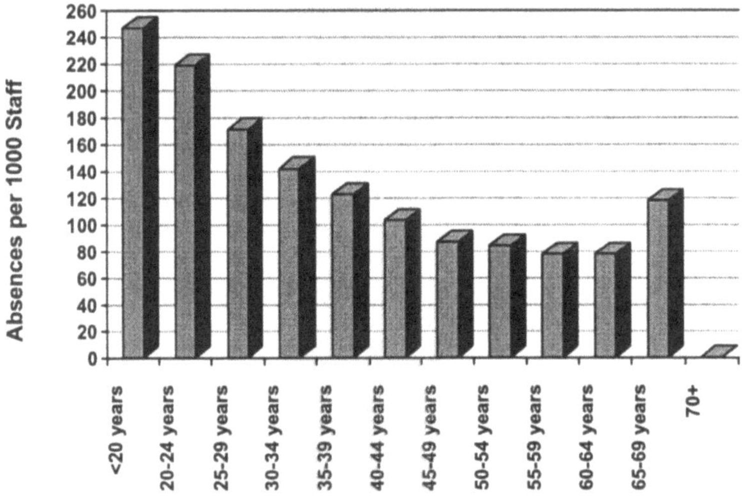

Figure 1.4. Consignia absences per 1000 staff against age group

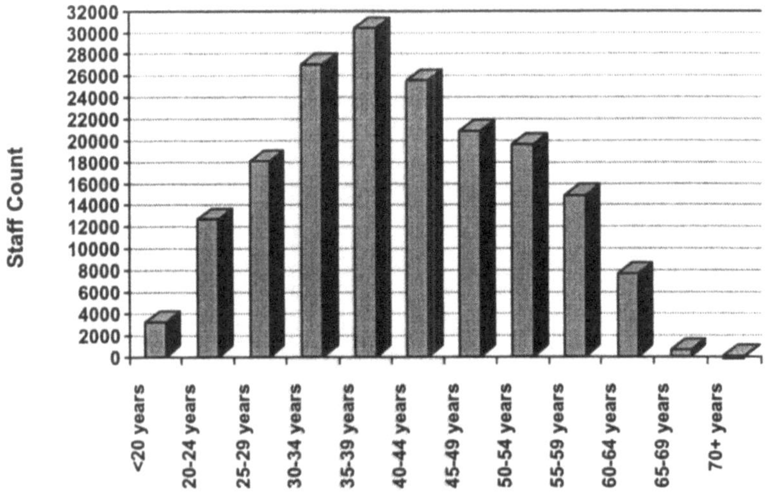

Figure 1.5. Consignia staff count against age

Figure 1.5 shows the age profile of Consignia's workforce. Despite their reliability, the over 50's still account for less than one quarter of the workforce. Demographic drivers aside, it is clear that there are gains to be accrued by employing and retaining more people in this age bracket where possible.

A remarkably similar effect can be seen in the employment of people with disabilities; it is established among employers that they show a higher level of commitment which is manifest in a reduced tendency to take time off and remain loyal to the company.

1.3.3 Technical Requirements

Accessibility of work encompasses:

- Accessibility of the workplace itself;
- Accessibility of the work tasks;
- Accessibility of procedures and information.

As the first of these aspects of accessibility is well accommodated by most employers, it is the latter two that concern us for the purpose of this chapter.

Ideally, the accessibility of work tasks should be considered at the specification stage, and decisions based upon real data regarding the intended user group (e.g. ADULTDATA, 1998) and well considered user performance models (Card, Moran and Newell, 1983). However in IT/computing related tasks, in reality, many organisations have a significant proportion of legacy systems, and therefore objective accessibility assessment procedures, veneers and retrospective adaptation also have an essential function (Coy, Keates and Clarkson, 2001). However, there are a great many options for improving accessibility of computing tasks, the array of input devices and specialised software on the market is bewildering. Among this plethora of options, it is difficult to ensure that the best solutions have been chosen for the employee. The interactive capabilities of computer users are unique to that individual, and it would be mistaken to develop a policy of standard solutions based upon basic categorisation by disability type. Consignia, realised the need for a different approach, by working with Cambridge University Engineering Design Centre to develop an objective interaction assessment process that could be implemented by company occupational health therapists, and ultimately, to minimise costs, by developing an automated procedure which could potentially be implemented over the company intranet.

1.3.4 Accessibility of Information and Communications

It seems obvious to state that the creation of a truly accessible workplace involves the consideration of far more than the accessibility of tasks: employees must be able to avail themselves of information regarding company policy and procedures and the support functions such as employee health services, training services etc. Failure to accommodate accessible information formats and communication channels in many cases results in sub-optimal personal development, a lack of appropriate on the job support and a sense of exclusion on behalf of the employee. Such a situation often results in a decision for the employee to leave the company. Again, the use of technologies such as deaf signing avatars (with appropriate computational linguistics), screen and document readers and flexible visual formatting must be viewed as a way forward.

1.4 Concluding Remarks

It is clear that service providers and employers are facing ineluctable legal requirements to ensure that accommodation is made for people with disabilities, and/or the functional limitations that accompany older age. However, Consignia is also aware of the positive opportunities that are afforded by a well considered approach to improving accessibility to its services and workplace, and that the use of appropriate technologies and design practices provide the means by which this potential can be realised, hence the commitment to support CWUAAT.

1.5 References

ADULTDATA (1998) The handbook of adult anthropometric and strength measurements Department of Trade and Industry, UK

ADA (1990) Americans with Disabilities Act (ADA) of 1990. US Public Law. pp 101-336

Ballabio E (1998) The Information Society Research Challenges for 2005 for People With Disabilities. CSUN, Los Angeles

Card SK, Moran TP, Newell A (1983) The Psychology of Human-Computer Interaction, Lawrence Erlbaum Associates

Coleman R (1993) A demographic overview of the ageing of first world populations. Applied Ergonomics 24(1): 5-8

Coy J, Keates SL, Clarkson PJ, Harrison L, Robinson P (2001) Design for Accessibility: The Personal Information Point. In: Proceedings of the Institute of Mechanical Engineers Conference on Mail Technology: Evolution to E-Revolution, pp 59-168

Coy J, Keates S, Clarkson PJ (2001) Improving accessibility in the workplace: Manual data entry in video coding. Proceedings of the Institute of Mechanical Engineers Conference on Mail Technology: Evolution to E-Revolution, pp 201-210

Disability Discrimination Act (1995) Department for Education and Employment, UK

DDA (1999) DDA Code of Practice (DDA COP), Rights of Access to Goods, Facilities, Services and Premises

Vanderheiden GC (1990) Thirty Something Million: Should They Be Exceptions? Human Factors 32(4): 383-396.

Part I

Design Issues for Universal Access and Assistive Technology

Chapter 2

Defining Design Exclusion

S. Keates and P.J. Clarkson

2.1 Introduction

It is known that many products are not accessible to large sections of the population. Designers instinctively focus on providing the necessary utility for someone with physical and skill capabilities similar to their own (Cooper, 1999), unless specifically instructed to do otherwise. They are either unaware of the needs of users with different capabilities, or do not know how to accommodate their needs into the design cycle.

One of the key steps to ensuring that designs are as genuinely inclusive as possible is to provide metrics for defining the level of inclusivity attained throughout the design process. By providing suitable metrics, designers should be able to measure the success of their designs and also identify accessibility shortcomings. The aim of this chapter is to discuss possible metrics for measuring the inclusivity of a design and to present a tool for the graphical representation of the population included by a design compared to the population excluded.

2.2 The Need to Avoid Exclusion

The motivations for wanting to design for a wider range of user capabilities and avoid unnecessary exclusion are easily identified. The demographic change to an aged population distribution in the developed countries is marked. Studies show that by 2021, half the adult population in the UK will be over 50 (Coleman, 1993). Ageing also brings increasing divergence in physical capabilities (Coy, Keates and Clarkson, 2001), so it will become increasingly necessary for products to support a wider range of physical capabilities.

There is also a legal imperative from legislation such as the UK 1995 Disability Discrimination Act (DDA, 1995), the US 1990 Americans with Disabilities Act (ADA, 1990) and Section 508 of the US 1998 Workforce Investment Act (WIA,

1998) all provide a case for designing for the widest possible population. However, in spite of the motivations for more inclusive design practices, industry has been slow to adopt them. There are a number of reasons for this:

- a lack of awareness of the issue;
- a lack of motivation for tackling it;
- a lack of methods for tackling it.

Each of these issues will need to be explored in detail, however first it is interesting to address the background behind the existing theories of designing for a wider population.

2.3 Designing for a Wider Range of Users

2.3.1 The Goals of Inclusive Design

According to Nielsen (1993) *system acceptability* is the goal that designers should be aiming for and can be achieved by meeting the *social* and *practical acceptability* objectives for the system. He further identifies *usefulness*, constituting *usability* and *utility*, as a key objective to providing practical acceptability. Most designers focus on providing the necessary utility, or functionality of the system required for the task, and the social acceptability, such as the aesthetic characteristics, for users who match their own capabilities and taste. There are two reasons for this. The first reason is that these are indisputably very important objectives. The second is that it a minimally effective solution can be obtained in the minimum of time.

However, as numerous usability texts will attest (e.g. Nielsen, 1993), such minimally effective solutions are increasingly unacceptable to the wider population. They argue that *usability*, that is the ability to use the utility, is also important and needs to be designed directly into the system. In principle, usability techniques should be applicable for the whole population. However, in practice, they still generally assume the same, able-bodied physical capabilities of the users.

Consequently, *accessibility* design approaches have had to be developed. These approaches are variably referred to as "design for all", "universal access" and "inclusive design." Accessibility practitioners believe that design for all practices need to be explicitly included in the design process to ensure that all user capabilities are considered.

2.3.2 Existing Approaches to Inclusive Design

There are several existing approaches for designing more inclusive products. However, there are shortcomings of each of these approaches that prevent each of them from being used to provide the definitive design approach that designers can use in *all* circumstances. The principal weaknesses stem from the targeted nature of the approaches.

Initially it was recognised that the disabled and elderly were the principal groups excluded from using most products. The solution appeared obvious - if the users could not use the products, then developing special products designed specially for them would solve the problem. Thus concepts such as Design for Disability were born.

While many good products were developed, they were outnumbered by those that were either expensive, inappropriate, or just did not offer the necessary utility. The focus of the products was often on very specific needs arising from very specific circumstances. Also, many of the products had to be designed from scratch. This made for very long development times, with resultant high costs. Frequently, the time that should have been devoted to improving the usability was spent on technical development (Buhler, 1998). In many cases, usability was often overlooked completely. The situation became so bad that many rehabilitation robotics products failed to even reach double figures for sales (Mahoney, 1997).

In parallel with the lack of attention paid to usability issues, the social acceptability of the products was often overlooked as well. Many products were developed with no thought of whether someone would actually want to use or be seen using them. As people rebelled against using ugly, stigmatising, expensive and unusable products, it was clear that new approaches to design was required.

A number of new design approaches were developed to overcome the shortcomings of the preceding methods. However, these newer approaches have their own shortcomings, for example often being targeted at specific population groups or impairment types. For example, Transgenerational Design (Pirkl, 1993) focuses on design for the elderly. Alternatively, they focus on specific impairment types, as for Rehabilitation Design (Hewer *et al.*, 1995). They can also be targeted at specific cultures. For instance, Universal Design (Bowe, 2000) dominates US/Japanese approaches to inclusive design, whereas Europe has generally tended to develop other methods, such as the User Pyramid Approach (Benktzon, 1993). In addition, the prescribed methods of application of the existing methods are often vague. For example, Universal Design is more of an ethos than a rigorous, systematic design approach. There are very few structured descriptions of the implementation of Universal Design in more detail than broad design objectives (Bowe, 2000). Consequently, while combined the existing approaches may offer complete coverage of the population needs, individually they do not.

2.4 A New Model for Supporting Inclusive Design

Having discussed that the existing approaches to design for all tend to cater for specific circumstances or populations, it would be helpful if guidance could be provided to designers to identify which approaches focus on which sector of the population. The most effective method of offering the guidance would be in the form of a visual tool. Such a tool would need to show both the population and the proportion addressed by the design approach in a single diagram. The population could be represented by almost any shape, whether a circle, square or pyramid, for example and the design approach shown as a sub-region of that shape. However, while such a representation would show how many people were included by a particular approach, it would not offer much information beyond that.

A more attractive proposition would be to replace the arbitrary shape with one that represented features of the population that would be of use to a designer. Such methods of dividing the population could be along lines of gender or age, for example. Such partitioning of the population is useful for marketing purposes, but not necessarily for designers. An alternative partitioning is suggested by studying the nature of human-product interaction, such as in the case of HCI.

2.4.1 Understanding Interaction

Human-computer interaction has been studied for a number of years and there is a wide range of user models that have been developed to describe interaction. One of the most versatile and straightforward models is the Model Human Processor (MHP), developed by Card Moran and Newell (1983).

The MHP provides a succinct method for distinguishing between functional impairments in a manner that affords useful information to interface designers and vocational assessors. It segments the interaction into three function types: the time to perceive an event; the time to process the information and decide upon a course of responsive action; and, finally, the time to perform the response. Consequently, total response times to stimuli can be described by the following equation:

$$\textit{Total time} = x\tau_p + y\tau_c + z\tau_m \qquad (2.1)$$

where x, y and z are integers and τ_p, τ_c and τ_m correspond to the times for single occurrences of the perceptual, cognitive and motor functions. On empirical and neurological grounds, the model assumes that it is only possible for each constituent of the cycle to occur in integer multiples of the base time.

2.4.2 The Inclusive Design Cube

The division of interaction into the three distinct stages identified above - perception, cognition and motor functions - suggests a method for dividing the population according to the ability to perform those functions. Applying equal weight to the capability to perform each of these actions implies a cubic representation of the population. Design approaches can then be represented according to which level of capability they address.

Building on the concept of the user pyramid (Benktzon, 1993) with its banding of users by impairment level, the authors have developed a model that relates capability level, population profile and design approaches in a simple graphical format. The resultant model, the inclusive design cube (IDC) (Keates *et al.*, 2000), is shown in Figure 2.1. Each axis on the cube represents user capability as in the MHP, and the enclosed volumes reflect population coverage.

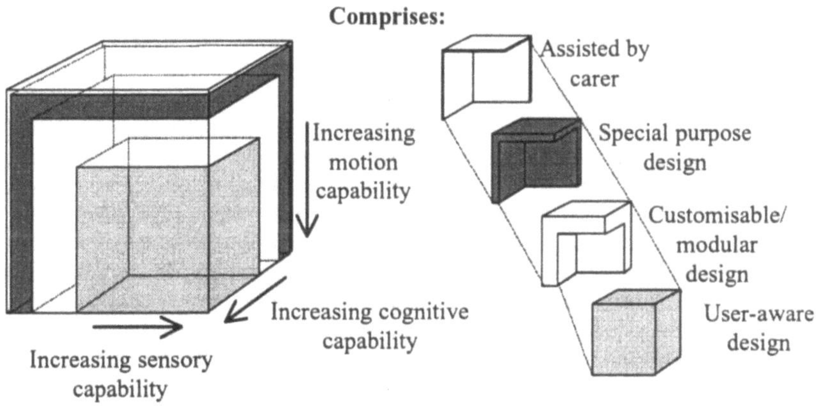

Figure 2.1. The Inclusive Design Cube (IDC) - mapping design approaches to populations

It was recognized that the principles of Universal Design generate products widely accessible to the population and hence having good population coverage. Consequently this approach, denoted *user-aware design*, dominates the cube. For severely impaired users, it may be necessary to adopt rehabilitation design approaches of custom products for specific users, *special purpose design* in Figure 2.1. In between the two approaches is an intermediary design approach with flexible boundaries. *Customisable/modular* design takes a base unit designed using the user aware design principles, but with a changeable interface that is either adaptable or can be swapped for one of a series of modular designs. The Inclusive Design Cube is a very potent visualisation tool and communicates the needs of different sections of the population.

2.4.3 The IDC and Exclusion

As can be seen from Figure 2.1, not only does the IDC show who is included by each design approach, but also who is excluded and, most importantly, begins to address the issues of why people are excluded.

This is an extremely important concept. While it is useful to know who and how many can use a particular product, that information will not provide guidance on how to include more. However, knowing who and how many cannot use the product immediately highlights the aspects of the product that need to be improved. For example, if a product excludes a significant proportion of the population because of the perceptual demands, this implies that users either cannot hear or see the output from the product.

The cube also begins to raise interesting issues, such as whether it is possible to compare one population with another, and consequently how one might define population types and describe exclusion. A working definition of inclusive design and a new measure, that of the *inclusive merit* of a product, are proposed.

1.5 A Working Definition of Inclusive Design

Design typically involves the creation of solutions and then a review to ensure that the design criteria are met. At the lowest level a design review process could involve a simple check to ensure that the resultant product offers the necessary functionality. At higher levels of sophistication, though, increasingly less quantifiable measures are required. The measures can range from whether the product is usable or accessible through to the outright qualitative, such as whether it is aesthetically pleasing and socially acceptable. Consequently, when developing a design approach for inclusivity it is necessary to consider the measure of success, i.e. the point at which the design is considered to have met the stipulated requirements. This shall be referred to as the *inclusive merit* of the product.

There are two important interpretations for defining the stipulated requirements of interaction for inclusive design. The traditional view of designers has been to specify the functional and/or aesthetic needs of the product and then, through the interface, place functional demands that the user must be able to meet. User-centred design practices put the emphasis on the user capabilities, wants and needs, driving the process in the other direction. These interpretations have led to the two principal strategies for the development of an interface for different user capabilities. The first is to take the existing interface and then tailor it retrospectively to different users. The second is to change the definition of the user at the very outset of the design process to include a wider range of capabilities. These approaches can be described as *reactive* and *proactive* respectively (Stephanidis, 2001).

Consequently the stipulated requirements of the application/product have the potential to exclude certain sections of the population who cannot meet the necessary functional capabilities. As another example, consider a kettle. If the kettle has to be able to boil a certain amount of water then there is going to be a minimum weight associated with the kettle when it has water in it. Therefore, users will be required to have the strength to move that minimum weight if they are to be able to use the kettle. Anyone not meeting that strength requirement will not be able to use the kettle, irrespective of other design decisions made or product requirements stipulated.

The recognition of fixed limits on the target user population set by the stipulated application requirements therefore leads to a possible working definition of an inclusive design:

> *An inclusively designed product should only exclude the end users who the product requirements exclude.*

The corollary of this is, of course, that the design fails to be inclusive if people are excluded from using it even though they possess the functional capabilities to meet the demands of the product. This implies that the designers have introduced new capability demands on the users that are not essential attributes of the product, but resultant from the designer's decisions.

The principle that only those who the product/application requirements exclude should be excluded by the product/application therefore provides the basis of a metric for measuring whether the design solution generated is successfully inclusive. However, this raises an issue that needs to be addressed at the strategic level of the design management, that of where the stipulated requirements should be set. Taking the example of the kettle, how much water should it hold? The smaller capacity decreases weight and increases inclusivity, but the marketability probably decreases. A managerial decision is therefore required between marketability of the product and the level of population exclusion, and hence potential market size.

In summary, one possible measure of *inclusive merit* of a product depends on two criteria: the merit of the requirements that define the product; and the merit of the product when judged against those requirements. However, such a definition is focused on only two possible population definitions. In practice there are a number of possible populations that can be considered.

2.5.1 Defining the Target Populations

The most obvious population to refer to is the *target population*. However, the problem is that the composition of the target population depends on the context of the discussion. It does not even always refer to the product users. It is possible, in the context of discussing design approaches, that the target population being discussed are the designers and managers, not even the people that will ultimately use the product. However, there are other populations that are fixed or directly measurable.

The most logical place to begin is defining the terminology for the global/geographical population being considered, i.e. the absolute maximum number of people who could use the product. This is referred to as the WHOLE POPULATION and it includes all people of all ages and capabilities.

The *whole population* is often thought of as the target population for the product. However, that is a very simplistic view. In reality, there will be certain limits on the number of people who may wish to use the product. For instance, legislative or safety requirements forbid people from using certain products, such as under-17's being forbidden from driving cars in the UK.

Another group that may be excluded are those who *even under the most optimistic assessment*, would be incapable of using the product for its intended purpose. This assessment should be completely solution-neutral. An example would be if the requirement was "to produce a product for making hot drinks." The exclusions under this requirement would be:

- *motor* – unable to lift/manipulate any cup-size container of hot liquid;
- *cognitive* – unable to understand how to handle any cup-size container of hot liquid safely;
- *sensory* – unable to distinguish correct cup-size container from other objects.

The resulting population following the removal of those who are prevented by law, safety considerations and irremediable lack of capability from using the product, shall be referred to as the IDEAL POPULATION. This is the maximum population that a product could possibly target under ideal conditions.

Within this *ideal population* sits the product itself and its requirements. Looking first at the product, as soon as anything physically tangible is produced, it can be assessed. This means that at any stage from initial concept through to the final product on the shelves, the inclusivity of the product can be assessed from its physical properties of its prototype. This is referred to as the INCLUDED POPULATION, i.e. the people who could actually use the product.

Sitting between the *included* and *ideal populations* is another population that reflects the product requirements. Under ideal conditions, if standard engineering practice is adopted, each new product will first be defined by a specification or set of requirements, before any product concepts are developed. This can be thought of as the *requirements population*. However, this definition is problematic because it is hard to define a particular stage of the product design cycle where the requirements are fixed and do not alter, short of the final product itself.

Consequently, explicit definitions of a requirements population are very difficult to specify. However, the concept of capturing something other than the product population is important. Therefore, we need to specify a population where it is acknowledged that the population will change, based on how the requirements develop and evolve. This is referred to as the NEGOTIABLE MAXIMUM POPULATION. 'Negotiable' implies that this population is not fixed and can change as the requirements change. It is the 'maximum' because by definition the inclusivity of the product cannot exceed that of the requirements/specification.

This is not immediately obvious, but arises from the difference between the likely method of assessing the requirements/specification and that of assessing the product. Any assessment of the requirements is likely to focus on the individual components in isolation, because the interaction between elements will be unknown and consequently unquantifiable. This can be thought of as an idealised assessment of the best possible product to meet those requirements. In practice, though, any attempt to design an actual product to those requirements will inevitable involve some trade-offs that will reduce the inclusivity of the product.

These populations can be mapped onto the IDC as shown in Figure 2.2.

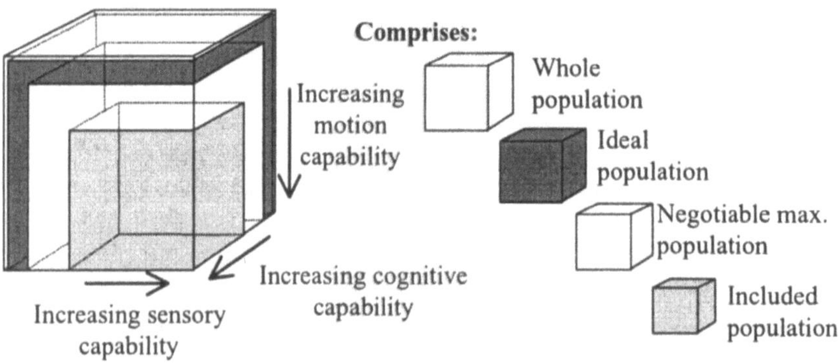

Figure 2.2. The IDC showing the WINI scales

At no point in the above definitions is the 'target' population referred to, because there are so many options that it can be mapped to. For example, the whole population is the utopian target solution, the ideal population is the best that can be achieved and the negotiable maximum may be what a product designer is happy to reach. Consequently the concept of a target population is difficult to specify without a clearly specified definition of who is defining the 'target' population and what the definition is.

One possible 'target' population that may be of interest is the INTENDED (SALES) TARGET POPULATION. We can add this to the above WINI categorisation, but with caution because it is an arbitrary definition, dependent upon the choices of the company management. For example, it could be particular age groups such as the over-75s, or particular marketing stereotypes. Mapping such populations into a population of real people with real variability in capability and then mapping this to the negotiated maximum and included populations will be discussed further in Chapter 3.

To summarise the defined WINIT populations:

- *Whole population* – everyone;
- *Ideal population* – the maximum achievable;
- *Negotiable maximum population* – everyone included by the specification;
- *Included population* – those who can actually use the product;
- *Target population* – those who were intended to use the product.

2.5.2 Defining Measures of Inclusive Merit

Having defined the different types of populations being considered, it is possible to enumerate the ratios between them. These can be used as measures of the inclusive merit of the product.

The ***ratio between the whole and ideal populations*** gives an indication of the level of exclusion associated with the concept task, irrespective of the solutions developed. Changing the position of the product being considered, so that it is subject to different health and safety regulations or different legislation, is the only option for changing this ratio.

The ***ratio between the negotiated maximum and ideal populations*** reflects the level of exclusion that has been generated by the refinement of the product requirements.

The ***ratio between the included and negotiable maximum populations*** indicates the level of exclusion generated by the particular configuration of the product at that point in time. As the design progresses and the requirements are refined more explicitly, the ratio should approach unity.

The ***ratio between the included and ideal populations*** is probably the most important as it provides a direct comparison of how good the product is at the moment compared to its theoretical maximum.

Finally, the ***ratio between the included and intended populations*** would show how successfully the product reaches the intended sales target population, while the ***ratio between the negotiable maximum and intended populations*** shows the success of the product requirements in meeting that same target population.

2.6 Summary

In summary, this chapter has presented a powerful graphical tool, the Inclusive Design Cube, that can be used to represent not only the level of population included, but also how many people are excluded. By developing the WINI concept of different populations, it is possible to measure the inclusive merit of the design against different target populations.

Such a tool also offers indications of how new design approaches can be developed based on an understanding of the elements of interaction. However, before such models can be applied widely, it is necessary to address the issues of assessment and quantification of the levels of capability required to use a design.

2.7 References

ADA (1990) Americans with Disabilities Act (ADA) of 1990. US Public Law 101-336

Benktzon M (1993) Designing for our future selves: the Swedish experience. Applied Ergonomics 24(1): 19-27

Bowe FG (2000) Universal Design in Education, Bergin & Gavey, Westport, CT

Buhler C (1998) Robotics for rehabilitation - a European(?) perspective. Robotica 16(5): 487-490

Card SK, Moran TP, Newell A (1983) The Psychology of Human-Computer Interaction. Lawrence Erlbaum Associates, Hillsdale, NJ

Cooper A (1999) The inmates are running the asylum. SAMS Publishing, Indianapolis

Coleman R (1993) A demographic overview of the ageing of first world populations. Applied Ergonomics 24(1): 5-8

Coy J, Keates S, Clarkson PJ (2001) Improving accessibility in the workplace: Manual data entry in video coding. In: Proceedings of the Institute of Mechanical Engineers Conference on Mail Technology: Evolution to E-Revolution, pp 201-210

DDA (1995) Disability Discrimination Act (1995) Department for Education and Employment, UK

Hewer S, *et al.* (1995) The DAN teaching pack: Incorporating age-related issues into design courses. RSA, London

Keates S, Harrison LJ, Clarkson PJ, Robinson P (2000) Towards a practical inclusive design approach. In: Proceedings of CUU 2000, ACM Press, New York, NY, 45-52

Mahoney R (1997) Robotic products for rehabilitation: Status and strategy. In: Proceedings of International Conference on Rehabilitation Robotics 1997, BIME, Bath, pp 12-22

Nielsen J (1993) Usability Engineering. Morgan Kaufmann, San Francisco, CA

Pirkl J (1993) Transgenerational Design: Products for an aging population. Van Nostrand Reinhold, NY

Stephanidis C (2001) User interfaces for all: New perspectives into human-computer interaction. In: User Interfaces for All, Lawrence Erlbaum, Hillsdale, NJ, pp 3-17

WIA (1998) Workforce Investment Act (WIA) of 1998. US Public Law 105-220

Chapter 3

Quantifying Design Exclusion

P.J. Clarkson and S. Keates

3.1 Introduction

Products make demands of their users which effect their utility and usability. As a result, those users who do not have the capability to use the product are denied access to it. For example, a kettle that is so heavy that a weaker user cannot lift it denies access to that user regardless of the cause of their weakness. There are many such products causing access problems with a wide range of users, particularly those who are *older* or *disabled*, and it is generally recognised that more inclusive approaches to design must be adopted to resolve this problem.

The aim of this chapter is to explore the link between *product demands* and *user capabilities* and, where possible, to quantify the number of users excluded by a particular set of demands. The chapter comprises three parts. First, the information requirements for inclusive design are reviewed, along with the availability of user capability and anthropometric data. Second, the development of a framework for accessibility evaluation is described. Finally, the new approach is evaluated through its application to a product case study.

3.2 Inclusive Design

In the year 2002, 1000 million of the world population will have a noticeable degree of functional impairment (WHO, 1998). It is well established that impairments such as reduced hearing, vision and motor capability are often of a degenerative nature and frequently associated with increasing age. In response to this increasing level of impairment, legislation has forced organisations to consider designing products for impaired users. In particular, the directives from the USA and the UK have been instrumental in encouraging an upsurge of initiatives in 'universal design' (Universal Design, 1998) and 'design for all' (Janssen and Van der Vegt, 1998).

More recently the concept of 'inclusive design' has emerged to provide a framework for the design of products better suited to a wider range of users. This has the potential to benefit disabled and/or elderly people who are expected to interact with an increasingly complex technological environment, where user interfaces are usually designed only with "able-bodied" users in mind (Stephanidis, 1997). Designers frequently impose limitations regarding product accessibility (HUSAT, 1996). Inclusive design aims to highlight and reduce such exclusion.

A description of inclusive design, along with and a number of metrics which may be used to quantify the level of inclusion achieved, are described in Chapter 2. Such metrics may be applied qualitatively based on user capabilities, but may have greater impact if they can be described quantitatively. This then requires knowledge not only of the capabilities demanded by the product, but also of the number of potential users with at least that capability.

3.2.1 Information Requirements for Inclusive Design

In order to confirm the accessibility of a product or product concept, it is necessary to verify that the intended users of a product are able to use it. This verification can take the form of user trials, expert assessment or systematic analyses of the product interface. The latter option is attractive since, in principle, it can offer a low-cost, comparatively quick evaluation. However, to achieve such an evaluation requires a suitable framework and assessment criteria.

The key requirement for an evaluation system is the ability to relate *users* to the *ergonomic features* of a product (Figure 3.1). In this context, *capabilities* refers to the users' sensory, cognitive and motion capabilities and *physical attributes* to the users' anatomical dimension related characteristics such as height, reach, grip strength, etc. The solid arrows in Figure 3.1 refer to relationships which may be derived from existing data, whilst the dashed arrow represents the mapping required for matching potential users to the ergonomic features of a product. This link does not currently exist.

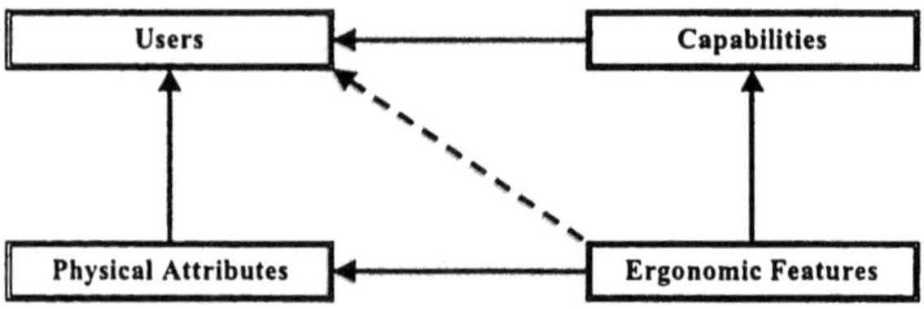

Figure 3.1. Information requirements for assessing inclusive design

3.2.2 Current Information Available for Inclusive Design

There are several sources of *capability* data, but perhaps the most obvious (for the UK) is the Great Britain Disability Follow-up Survey (Grundy *et al.*, 1999). This source recognises thirteen capability scales of which seven are particularly pertinent to product evaluation, namely: motion, dexterity, reach and stretch, vision, hearing, communication, and intellectual functioning. Each of these scales, ranging from 0 (fully able) through 0.5 (minimal impairment) to 12.5 (most severe impairment), have been aligned to ensure that equal scores broadly relate to equivalent levels of disability (Martin, 1988). As an example, definitions for the locomotion scale are shown in Table 3.1.

Table 3.1. Assessment scale for user locomotion capability

LOCOMOTION		Severity score
L1	Cannot walk at all	11.5
L2	Can only walk a few steps without stopping or severe discomfort/Cannot walk up and down one step	9.5
L3	Has fallen 12 or more times in the last year	7.5
L4	Always needs to hold on to something to keep balance	7.0
L5	Cannot walk up and down a flight of 12 stairs	6.5
L6	Cannot walk 50 yards without stopping or severe discomfort	5.5
L7	Cannot bend down far enough to touch knees and straighten up again	4.5
L8	Cannot bend down and pick something up from the floor and straighten up again	4.0
L9	Cannot walk 200 yards without stopping or severe discomfort/Can only walk up and down a fight of 12 stairs if holds on and takes a rest/Often needs to hold on to something to keep balance/Has fallen 3 or more times in the last year	3.0
L10	Can only walk up and down a flight or 12 stairs if holds on (doesn't need a rest)	2.5
L11	Cannot bend down to sweep up something from the floor and straighten up again	2.0
L12	Can only walk up and down a flight of stairs if goes sideways or one step at a time	1.5
L13	Cannot walk 400 yards without stopping or severe discomfort	0.5

It can been seen from the locomotion example that the severity scores are not evenly spaced, nor are the definitions consistent in their language of description. This is typical of all the scales and presents some interesting challenges that are discussed later. The alignment of the severity scales allows for the combination of scores to give an overall severity category. This is derived in the survey report (Martin, 1988) as a weighted sum where:

$$\textit{Weighted disability score} = \textit{worst} + 0.4 \times (\textit{second worst}) + 0.3 \times (\textit{third worst}) \quad (3.1)$$

This weighted sum is then translated into an overall severity category using the mapping shown in Table 3.2.

Table 3.2. Correspondence between disability scores and severity category

Severity category	Disability score
10 (most severe)	19-21.4
9	17-18.95
8	15-16.95
7	13-14.95
6	11-12.95
5	9-10.95
4	7-8.95
3	5-6.95
2	3-4.95
1 (least severe)	0.5-2.95

The survey data also allows the GB population to be segregated by age and gender. There is, as might be expected, an increasing prevalence of higher severity scores with age. This is illustrated in Figure 3.2 which shows the percentage of GB population, in a number of age bands, with any loss of capability (severity category 1 through 10). This use of a number of capability scales and bands differentiates the approach taken in this chapter from standard inclusive design practice (Benktzon, 1993; Hewer *et al.*, 1995), which focuses on one capability.

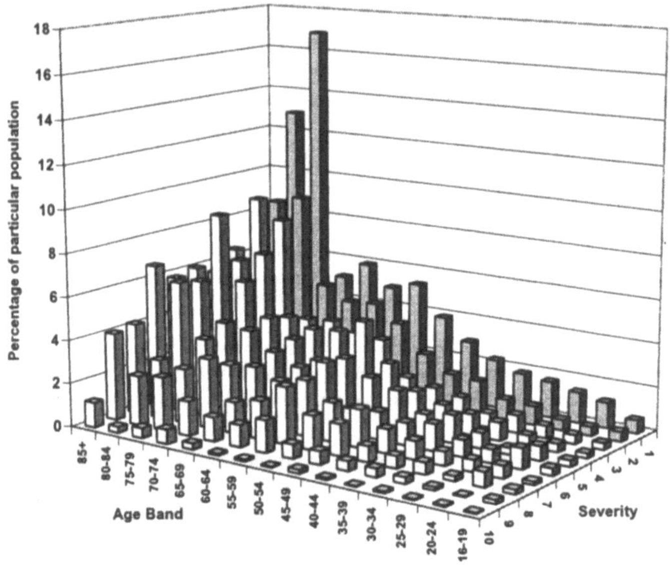

Figure 3.2. Severity category as a percentage of specified GB population age bands

Again there are several sources of *physical attribute* data, but the most useful single source is provided by the Department of Trade and Industry which distinguishes between child data, adult data (Peebles and Norris, 1998) and older adult data (Smith *et al.*, 2000). These data are divided into static anthropometry, functional anthropometry and strength categories. As with the capability data they show a variation with age. For example, the average height of adult females in the UK ranges from 1620 mm for those aged 18-50 to 1521mm for those aged 85+.

There are a number of sources of *ergonomic* data, mainly in the form of standards, ranging from the generic to the product specific. For example, British Standard BS 4467, provides a guide to dimensions in designing for elderly people, ISO 1007 provides ergonomic principles related to mental workload, ISO 6440 is essential for wheelchair design and ISO 12756 standardises ball point pens design.

Despite the availability of the aforementioned data there remains a need to relate potential users to a product's ergonomic features (the dashed arrow in Figure 3.1). It is proposed that this be achieved by considering the indirect links (solid arrows) via user capabilities and physical attributes. The following sections describe this approach.

3.3 Product Assessment for Inclusive Design

The *inclusive merit* of a product is dependent upon its physical and functional attributes, and how they are expected to interact with the user. It is tempting, therefore, to define an absolute scale where merit is based directly on the number of users able to use the product. However, this would not account for the fact that some products are, by definition, exclusive. For example, those with severe visual impairments are prohibited from driving motor vehicles and as a result cars are not designed for this group of users. Judging the inclusive merit of a car against the whole population therefore would be harsh when it is the legislative requirements for the vehicle that exclude the visually impaired users.

Any order of merit must therefore have at least three parts: the merit of an *ideal product*, i.e. the best design that meets the users' needs; the merit of the *product requirements* compared to the ideal design; and the merit of the *actual product* when judged against the requirements or the ideal design. A design review process for inclusive design, based on this three level approach, is illustrated in Figure 3.3.

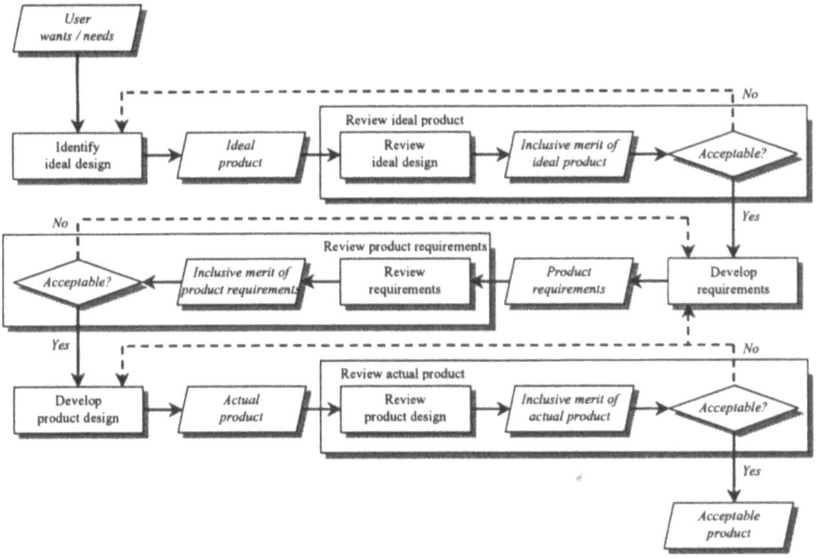

Figure 3.3. A design review process for inclusive design

The core of the review process is the same for the *ideal product*, *product requirements* and the *actual product*, each following a four-step approach:

- Step 1 – *specify the context of use*. State any assumptions regarding the environment in which the product is used and the sequence of actions encountered when using the product.
- Step 2 – *assess capability demands* imposed by the product, subject to its defined context of use. Determine the number of users excluded from using the product and the reasons for their exclusion. Assessment methods

include population-based assessment, simulation assessment, observational studies, user group evaluations, expert analysis, envisaging, and analytical approaches.

- Step 3 – *assess the physical attributes* required by the product, subject to its defined context of use. Determine the number of users excluded from using the product and the reasons for their exclusion. Assessment methods are the same as those listed for step 2. In addition, the number of users disadvantaged, but not excluded, when using the product should be identified.
- Step 4 – *eliminate multiple counting* from the results of the capability and physical attribute assessments. Identify the number of users who may be excluded or disadvantaged for more than one reason.

To assess the ideal product, it is sufficient to judge a conceptual product which meets the widest range of users' needs. Similarly, to assess the requirements, it is sufficient to judge a conceptual product which best meets the product requirements.

Orders of *inclusive merit* should then be established. The inclusive merit of the *ideal product* is the maximum proportion of the total population who could be expected to be able to use an ideal product. The inclusive merit of the *product requirements* is the maximum proportion of the ideal population who could be expected to be able to use a product derived from the requirements – this is negotiable. Finally, the inclusive merit of the *actual product* is the maximum proportion of the population included by the requirements or the ideal design that could be expected to be able to use a particular product, where the later definition is probably more useful as a measure of the goodness of the product. Rework of the product design, or in extreme cases the requirements, may be necessary if inclusive merit targets are not met. This is shown by the dashed arrows in Figure 3.3.

The following section describes in more detail how this review process may be conducted, with reference to a specific case study. The assessment methods used for the capability and physical attribute reviews were based on expert analysis.

3.4 A Case Study of Product Evaluation

Consider again the example of the kettle. Early kettles were made of metal and suspended over an open flame. They had a large handle, which doubled as the means of suspension, mounted above the body of the kettle (Figure 3.4a). Such kettles required limited dexterity and were well balanced for carrying and pouring, but care had to be exercised when using them close to the open flame. The corded electric kettle, as described above, initially retained the shape and balance of the earlier models (Figure 3.4b) and removed the open heat source, but with the disadvantage of the additional dexterity required to insert and remove the cord.

In contrast, the early plastic cordless jug kettles, although eliminating the need to remove the cord, introduced a new problem. The side mounted handle changed the balance of the kettle making it more difficult to use for those with limited upper-body strength. The more recent arrival of the traditional shaped cordless kettle (Figure 3.4c) has partly resolved this issue although the overall weight of these metal kettles remains a problem for weaker users. This example illustrates the difficulty of inclusive design. No sooner had one problem been resolved (detaching the cord), than another was introduced (poor balance).

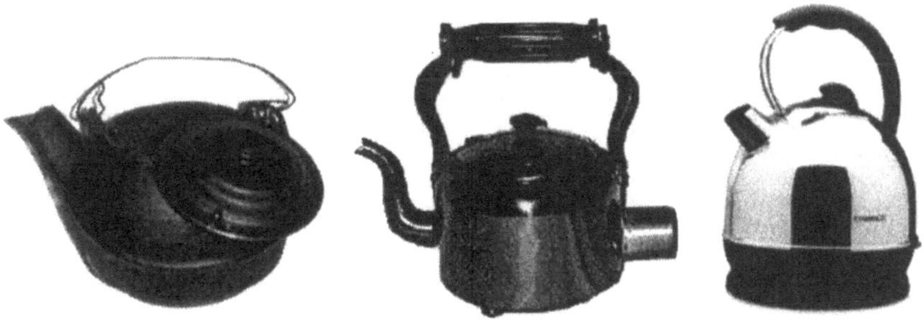

(a) The early kettle (b) Corded kettle (c) Cordless kettle

Figure 3.4. A range of kettles

3.4.1 Specify Context of Use

The cordless kettle will be assessed in the following sections. The first step of the review process is to state any assumptions regarding the environment in which the kettle is to be used and the sequence of actions encountered when using it. In this case it will be assumed that the kettle will be positioned to suit the height and mobility of the user and the actions required will be to fill the kettle with water, switch it on and to pour the boiling water into a cup.

3.4.2 Assess Capability Demands

The second step of the review process requires the determination of the number of users excluded from using each product as a result of their comparative lack of capability. This may be concluded by assessing the level of capability required to undertake the actions listed above.

Consider first the *ideal* product: this device should demand no more of the user than the action of drinking from a cup. Hence, those users who could not safely drink from a cup are excluded from the analysis. In practice, this 'kettle' would have to be more like a drinks machine where no filling and pouring are required.

The *actual* product may resemble that shown in Figure 3.4(c); a device which is relatively heavy when full with a non-illuminated switch. The product requirements may, however, suggest the design of a lighter, smaller kettle with a simple lid-opening mechanism and a clearly marked and illuminated switch.

The results of a capability assessment for the seven capabilities identified in Section 3.2.2 are shown in Table 3.3 for the ideal product, product requirements and actual product. Significant increases in the number of users excluded in response to each capability demand are evident in moving from the ideal to the actual product.

Table 3.3. Great Britain population aged 16+ excluded as a result of capability requirements

Capabilities	Ideal product		Product requirements		Actual product	
	Minimum requirement	Total 16+ excluded	Minimum requirement	Total 16+ excluded	Minimum requirement	Total 16+ excluded
Locomotion	n/a	0	n/a	0	n/a	0
Reach and stretch	8.0	116,000	5.5	495,000	4.5	654,000
Dexterity	9.5	211,000	7.0	945,000	5.5	2,105,000
Vision	8.0	137,000	5.5	198,000	4.5	387,000
Hearing	n/a	0	n/a	0	n/a	0
Communication	n/a	0	n/a	0	n/a	0
Intellectual Functioning	9.5	115,000	8.0	188,000	7.0	305,000

Note: the total Great Britain population for 16+ may be taken as 46,907,000

3.4.3 Assess Physical Attributes

The third step of the review process requires an assessment of the number of users excluded or disadvantaged from using each kettle as a result of their physical attributes. This may be concluded by assessing the range of attributes that affect the filling, switching and pouring tasks. In this case it may be assumed that hand and finger size have no significant impact on the users' ability to use the products.

3.4.4 Eliminate Multiple Counting

The analysis presented above does not consider the fact that an individual may exhibit more than one loss of capability or be affected by more than one physical attribute. Whilst this is not significant when assessing particular shortcomings of a product, it is important in determining the total number of users excluded from using the product. In addition, when aiming to improve products it is important to know if the changes proposed will indeed include more users, or whether they will still be excluded for some other reason. However, this is a task made very difficult by the lack of a single coherent data source describing capabilities and physical attributes. Current efforts are focused on extracting data from the disability survey (Grundy *et al.*, 1999) to account for multiple instances of capability loss.

The prevalence of multiple capability loss is illustrated in Figure 3.5 for combined measures of motion capability (a weighted score derived from reach and stretch, locomotion and dexterity capabilities) and sensory capability (a weighted score derived from vision and hearing capabilities). Here the area of each circle represents the number of individuals exhibiting a particular combination of capabilities. In this example it can be seen that there are many users with either full sensory capability (i.e. capability of 0) or a limited loss (capability of 1) coupled with a loss of motion capability (1-10). Hence, if the sensory demands of a product are intended to be set to include users with lower capability (capability of more than 0), such users will only be included if their motion capability is also accommodated.

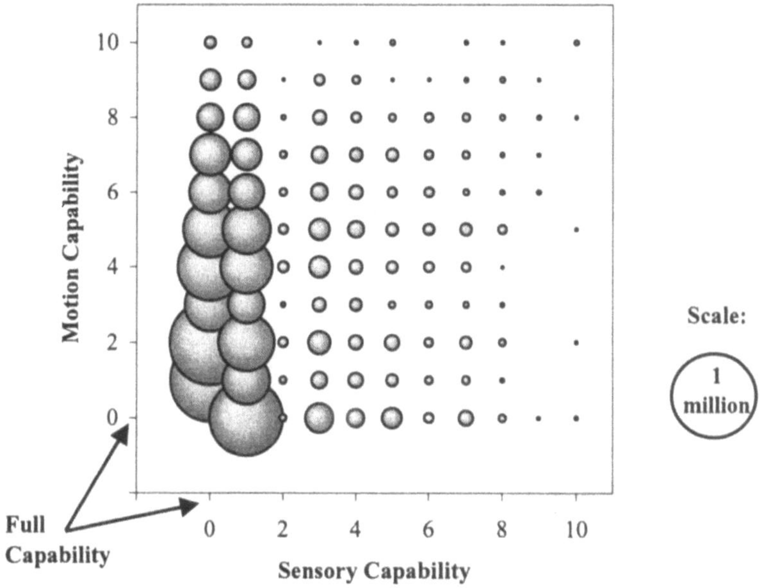

Figure 3.5. Great Britain population aged 16+ showing multiple capability loss

In summary, design changes do not always provide the benefit that may be expected.

3.4.5 Summary of Analysis

In the case of the kettles, no users are disadvantaged as a result of their physical attributes. Hence, the determination of *inclusive merit* is possible. Indices are shown in Table 3.4 for all users aged 16 and over and for users aged 75 and over.

Table 3.4. Inclusive merit for the ideal product, product requirements and actual product

Inclusive merit	Whole population		Ideal product		Product requirements	
	16+	75+	16+	75+	16+	75+
Ideal product	**99%**	**95%**	100%	100%	-	-
Product requirements	96%	85%	**97%**	**89%**	100%	100%
Actual product	93%	74%	**94%**	**78%**	96%	86%

It can be seen in Table 3.4 that the ideal product includes nearly the whole population for all users aged 16 and over, whereas the actual product includes only 94% of possible users. This situation is worse for users aged 75 and over where

22% of possible users are excluded from using the actual product. Yet the product requirements suggest there is much room for improvement without compromising the basic concept of a kettle. A lighter, smaller kettle with a clear and illuminated switch would only exclude 11% of possible users in the same age range.

3.5 Conclusion

Inclusive design will only be encouraged when managers and designers are able to see more clearly the impact that their specification and design decisions have on the usability of their products. An approach to reviewing product requirements and concepts has been presented which can be used to highlight areas of particular concern in an emerging product. Contrary to many Universal Design and Design for All approaches, this Inclusive Design approach incorporates a user capability range that does not configure an "average user". This has the advantage of enabling the manager and designer to consider all potential users with multiple combinations of impairment capabilities.

3.6 References

Benktzon M (1993) Designing for our future selves: the Swedish experience. Applied Ergonomics, 24(1): 19-27

Grundy E, Ahlburg D, Ali M, Breeze E, Sloggett A (1999) Disability in Great Britain. Department of Social Security, Research Report No. 94, Corporate Document Series

Hewer S, *et al.* (1995) The DAN teaching pack: Incorporating age-related issues into design courses. RSA, London

HUSAT (1996) Usability Assessment. European Usability Support Centre, INUSE D313v1.2

Janssen TJ, Van der Vegt H (1998) Commercial Design For All (DFA). In: Proceedings of the 3rd TIDE Congress, Marina Congress Center, Helsinki, Finland

Martin J, Meltzer H, Elliot D (1988) The Prevalence of Disability Among adults. Office of Population Censuses and Surveys, Social Survey Division, HMSO.

ONS (1997) Census - Samples of Anonymised Results (SARs). Office of Population Censuses and Surveys, Social Survey Division

Peebles L, Norris B (1998) Adultdata: The Handbook of Adult Anthropometric and Strength Measurements – Data for Design Safety. UK Department of Trade and Industry

Smith S, *et al.* (2000) Older Adult: The Handbook of Measurements and Capabilities of the Older Adult – Data for Design Safety. UK Department of Trade and Industry

Stephanidis C (1997) Editorial: Disabled and Elderly People in the Information Society. ERCIM News, No 28, Special Issue on Information Technology empowering Disabled and Elderly People, pp 4-5

Universal Design (1998) Principles of Universal Design. The Center for Universal Design, NC State University, School of Design, USA

WHO (1998) Population Ageing - A Public Health Challenge. Fact Sheet No. 135, World Health Organisation, Geneva

Chapter 4

Countering Design Exclusion

S. Keates and P.J. Clarkson

4.1 Introduction

Conventional product interfaces present serious difficulties to users with functional impairments. Conditions causing such impairments can occur throughout the life course, affecting all age groups. Certain symptoms, such as reduced hearing, appear with increasing frequency with advancing age, whilst other such as spasms are often associated with particular medical conditions, such as Cerebral Palsy. This has led to the common concept of "*the disabled and elderly*" as being groups requiring separate attention. Consequently, many design approaches for allowing accessibility by members of either group focus on *disabilities*. However, the principal concern for should be physical *capabilities*, irrespective of cause.

This paper presents a 7-level approach to inclusive design, building on existing usability techniques, user-centred design practices and user modelling methods, and is illustrated through the use of a case study. When designing a new approach, it is necessary to define the requirements that it has to meet, develop the approach and then evaluate it. This raises the question of how to define successful inclusive design. The answer offered is that inclusive design should only exclude those in the population who the product requirements exclude. Effectively, successful inclusive design can be thought of as countering design exclusion.

4.2 The Need For A New Design Approach

As described in Chapter 2, there are several existing approaches for designing more inclusive products. However, there are shortcomings of each of the above approaches that prevent each of them from being used to provide the definitive design approach that designers can use in *all* circumstances. The principal weaknesses stem from the very targeted nature of the approaches, both in terms of context of use and application.

Looking first at the context of use, the existing design approaches are often targeted at specific population groups. For example, Transgenerational Design focuses on design for the elderly (Pirkl, 1993). Alternatively, they focus on specific impairment types, as for Rehabilitation Design (Hewer *et al.*, 1995). They can also be targeted at specific cultures. For instance, Universal Design (UD) dominates US/Japanese approaches to inclusive design, whereas European countries have generally tended to develop their own particular methods, such as the User Pyramid Approach (Benktzon, 1993).

The prescribed methods of application of the existing methods are usually either left vague or alternatively are very tightly defined. UD is more of an ethos focused on a particular objective, that of making everyday objects more accessible. However, there are very few structured approaches that describe the implementation of UD in more detail than broad design objectives (Bowe, 2000).

Consequently, while combined the existing approaches may offer complete coverage of the population needs, individually they do not. Therefore, there is a need for a new approach that draws on the strengths of the existing inclusive design approaches and offers practical and measurable design criteria.

4.3 Developing a New Inclusive Design Approach

When designing any new product, it is necessary to adopt a three-stage development strategy (Blessing, Chakrabati and Wallace, 1995):

- *Stage 1 – define the problem* – gain an understanding of the system requirements;
- *Stage 2 – develop a solution* – develop a system that includes consideration of able-bodied and motion-impaired users;
- *Stage 3 – evaluate the solution* – make sure that the solution is effective.

These stages are also applicable for designing an interface. The inclusion of a broader range of user capabilities affects all three of the above stages:

- *Stage 1* – include explicit reference to the intended target users in the problem definition;
- *Stage 2* – adopt an appropriate design approach for the target users;
- *Stage 3* – include the target users in the evaluation process.

In order to produce a usable and accessible product or service, it is necessary to adopt strongly user-centred design practices. It is important to be able to modify and refine the interface iteratively, combining both design steps and usability evaluations. Such evaluations typically involve measurement against known performance criteria, for example Nielsen's *heuristic evaluation* (Nielsen, 1993).

Developing a usable interface for a wider range of user capabilities involves understanding the fundamental nature of the interaction. Typical interaction with an interface consists of the user perceiving an output from the product, deciding a course of action and then implementing the response. These steps can be explicitly identified as perception, cognition and motor actions (Card, Moran and Newell,

1983) and relate directly to the user's sensory, cognitive and motor capabilities respectively. Three of Nielsen's heuristics explicitly address these functions:

- *Visibility of system status* – the user must be given sufficient feedback to gain a clear understanding of the current state of the complete system;
- *Match between system and real world* – the system must accurately follow the user's intentions;
- *User control and freedom* – the user must be given suitably intuitive and versatile controls for clear and succinct communication of intent.

Building on these heuristics, a design approach has been developed that expands the second stage of the design process, solution development, into three specified steps (Clarkson and Keates, 2001). Each level of the resultant design approach, shown in Figure 4.1, is accompanied by user trials throughout and a final evaluation period before progression to the next level, thus providing a framework with clearly defined goals for system usability.

The 7-level approach addresses each of the system acceptability goals identified by Nielsen (1993). The approach has been applied to a number of case studies including the design of a software interface for an interactive robot (Keates, Clarkson and Robinson, 1999) and the case study presented in this chapter.

4.3.1 Applying the 7-Level Approach

The 7-level approach has been structured as a high-level model, so each level represents an aim, but the method of achieving that aim can vary according to the expertise and knowledge of the designer.

Level 1 defines the user needs, that is the social motivation for designing the product. This can be identified through softer, sociological assessment methods. Questionnaires and interviews are good methods for identifying the user needs.

Level 2 focuses on specifying the required utility of the product. Traditional engineering requirements capture techniques (Beitz and Kuttner, 1994) can be used, as can task analysis (Nielsen, 1993). Alternatively, assessments of rival products or user observation can provide insight into the necessary functionality.

Levels 3 to 5 focus on the stages of interaction. Usability and accessibility techniques can be applied directly to these levels, as can anthropometric and ergonomic data. Prototypes of varying fidelity play a key role in these levels.

Level 3 addresses how the user perceives information from the system. This involves assessing the nature and adjustability of the media used, their appropriateness for the utility, and the physical layout. Anthropometric data are important to ensure that the output is in a position that the user can perceive it. Ergonomic and empirical data from trials are also necessary to ensure that the stimuli are intense enough to be perceived. Ideally, environmental conditions, such as lighting and noise, also need to be identified and modelled.

Level 4 assesses the matching of the system contents and behaviour to the user mental model. Once the output channels are defined, the content/utility can be added to the system and evaluated because the functionality for monitoring the system is in place. Literally the user can see/hear/etc. the data. Common techniques to map the user system behaviour to user expectations include cognitive walkthroughs.

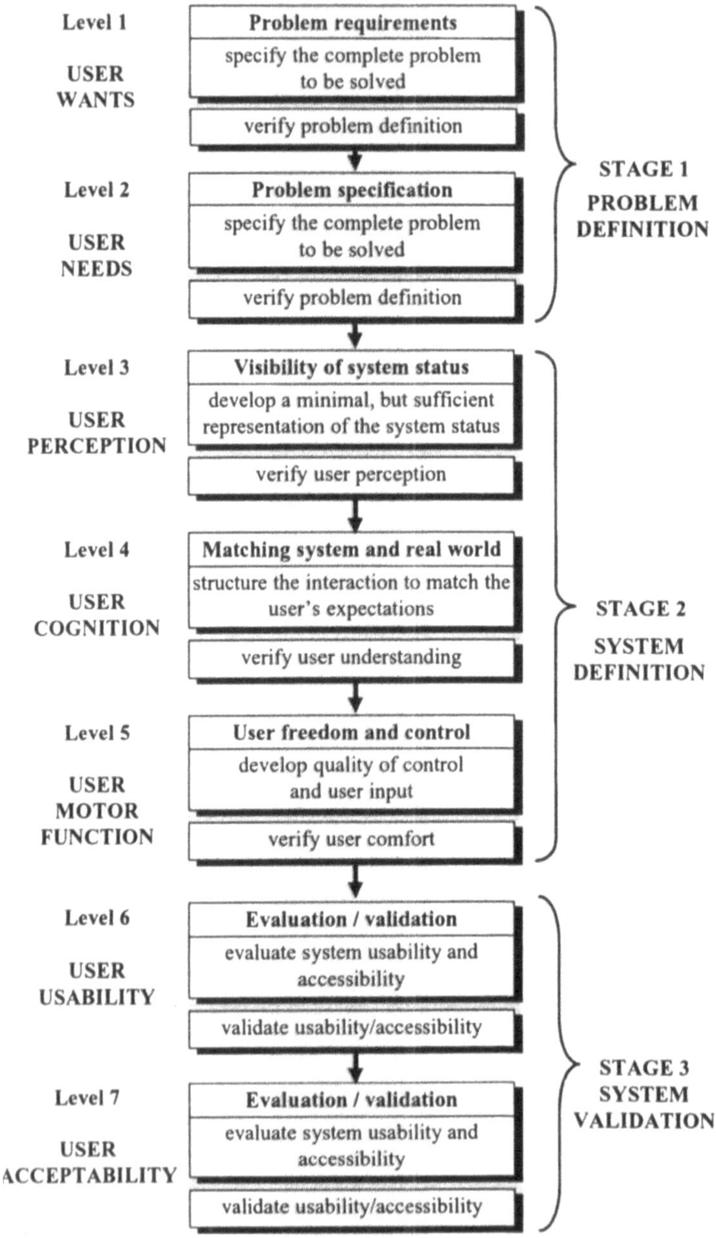

Figure 4.1. The 7-level design approach

Level 5 focuses on the user input to the system. As with level 3, this involves assessing the nature and adjustability of the media, their appropriateness for the utility, and the physical layout. Again anthropometric measures are important to ensure that the input media are within the operating range of the user. Ideally, empirical data from user trials needs to be gathered to evaluate the effectiveness of the input solutions. These can be supported by adopting user modelling techniques. Where user trials are impossible, suitably calibrated user models can be used to provide design data.

Level 6 involves the evaluation of the complete system to ensure satisfactory practical acceptability, i.e. utility, usability and accessibility. Formal user trials are essential at this point, before the design can progress to the final level.

Level 7 assesses the resultant system against the user needs. This mirrors Nielsen's social acceptability requirement. Softer, more qualitative approaches are generally needed, such as surveys, interviews and questionnaires.

Although the 7-level approach is presented as a flow diagram, in practice each of the stages can be applied in an iterative manner. Indeed, in many circumstances, it may prove essential to iterate within and between levels. However, the general order of levels should be applied in the order shown in Figure 4.1.

4.3.2 The 7-Level Approach and the Inclusive Design Cube

Both the 7-level approach and the Inclusive Design Cube (Chapter 2) share the same inherent emphasis on the interaction consisting of perceptual, cognitive and motor actions. Consequently, if the 7-level approach has been adopted as the framework for the development, then the Inclusive Design Cube (IDC) can be adapted to monitor the population coverage achieved by different design choices. Effectively, the 7-level approach can be thought of as designing for each axis on the IDC. The modification necessary to use the IDC for this is a straightforward re-labelling of the axes to reflect Levels 3 to 5 of the 7-level approach, Figure 4.2.

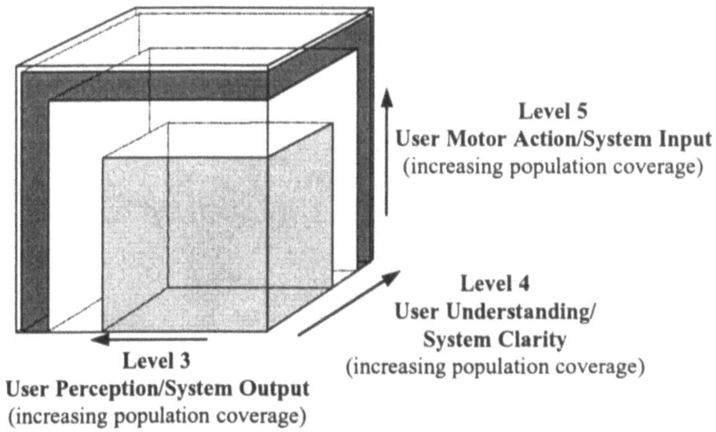

Figure 4.2. The IDC for use with the 7-level approach

4.4 Case Study: Auditing an Information Point

Consignia is one of the UK's largest employers. As with all large UK companies, Consignia is expected to comply with the Disability Discrimination Act (DDA, 1995), which stipulates that all companies offering services to the public should not bar use of those services on the grounds of disability. The age profile of Consignia customers is biased towards the over-65's, with a large proportion of customers visiting post offices to collect their pensions. With the increased variability in capability associated with ageing, the incentive for inclusive design is very great. Consignia is aiming to introduce automated customer information points (IPs) into post offices to augment the current range of services.

Consignia is also very keen to ensure that the product is as usable and accessible as possible, not simply for DDA compliance, but also to engender customer satisfaction. An initial concept system, Figure 4.3, has been developed by a design company for review as a possible solution to Consignia's requirements.

The concept IP consists of three display heads mounted on a central free-standing pedestal of fixed height. Each unit head has a small LCD panel mounted at a fixed angle, with three buttons on either side of the screen for input and a telephone handset for audio output. The output is primarily recorded video footage with accompanying soundtrack. The purpose of the case study here is to examine the usability of the prototype and how this would have been affected by the use of the 7-level approach.

The 7-level design approach can be divided into the following steps for the IP:

- **Level 1** What is the aim of the IP?
- **Level 2** What are the IP system requirements?
- **Level 3** How does the user receive information from it?
- **Level 4** Does the user understand what is happening?
- **Level 5** What are the physical demands on the user for entering inputs?
- **Level 6** Does the IP meet the functionality and usability requirements?
- **Level 7** Does the IP meet the stated aim?

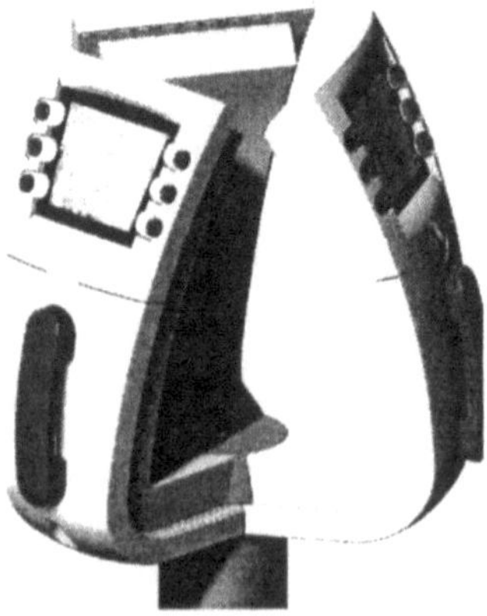

Figure 4.3. The concept Information Point

4.4.1 Level 1 – System Aims

The aims of the IP are more sociological than functional and consequently open to interpretation. One of the aims is to provide Consignia customers with an introduction to modern technology as a precursor to post office transactions becoming increasingly automated. the subsidiary aim is to reduce queue length for the counter service in a cost-effective manner. These aims must be achieved in such a way that meets legislated accessibility requirements. No explicit usability or performance criteria were stipulated.

4.4.2 Level 2 – System Requirements

The target user of the new Information Point is the typical post office customer. Owing to the age profile of typical post office customers, the real target person is likely to be older and have at least one major impairment, most likely visual, auditory or motor. The user are likely to be more resistant to change and to new technology.

The concept IP was designed to be bright, open and attractive to tempt customers to use it. However, to be of real use, the IP also needs to offer easy access to significant content, with sufficient bandwidth for the interaction. For maximum accessibility and legislative compliance, the design process should be entirely driven by user needs and product objectives. The concept IP was developed to meet the broad aims identified in Level 1. This implies that the concept IP may not offer the necessary functionality or usability because these issues have not been explicitly defined by Consignia at this stage.

4.4.3 Level 3 – User Output

The concept IP used a combination of video footage displayed on the screen and accompanying soundtrack on the telephone handset. Neither output mode was sufficiently complete to provide all the information on its own. Consequently, the 1.7 million adults in the UK with visual impairments and the 4.5 million hearing impaired adults (Martin, Meltzer and Elliot, 1988) would be unable to use the system successfully. This does not include those who are environmentally impaired through background glare or noise.

The other major concern when addressing user output is that the output solution chosen is positioned in an accessible manner. The number of people excluded by the fixed height and angle of the concept IP display is a good example of this. The display viewing height is set rather high at 1610 mm, with a lower bound on the viewing height of 1451 mm. This excludes half of women of 65 and approximately a quarter of all adult women, rendering 6 million women unable to view the display (Peebles and Norris, 1998).

4.4.4 Level 4 – User Understanding/Cognition

With the concept IP not having any real content at this stage, detailed evaluation of the user understanding of the system was not possible. However, it was possible to estimate the likelihood of good user understanding being attainable by the IP. The structure of the interaction, and hence of the interface, is partly dependent upon input and output modes chosen. Under the 7-level approach, only the output modes will have been specified by this stage. Looking only at the output capabilities, the small IP screen limits the richness of content that could be achieved compared to larger display. It requires many more levels of searching to reach a target goal because fewer options and less information can be displayed simultaneously. However, with the focus on the technology in the design of the concept IP and the decision to include only six buttons for input, the functionality of the software interface is arbitrarily limited to selection from a list. If the list is well designed, though, then the system has the potential at least to be easy to learn.

4.4.5 Level 5 – User Input

The prototype IP only offers button input through a limited number of buttons. Text entry is impossible without the use of voice recognition technology or scanning input to a keyboard emulator. The other issue of concern is the physical positioning of the input for user comfort. The free-standing design of the prototype is likely to affect anyone who has difficulty standing for extended periods of time. The requirement that both hands be used eliminates anyone who needs to use a walking stick for support. Similarly the requirement to stand for extended periods of time excludes anyone who has difficulty standing. The associated reaching and dexterity requirements for operating the buttons and the handset also excludes a further 3 million people (Martin, Meltzer and Elliot. 1988).

4.4.6 Levels 6 & 7 – Evaluation

This review process represents the first stage of the evaluation of the concept IP. The IP is currently undergoing a re-design to take into consideration the accessibility flaws revealed by this analysis. The first evaluation prototypes of the new design should be out later this year for trial periods in three local post offices.

4.4.7 Summary of the Information Point Review

Having applied a first pass of the 7-level approach as a review, a number of pointers for the re-design of the prototype have been identified. Starting with Level 1, it is clear that the existing design does not offer sufficient functionality to meet Consignia's requirements.

Levels 3 to 5 illustrate the importance of being aware of the user needs throughout the design process. Assuming that impairments are independently distributed across the population and that the presence of one impairment does not alter the probability of another impairment being present, up to 45% of the UK adult population could have been excluded from using the IP because of the failure to consider different user physical capabilities, environmental impairments, or temporary impairments, e.g. through injury.

The Inclusive Design Cube (IDC) in Figure 4.4 shows the *Negotiable Maximum population* and the *Included population* (Chapter 2) for the IP. The Included population reflects the number of people who can use the concept product/prototype, whereas the Negotiable Maximum population represents the number of people who should be able to use the product based on the capability demands of the product requirements/specification. Consequently, the difference between the two volumes represents the level of exclusion that has arisen from choices made in the design and implementation of the concept product. In this example, the Negotiable Maximum population shown should be considered the *theoretical* maximum as no product specification or requirements were available.

The arrows indicate the direction of increasing population inclusion from the most capable users to the least capable. The volumes are derived by plotting the levels of exclusion identified in the assessment of the IP on each axis. Note that the volume therefore reflects the population coverage. A general discussion on how to populate the Inclusive Design Cube is presented in Chapter 3.

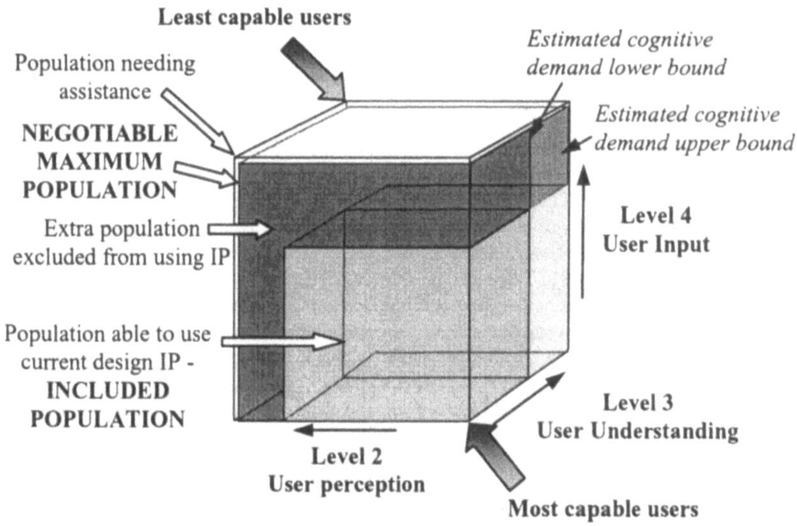

Figure 4.4. The current design compared to the revised user-aware design

Fortunately, potential, and often simple, remedies for decreasing the level of exclusion can also be identified. For instance placing the unit at desk height and having chairs nearby would remove almost all of the difficulties related to user height or the need to stand for periods of time.

4.5 Overall Summary

The information point case study illustrate the successful use of the 7-level approach and the Inclusive Design Cube. However, to be of genuine use, both tools should be usable by designers with varying backgrounds and expertise, and also in different circumstances.

With this in mind, the 7-level approach is envisaged as being a framework, rather than a string of rigorously defined steps, and offering designers the freedom to select which design tools they deem most appropriate for each level and for the product being considered. The underlying strength of the 7-level approach is that because it was derived from a model of interaction that was not product-specific, the approach itself is not product-specific either. Consequently, there are no philosophical reasons why it should not be applicable to a wide range of products.

As a final note, this paper has shown the level of exclusion that can be avoided through the application of a methodical user centred design approach such as the 7-level model and highlights areas where the greatest benefit can be achieved. Therefore, the real challenge that this research identifies is how to make industrial designers more aware of these potential benefits.

4.6 References

Beitz W, Kuttner K-H (1994) Handbook of Mechanical Engineering. Springer-Verlag, London

Benktzon M (1993) Designing for our future selves: the Swedish experience. Applied Ergonomics 24(1): 19-27

Blessing LTM, Chakrabarti A, Wallace KM (1995) A design research methodology. In: Proceedings of the 13th International Conference on Engineering Design, Glasgow, UK, pp 502-507

Bowe FG (2000) Universal Design in Education, Bergin & Gavey, Westport, CT.

Card SK, Moran TP, Newell A (1983) The Psychology of Human-Computer Interaction. Lawrence Erlbaum Associates, Hillsdale, NJ

Clarkson PJ, Keates S (2001) Towards an inclusive design approach. In: Proceedings of the 13th International Conference on Engineering Design, Glasgow, UK, pp 355-362

DDA (1995) Disability Discrimination Act. Department for Education and Employment

Hewer S *et al.* (1995) The DAN teaching pack: Incorporating age-related issues into design courses. RSA, London

Keates S, Clarkson PJ, Robinson P (1999) A design approach for accessibility. In: Bullinger HJ, Ziegler J (eds.) Human-Computer Interaction, Lawrence Erlbaum 2: 878-882

Martin J, Meltzer H, Elliot D (1988) OPCS surveys of disability in Great Britain. Report 1: The prevalence of disability among adults, HMSO

Nielsen J (1993) Usability Engineering. Morgan Kaufmann, San Francisco, CA

Peebles L, Norris B (1998) Adultdata: The Handbook of Adult Anthropometric and Strength Measurements – Data for Design Safety. UK Department of Trade and Industry.

Pirkl J (1993) Transgenerational Design: Products for an aging population. Van Nostrand Reinhold, NY

Chapter 5

Inclusive Design – Developing Theory Through Practice

R.R. Gheerawo and C.S. Lebbon

5.1 Introduction

This chapter focuses on applied research projects run by the Helen Hamlyn Research Centre (HHRC) at the Royal College of Art (RCA) where an empathic approach is taken to the design process. The chapter is a description of the practical manner in which this method can be used and the emphasis is on how this and other user-centred design research methods can feed into the disciplines of engineering and design. The methodologies are not tied to one discipline, but have the ability to be transferred and adapted to suit any part of the design or engineering processes.

5.2 Design and Engineering

5.2.1 Are They So Different?

Design and engineering are closely related professions that seem to have grown apart over the past century. In terms of language, culture and education, the two disciplines now appear separate and exchange of ideas and experience between the two is constrained. In the academic sphere, design, broadly including the areas of products, furniture, transport, graphics and human computer interaction tends to be confined to the studios and galleries of art and design institutions; engineering, whether mechanical, civil, electrical, aeronautical or robotic, is firmly situated in the science block.

Historically, the links are stronger than they appear today. Leonardo Da Vinci, Michelangelo and Brunelleschi were polymaths, as were Wren and Brunel. Da Vinci, for example, is primarily known as an artist. However, he was also an architect, an engineer and a scientist and exemplifies the need to ask the question:

should lines be drawn or limits made as to where one part of the creative process begins and another ends?

The truth is that design and engineering have to be reconciled in the production of manufactured objects. Nowhere can this be more clearly seen than in the automotive industry. Major car manufacturers are now integrating working practices in a holistic process of design engineering instead of separate processes of design, then engineering. People work in teams on the same car, rather than in sections grouped by discipline. During employment as a concept engineer at Rover, one of the authors experienced the cultural changes taking place in the company leading to, the recent recovery of Rover as a brand and as a range of products. This was, in part at least, due to this type of internal reshaping within the company structure, with design playing a central role in pulling together the disciplines.

5.2.2 Culture and Language

Language also reveals some interesting commonalities between engineering and design. The word 'engineer' derives from the Latin 'ingenium', meaning 'cleverness, ability or talent – concepts linked very much to creativity, usually considered to be more an aspect of design than of engineering. The word 'design' originally means to 'mark out' or 'trace out', a linear activity much used in engineering (Oxford English Dictionary).

Language can also act as a powerful isolator – words take on different meanings between the disciplines and can project potent stereotypes. Creativity is a word with positive meaning within the design industry yet it can have negative connotations within an engineering context – 'creative' use of data suggests the doctoring of results. Language entrenches itself deeply and stereotypes are carried forward, ingraining themselves both in academic culture and company policy.

5.2.3 Where Can They Meet?

Engineering and design are better understood as part of a single process, and approaching the design of products, systems or services with this in mind could yield improved results and open up new opportunities. One area where sharing could be of enormous benefit is in design methodologies.

Some work is being done within both the design and engineering communities on developing suitable methodologies to ensure a product is designed and engineered with the end user at the centre of the process, but often, this work is not taken up in practice. In reality, the end user should be considered at every point in the design process, as products that fail to satisfy user need effectively exclude, to the disbenefit of both the producer and consumer. In rehabilitation robotics the end user can have an extreme variation in ability and therefore in need. Methodologies that focus attention on such users to draw out solutions can bring considerable benefit in increased usability and therefore in market potential going beyond the compass of rehabilitation:

> *"... an expansion of the concept of average leads towards a newer concept of universal design which ... results in a design outcome that is better suited to the majority of people. Such an approach has important implications for marketing of new products which will help to move design for old people from the margins to the mainstream of product development in the future."*
>
> (Benktzon, 1993)

Bringing extreme users into mainstream product and service development could offer real benefits to both producers and consumers, and in particular, those currently excluded by inconsiderate and user unaware design. Meeting this goal through design research collaborations with industry and voluntary sector partners has become a key focus of the HHRC's Research Associate Programme.

5.3 The User

5.3.1 Design Exclusion

Designers generally design for themselves, to their own aesthetic values and to their own likes and dislikes, and this often leads to design exclusion:

> *"We all find it much easier to develop products and services for ourselves than for other people. Entrepreneurs, marketing people, designers and engineers are often selfish in this way."*
>
> (Moggridge, 2001)

The are many groups who are presently excluded in the design process. These range from women with children struggling through today's transport system to older people ignored by an increased focus on the youth market. Disabled people and those recovering from an illness or an accident are rarely considered in mainstream design. The list is long and the lack of design input can have a severe effect on their quality of life. Ignoring users can also mean that important opportunities are missed:

> *"This design exclusion takes several forms: Older and disabled people suffer from it; so do those marginalised by changing technologies, work practices and economic structures. In a period of rapid change, bringing people from the margins to the mainstream through inclusive design is important not just from the perspective of social equality but also for business growth through new products and services."*
>
> (Myerson, 2001)

5.3.2 Countering Design Exclusion

Ergonomics, originating in the need to plan for military production, has only recently responded to the requirements of older and other marginalised users. The Department of Trade and Industry (DTI) in the UK commissioned a series of ergonomic studies including 'Older Adultdata', a handbook of measurement and capabilities of older people containing exhaustive physical measurements throughout the age range. Also included is data on the physical strengths, reaction times and flexion of various parts of the body:

> *"The need for data when designing for the older adult is becoming more important as the population ageing process continues in the world. The number of people in the world over 65 years of age is predicted to grow by 88% over the next 25 years."*
>
> (DTI Older Adultdata, 2000)

This is a direct and correct response to demographic data, but whilst groundbreaking and extremely useful, it still has its limitations.

Ergonomics has played an important part in helping the designer and engineer understand and respond to user characteristics, but there is a danger of seeing ergonomic data as sufficient, when in fact human beings have aspirations, spiritual dimensions and cultural characteristics, that design should address. Again, the car industry provides a clear example; plastic dummies and painstakingly detailed drawings are used to create interiors and seating positions to fit all but the extremes of physical size, but manufacturers have paid little attention to the dynamics of getting in and out of the car which can cause considerable problems for a large group of drivers. The Department of Transport has even had to write a guide for older people and those with disabilities in order to advise them on choosing a vehicle – problems faced when getting in and out of the vehicle was a key part of this publication (Department of Transport, 1985). The average new sports car buyer is aged about 55 years old and therefore likely to have reduced joint flexion and strength; the question has to be asked – are designers and engineers accommodating their target users?

How do we look past physical dimensions, and tap into the needs and aspirations of users? By taking a more holistic approach in which quantitative data and qualitative user insights are combined. The 'i~design' project (Clarkson *et al.*, 2000), due for completion in 2003, is a positive move in this direction and seeks to provide inclusive tools for designers and engineers that combine quantitative aspects of population data and qualitative aspects of user preference and lifestyle.

5.3.3 Inclusive Design

'Inclusive design', the focus of the 'i~design' project, is a relatively new term, yet it is quickly emerging as a potentially important driver of change within the broad field of design. Increasingly recognised by the UK government, inclusive design is described as a process whereby:

> *"designers ensure that their products and services address the needs of the widest possible audience."*
>
> (DTI Foresight, 2000)

Nevertheless, difficulties still remain in terms of definition. What does designing inclusively mean and what does it include under its banner? To open up discussion and debate around the subject HHRC and the Contemporary Trends Institute staged the 'INCLUDE 2001' conference in April 2001 at the RCA. The conference allowed an international audience from diverse communities to meet and debate these issues, and share best practice and research results. Engineers, designers, social scientists, researchers, ergonomists, students and members of the business community all participated in three days of workshops, presentations and plenary discussion, creating a pool of knowledge and a network of practitioners spanning disciplines and continents.

> *"Many came to the conference with the goal of finding better ways to integrate the disabled and the elderly into the socio-economic fabric of Britain and other countries. Yet in discussions, it became clear that the disabled and the elderly fall into a much wider continuum of differently abled people. Products and services that were better designed in general helped all consumers."*
>
> (Nussbaum, 2001)

What is clear is that user unaware design can have serious consequences. For example, the push-button London Transport ticket machine was designed and engineered under a tight brief and with limited technology. The result was a machine with a plethora of buttons and no obvious place to start the process of ticket buying. In a study sponsored by London Transport and carried out in 1997 by one of the authors, it was observed that nearly 70 percent of people who approached the machine, regardless of age or ability, found it difficult, and even impossible, to use – a clear example of design exclusion. The newer, touch-screen machine commissioned by Transport for London and developed by IDEO and Andrew Parker of CTS, is a testament to companies trying to design inclusively within tight practical and financial constraints. It was observed in a subsequent study that nearly 90 percent of users, including foreign language speakers and older people, could make a transaction on the machine without undue difficulty.

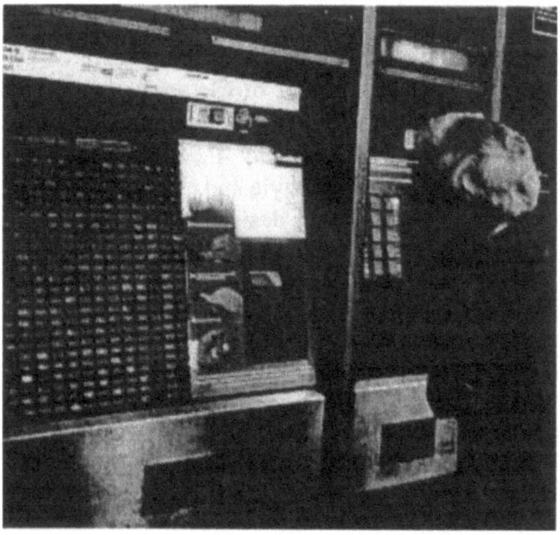

Figure 5.1. Push-button London Transport ticket machine

5.4 Theory Through Practice

5.4.1 The Helen Hamlyn Research Centre

At the HHRC, the focus is on encouraging young designers to design for people other than themselves. Design research is carried out with small groups of critical users selected on a project-by-project basis to reflect tensions between changing demographics and resulting extremes of capabilities, and the rapid advancement of technology. Including groups of critical users in the design process has had a positive influence on RCA students and recent graduates, and on design professionals who have engaged in collaboration with the Centre. In particular, regular user-forums bring older people and other marginalised users into the RCA design studios.

By working with users such as these, new insights have been gained and new design solutions proposed. The main vehicle for this is the Research Associates Programme where new RCA graduates collaborate with industry and voluntary sector partners on year-long design research projects. Each project addresses an area of concern or interest for the research partner, where an inclusive design approach can be practically implemented and evaluated.

In 1999, ten RCA MA graduates were teamed up with ten research partners including Levi Strauss, British Airports Authority and the Laura Ashley Foundation. In 2000, 14 graduates joined the programme and a further 13 joined in October 2001 from a range of disciplines including architecture, product design, transport design, communication design and design engineering. The projects employed a range of design research methodologies tailored to identify and include the needs and requirements of diverse and often marginalised groups of users in the design process including questionnaires, expert consultation, user diaries, interview, observation 'in situ', testing with prototypes, and research 'kits' requiring a range of responses from photographic to emotive.

By working closely with small groups of users, often with capabilities towards the extremes of the bell-curve, empathic bonding stimulates creative thinking and user-facilitated innovation. Bonding with the user helps identify assistive technology products and understand lifestyle and aspirational factors that are all too often overlooked in 'rehabilitation' design. Many people cover up their dissatisfaction with products when questioned or interviewed. The technique of iterative engagement and testing with select users, overcomes this problem as the designer moves from passive observer to active promoter of the user's interests. The following case studies illustrate this process.

5.4.2 Case Study 1 – The Abilizer: Aiding Rehabilitation for Disabled People

An applied research study leading to a wheelchair accessory to aid standing by people with limited lower body control and to facilitate treatment by Functional

Electrical Stimulation (FES). The aim being to design and manufacture a production-ready prototype with full engineering specification.

An initial focus group of paraplegics undergoing FES at Salisbury District Hospital, was expanded to include elderly people with degenerative muscular and neurological conditions, and people in need of ambulant care. The Department of Medical Physics and Bio-medical Engineering at Salisbury District Hospital collaborated with the HHRC to provide both project support and groups of users, with project funding coming from the Laura Ashley Foundation.

The researcher, Judith Anderson, worked closely with this key user group throughout the project. The research showed that apart from the recognised need for wheelchair users to stand if at all possible in order to exercise and increase blood flow, there were key self-esteem issues at stake. In any social gathering, wheelchair users often found themselves left out of conversations that took place whilst people were standing. To be able to stand in a social situation was seen to be of enormous benefit.

Further user studies emphasised the need for the wheelchair user to operate the whole mechanism independently. This prompted important changes in the way the mechanism was to work. The users wanted to be able to operate it efficiently and as quickly as possible and in a variety of situations, from standing up to greet a friend to reaching to close a window. The mechanism therefore had to be attached to the wheelchair and stow away neatly when the chair was in use. The final proposal consisted of two telescopic supports connected to either side of the wheelchair by two mounting units designed to fit most types of wheelchair. The mounting unit could be adapted to a variety of additional functions – for instance the attachment of a buggy or pram for wheelchair-bound mothers.

This kind of concentrated investigation with small groups of extreme users has considerable potential to fuel creativity and the Salisbury District Hospital team saw the project as a very positive response to the problems that wheelchair users have in addition to the specific needs of FES patients.

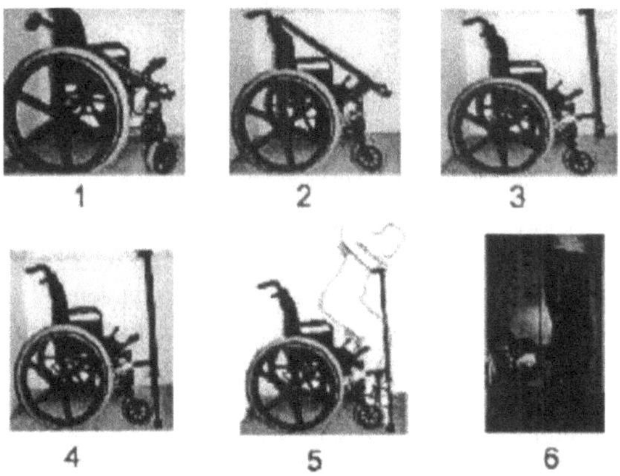

Figure 5.2. Early prototype for user testing

5.4.3 Case Study 2 – Power to the People: DIY Tools Made Easier for All

This project stemmed from B&Q's interest in extending its diversity initiative which is focused on access provision, to encompass the tools and equipment on sale within the store by including the needs and requirements of older users.

Researcher Matthew White, started by carrying out an audit of existing products. Interviews were not only conducted with the users and buyers of the products, but also with shop floor staff and suppliers – people who were not necessarily end users of the product. The information gained from these 'supporting' users was invaluable, as it tapped into long-term, product-related experience based on formal complaints and casual consumer comment and reaction, as well as giving an insight into customer choice as defined by age and other factors.

This helped Matthew focus his research around a user group of retired people with more time and inclination to indulge in DIY, but who might be put off by the bulk and industrial feel of available tools, and by other factors such as weight and complicated functionality.

Focus groups were conducted with older users with varying degrees of DIY experience. They were asked to perform simple functions on existing tools, such as switch operation or changing attachments, and subsequently to comment on design proposals during the concept creation stage. In-depth discussion on the DIY experience and the personal needs and reservations each had about using tools gave further focus to the design development process.

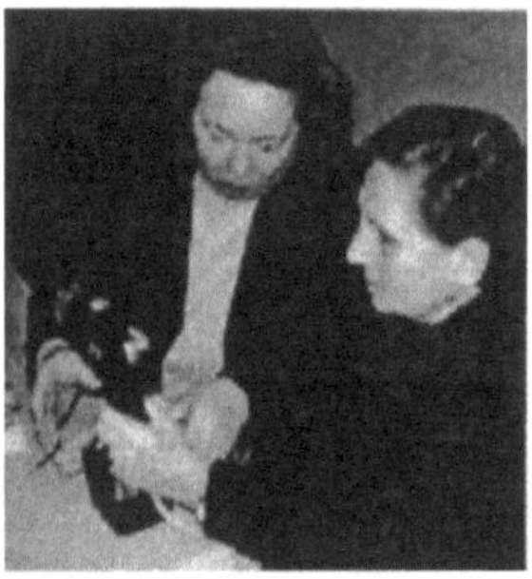

Figure 5.3. Focus group in progress

Short-term testing was carried out by 'expert' users – retired and active tradespeople – as well as amateurs. Tests lasted from two weeks to two months and were centred specifically on task-based work. Observation of tools in use in different situations, plus informal interviews added more realism to the user response noted in the focus groups, and specific aspects of a design such as ergonomics, usability or aesthetics could be assessed.

Long-term testing was carried out with a group of nine users ranging from a professional carpenter, to a retired businesswoman, a bank manager, and a design student, the object being to better understand a broad range of user need and preference and further inform the design process. Each was given tools to use over eight months, and a diary to record activities and responses to the tasks set and the tools used. The researcher deliberately chose some professional workmen to act as expert users, to encourage a more detailed level of user analysis and feedback. The one-to-one relationship that resulted allowed deeper interaction between designer and user. As a result, key physical problems, mindsets and cultural issues linked to performing DIY were revealed.

The project audited the current range of B&Q power tools against criteria developed from user tests and ergonomic studies. The resulting document is being used as a quick reference guide for B&Q power tool buyers and own brand manufacturers. Combining this guide with findings from long-term user tests generated several products. Four were selected and prototyped – a compact cordless screwdriver fitting into the palm of the hand, a palm sander with a securing hand strap, an ergonomic reciprocating/jig saw and a weight-saving extension for a cordless drill.

The researcher used different approaches to suit different stages of the design process, but kept the user central throughout the design development. The products and adaptations that resulted from this inclusive approach were so well received by B&Q that the designer has been asked continue his work through to production. In all, five patents have been taken out by B&Q and a new range of hand tools is expected to be on the shelves in 2002.

In both the case studies presented, the researcher became a trusted part of the user's life. The aspirations and needs, and most importantly the hidden difficulties that the users encountered, were frankly talked about. Feedback was honest and direct, and invaluable when used to generate ideas and focus the project direction.

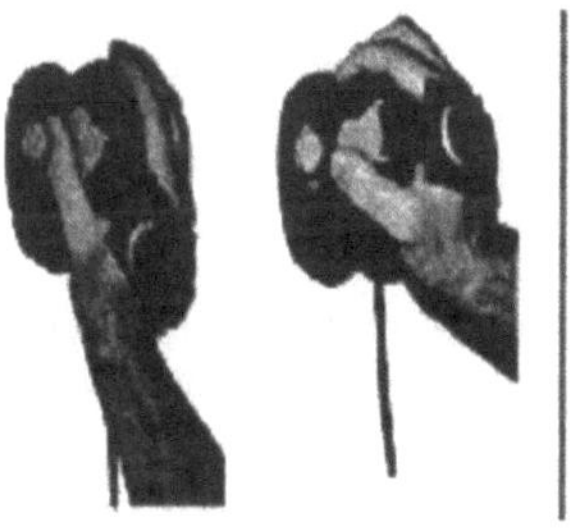

Figure 5.4. Hand-held sander – product of user-led design

5.4.4 Conclusion – The Value of Empathy in the Design Process

Combining engineering approaches centred on secure, factual information, with design approaches that seek to draw out more subjective information can help to build bridges between design and engineering whilst delivering real benefits to both end users and industry. Allowing an empathic relationship to develop between designer and user, though clearly non-objectives methods of inquiry, can open up a creative space in the process and facilitate innovation.

Such empathic design approaches could enhance current rehabilitation practice, by combining design-led information gathering with more conventional problem-solving. Rehabilitation designers already have a close working relationship with individual users. However, by embedding the empathic approach in design and engineering practice, and working at a more involved level with select critical users, new and unexpected solutions may emerge, enabling the resulting products to meet the needs of a wider population and increase the overall benefits to the companies manufacturing and selling the end product.

Benefits can also accrue to the research partner or client through greater user satisfaction and market share. Research partners on the HHRC Research Associate Programme have identified benefits over and above their original expectation. Importantly, companies and voluntary sector partners have been encouraged to adapt an inclusive approach to key areas of their business as a result of involvement with the programme. Raymond Turner, Group Design Director for Terminal 5 at Heathrow Airport remarked after two Research Associates proposed solutions to counter way-finding problems in airport terminals:

> *"We're involved in the Research Associates Programme not because it is the politically correct thing to do but because it is the economically sensible thing to do."*
>
> (Myerson (ed.), 2001)

5.5 References

Anderson J (2000) The Abilizer: Aiding Rehabilitation for Disabled People – Final Report. The Helen Hamlyn Research Centre, London

Benktzon M (1993) Designing for Our Future Selves: the Swedish Experience. In: Coleman R, Pullinger DJ (ed.) Applied Ergonomics: Human Factors in Technology and Society, Butterworth-Heinemann 24(1): 20

Clarkson PJ, Keates S, Coleman R, Lebbon C, Johnston M (2000) A model for Inclusive Design: Proceedings of Engineering Design Conference 2000

DTI Foresight (2000) Making the Future Work for You. Department of Trade & Industry, London

DTI Older Adultdata (2000) The Handbook of Measurements and Capabilities of the Older Adult. Department of Trade and Industry, London 1: 2-3

Department of Transport (1985) Ins and Outs of Car Choice: A Guide for Elderly and Disabled People. Department of Transport, UK

Moggridge B (2001) i Magazine: Magazine for the Design Council. The UK Design Council, UK, Issue 6, pp 12-13

Myerson J (2001) Design DK: Inclusive Design. Danish Design Centre, Denmark, p 3

Myerson J (ed.) (2001) The Helen Hamlyn Research Associates Programme Show and Symposium Catalogue 2001. The Helen Hamlyn Research Centre, London, p 63

Nussbaum B (2001) Breaking Boundaries. In: Include 2001: newsletter for the Include 2001 Conference. The Helen Hamlyn Research Centre, London

White M (2001) Power to the People: DIY Tools Made Easier for All – Final Report. The Helen Hamlyn Research Centre, London

Chapter 6

A Systematic Basis for Developing Cognitive Assessment Methods for Assistive Technology

R. Adams, P. Langdon and P.J. Clarkson

6.1 The Need for Systematic Assessment

We address the development of new assessment techniques for people of an employable age with acquired physical disabilities, such as head injuries and musculo-skeletal injuries. Specifically, we focus on cognitive function, which is fundamental to Assistive Technology and Rehabilitation engineering.

The approach described is aimed at organisations that carry out assessments as part of a programme of progression, or match adaptive technology and products to populations on the basis of individual profiles. The principal aims of the techniques will be to provide an assessment that yields information that enables the individual to (1) progress towards better employability or employment (2) to foster independence of living and enhanced lifestyle (3) pursue further education and training, as well as to aid organisations in the retention of employment. The main goals of the approach will be to develop new methods of assessment, with specific reference to cognitive factors, adaptive Information Communication Technology (ICT) issues and their interaction. This chapter outlines the basis of a systematic approach that will be implemented in the form of a set of techniques for assessing assistive technology and will be evaluated in use in a day-to-day assessment context.

6.1.1 The Context of Post-clinical Assessment

Improved post-clinical assessment of people with acquired physical disabilities is necessary for a number of reasons. There are over 6.6 million people with disabilities in Great Britain. Disabled people are twice as likely as non-disabled people to have no qualifications. They are only half as likely as non-disabled people to be in employment. There are around 1 million head injuries admitted to Accident or Emergency departments every year, many of these with brain injuries and acquired physical injuries. This implies that there will be an increasing need for better assessments of cognitive and psychomotor factors which are important for an individual's progression. Assessment centres practices are often out of date using outmoded methods based upon limited psychometric models. These approaches often do not address cognitive deficits such as those involving memory or attentional problems. Overall, existing assessment approaches can be characterised as employing an arbitrary collection of methods whose output may not be complete and that may lack rigour, objectivity and accuracy.

There is also a need for more cost-effective use of resources in assessment. For example, the time spent during assessment could be reduced with a more systematic approach and the cost of equipment could be reduced by updating techniques to use more ITC computer-based methods, which can be adapted to the assistive needs of the clients. The practical concern here on cognitive aspects of vocational assessment.

6.2 A Systematic Model for Assessment

There is therefore a need to develop a simplistic model or framework upon which to base research into systematic methods and tools. Such a model is important for the following reasons. First, when conducting a vocational assessment of an individual, the aim is to enable that individual to make significant progress while minimising subjective bias. Outcomes of such an assessment are measured in terms of either achievement of or distance travelled towards goals. It is important to define the objectives of the assessment since this aim itself helps to define the most appropriate methods to be selected. Second, the selection of the most suitable methods is also aided by a consideration of the assessment process itself and how it may be optimised. Since no two individuals are identical, the assessment process must be sensitive to individual differences and lead to the deployment of the most appropriate methods.

6.2.1 A Hypothesis Testing Approach

An important issue is the extent to which the assessor should take into account the disabilities of the individual. One approach to achievement of a good quality assessment is to view it as a process of hypothesis development and testing. Whilst it is possible to form rapid impressions and assumptions, the hypothesis testing approach has the dual advantages of being both rigorous and client centred. Pre-morbid information plus evidence from any source can thus be seen as potential basis for hypotheses information and allows the assessor to take such evidence into account, whilst also taking note of the varying quality of such information from different sources. In practice, the selection of methods with which to evaluate hypotheses has often been ad-hoc, reflecting their availability and the experience of the assessor. A much better approach would be to be guided by a systematic model or framework which provide both a comprehensible overview of the options and issues but, also provides a comprehensive reflection of the methods which should be considered at any one time.

6.2.2 The Simplistic Model

The purpose of a simplistic model in this context is to provide an overview of the range of psychology relevant to cognitive assessment for assistive technology. This model can also be used as a framework to derive a number of detailed alternatives for specific assessment methods. The notion of the simplistic model follows Broadbent (1984) who suggested the use of a model which was simply enough to satisfy the demands of parsimony and yet capable of guiding the application of psychology to the solution of practical problems. The equal emphasis upon both theory and practice is important in order to understand better the processes of assessment as well as to achieve higher levels of performance in practice.

6.3 The Components of the Simplistic Model

Cognitive skills are clearly important for effective, vocational assistive technology models (Argyris, 1991). Conversely, vocational assessment provides realistic data and settings with which to improve the validity, content and applicability of cognitive theories (Rabbitt, 1981). A model also needs to be developed with clear objectives in mind, so that others may consider its potential relevance.

Our main aim is to provide a model with at least two functional levels (Figure 6.1). The first and simplistic level is to provide us with an overall map to guide the implementation of a psychological assessment of an individual. The second level is to act as framework in which more complex models for specific problems or issues can be developed and sited. Furthermore, since we are often working with people with brain injuries, it is important to consider the need for cognitive factors like knowledge, awareness, sensory impairment, perception, thinking, and memory. The intention is to use this model framework to identify the selection of suitable assistive information technology that is capable of supporting skill and providing compensation.

6.3.1 Basis in Research

Cognitive psychology can provide a rich variety of architectures for working models. For example, simplistic architectures like Broadbent's Maltese Cross (Broadbent, 1984) capture an overview of cognition but do not attempt to be complete, whereas more complex models like the Interacting Cognitive Subsystems approach (Barnard, May, Duke and Duce, 2000) consists of an information processing, parallel approach that attempts to be complete and to address the complexity of realistic cognition. In addition, there are neural networks (Rumelhart, McClelland *et al.*, 1996) which aim to mimic the human brain and provide a computer instantiation; production systems such as ACT (Anderson, 1983) which reflect both cognitive psychology and computer simulations of cognitive processes. There are also approaches such as Marr's computational model and broader framework (Marr, 1982) which derive from research into Artificial Intelligence, exploiting nerurophysiology, engineering, and computer science. Whilst any of these could be used to model the assessment of cognitive skills, we adopt a parsimonious approach based on Broadbent's (1984) simplistic model.

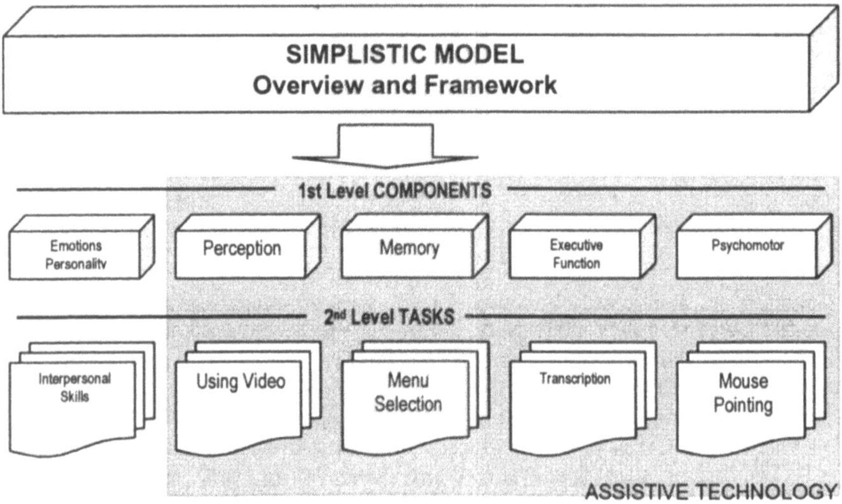

Figure 6.1. Unpacking the simplistic model for practical application

The aim of this is to develop a simplistic framework, which provides a first approximation for a model of cognition. It should be possible to show that the model of cognition can be unpacked to act as a framework for highly detailed sub-models such as a model of memory processes (Lee and Anderson, 2001). Specific tasks and settings should be addressable but the essential economy and simplicity of the framework is retained as would be required for an initial AT assessment of a potential computer user.

6.3.2 The Model Structure

The overall structure adopted in shown in Figure 6.2. It consists of a set of four memory stores that are linked by a central processing system. One of the roles of this central system is to transfer or copy memory traces from one store to another. The processing system also acts as a selection filter. This initial formulation (Broadbent, 1984) leaves out any indication of input and outputs, implying some form of selection or filtering before the sensory memory store. More recent adaptations of this model (Revelle and Loftus, 1990) incorporate a selective filter before sensory memory. However, the present model also allows for more advanced forms of selection when information is transferred between memory stores. The model allows for memories to be present in one or more stores, either partially or fully.

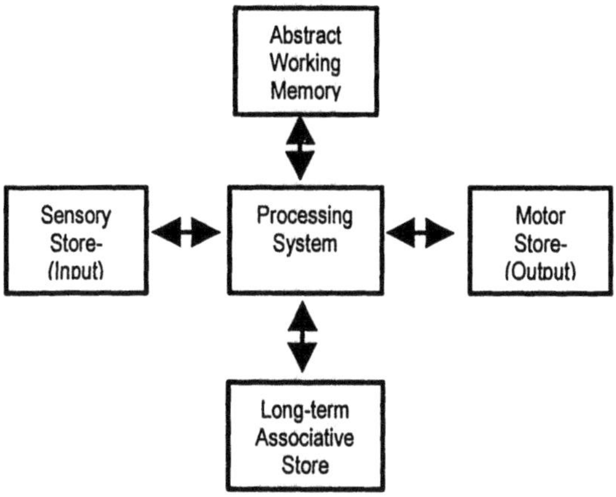

Figure 6.2. The overall structure of the simplistic model

6.3.2.1 Sensory Store

This is a limited capacity memory store which accepts transfers from the other stores as a translation or change of code. This store mainly receives a relatively raw input from the senses. It is divided up in terms of the physical dimensions which describe sensory inputs. A key feature is that a fresh input in the same region of store makes it difficult to retrieve items that are already there. The sensory store is not passive but a constructive encoding of the original sensory stimulus. The defining quality of this store is the presence of interference between memory events which share common physical qualities. In particular, where a memory is abolished or reduced by subsequent items, it would only occur where the subsequent items shared physical qualities. The reference experiment for this store would be (Coltheart, 1984) who explored the "stimulus suffix" effect where recall of memory test items is impaired by the presentation of a following item

6.3.2.2 Motor Output Store

This store holds sequences of motor output programmes, including sub-vocal speech sequences and is normally the last stage before responding. However, these programmes need not issue into overt actions but can feed back into another store. This it would include the coding of a sequence of inputs into an internal series of articulatory commands such as internal speech. Interference will be produced where a person undertakes actions using the same motor system. Thus, "articulatory suppression" occurs where the speaking of unrelated material impairs performance on an unrelated recall task (Baddeley, 1996). The Stroop effect, discussed below, can be due to interference between two stimuli which are appropriate to the same output categories (Stroop, 1935).

6.3.2.3 Abstract Working Memory

Interference between memories may not depend on similarity of later input, but rather on the sheer numbers of items. It is a temporary, limited capacity memory. Memories could be crowded out by a very large volume of information, if a large amount of central processing is performed. Thus memory for letter trigrams such as XDB may be more difficult than memory for familiar acronyms such as USA because of memory chunking of familiar material (e.g. Broadbent and Broadbent, 1981).

6.3.2.4 Long-term Associative Store

This is not concerned with events themselves but with the running totals of the co-occurrence of stimuli e.g. the number of times Event A and Event B have occurred together in the experience of the person. It is not a temporary store and may be used to explain practice effects and automaticity. The model assumes that with practice the individual builds up stronger associations between the relevant items in the task being learned. There is no sudden change from deliberate to automatic processing. As the task becomes more practised, the individual · leans the associations better. This would occur when someone learns to associate two items (A – B) and subsequently has to learn a new association (say A and C). The subsequent association impairs recall of the former association. This is known as retroactive inhibition. It should be noted that this is not the only long-term memory facility in the model as the processing system needs to store long term changes in procedures. These would not themselves be held in the long-term associative store.

6.3.2.5 Processing System

The processing system has the principal role of transferring information from one memory store to another. For example, on presentation of a symbol e.g. "2", then this leads to an identification of the name as "two". Thus the system must retain rules for transition on a long-term basis, in order to transform "2" into "two". Thus this system need to have its own long term memory, since these rules are not stored in the long term associative store. The Processing System must also have some form of shorter-term memory to keep track of current and recent actions.

6.3.2.6 Extensions to the Model

It has already been found necessary to enhance the framework, adding significant functions whilst retaining simplicity. In addition to the above, there should be an ability to model the environment; for selective filtering; and for storage of specific domains of knowledge. Models of the environment are important in a number of situations. For example, when solving problems, we often use a simple model of the problem rather than resorting to formal logic. Selective filtering of information is important in the computerised working environment. Our model allows for at least two types of selection. There first is input selection. For example, you might select all envelopes with the words "Confidential" before all others. This occurs at the input stage of the model. The second type of selection is content driven, as when you select all items which are related to financial planning, since that is the area you are working on at present. This occurs when transferring information within the model. It is also important to distinguish between declarative knowledge (knowing that...) and procedural knowledge or skill (knowing how...) as research demonstrates that recall from memory may itself be a learned skill (Adams and Berry, 1981; Baddeley, 1996; Lee and Anderson, 1998).

6.4 The Practical Use of the Approach

It is important to demonstrate that we can use our simplistic model to guide the implementation of an assessment in practice. The model is used in two ways. First it provides an overall view of the main areas of an assessment, setting out the main options for consideration. For example, an individual's varying capabilities may be compared with the components of the model. Let us suppose that problems with attention are identified. The model would then signpost areas for further investigation. The model also acts as a framework within which to deploy more complex sub-models without losing sight of the overall picture. Following the above example, consider the individual who has problems of selective attention. Unpacking the overall model to focus upon a sub-model of attention, we would then be able to explore this area more with a more complex model as a basis for understanding. In this case, this sub-model then points to suitable methods of assessment as will now be outlined.

6.4.1 Assessment of Attentional Requirements

Individuals must be highly selective in their responses to potential information overload but without missing vital new information or sources. The research literature identifies several important dimensions of selective attention which are relevant. For example, there is an important distinction between active (goal driven) attention and passive (externally driven) attention (Handy, Hopfinger and Mangan, 2001). Active attention requires more resources than does passive attention, even though the former is more typical of the tasks that individuals face. Similarly, divided attention (responding to more than one type of item) is more taxing than focused attention (responding to one type of item only). Effective selective attention also appears in the vocational literature in reference to such factors as being able to respond positively to feedback and having good interfacing skills (Myers, Kakabadse and Gordon, 1995). The failure of effective selectivity is found in information overload, a major factor in the experience of work stress (Cooper and Williams, 1994).

Mechanisms of selective attention can be explored by means of the Stroop test, a well-known task in which colour names are printed in different colour inks (Stroop, 1935; Hartley and Adams, 1974). The inks and the names present a problem of attention. Individuals find naming the ink colours of such items to be more difficult (and slower) than the reading the ink colours of neutral items like rows of XXX's. Such problems of attention can be due to either difficulties in attending to the correct aspects of the display (an input problem) or difficulties in selecting the correct responses (an output problem). On this basis, we have developed an assessment version of the Stroop test that allows us to distinguish between input and output problems of attention (Hartley and Adams, 1974). This result, in turn, enables the recommendation of appropriate Assistive Technology and user training solutions. A similar strategy can be adopted for other memory, perception, motor and reasoning capabilities.

6.4.2 The Simplistic Model and the Inclusive Context of Assessment

The development of a systematic basis for cognitive assessment for the purposes of matching individuals to ICT should make reference to an overall approach to accessibility and disability in the population at large. The simplistic model, outlined above, is intended to tackle in more detail a number of specific issues more generally addressed by the Cambridge Inclusive Design Cube (Keates, Langdon, Clarkson and Robinson, 2001). The Design Cube is a representation used for analysis of human interaction with computers, such as may take place while using computer–based assistive technology. The three axes of a 3D cube are used as imaginary scales of degree of capability with the fully able user being represented as the nearest bottom corner (Figure 6.3). Clearly, in this representation, the cognitive scale is a summation of the effects on the individuals capability of a range of fundamental cognitive competencies. The simplistic model, outlined above, allows the nature and relative importance of those competencies to be examined at a general level. Furthermore, the simplistic model allows interactions between sensory, motor and core cognitive functions to be specified in order to address specific tasks and skills.

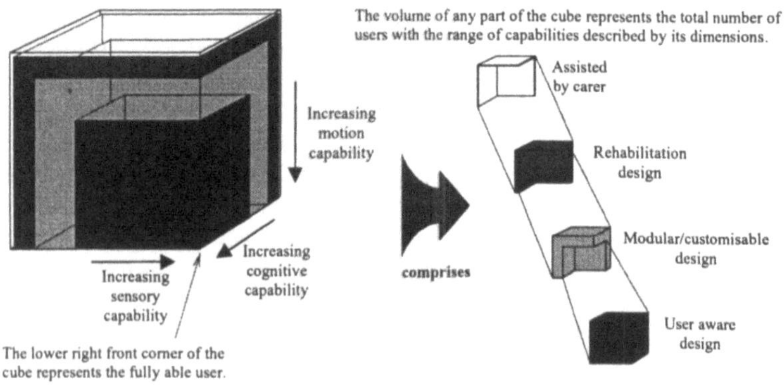

Figure 6.3. The Design Cube representation of human capability

It also follows that the cognitive simplistic model can also be used to unpack the detailed considerations that correspond to user perception, cognition, and motor function. For example, methods of verifying the users' perception of a computer–based AT display in an accessible interface can be derived from standard tests of visual cognition, such as visual search tasks that measure the relationship of the features of a target object in a visual display field to the time taken to detect that object (e.g. Treisman and Gelade, 1980), or figure-ground detection tasks that relate the time to detect a target to the visual grouping properties of clusters of 2D features. The simplistic model can therefore be used to specify the detailed content of the design of assessment methods for assistive technology. In particular, it is aimed at the cognitive elements of such an assessment, such as memory, attention and reasoning.

6.4.3 Evaluation in Practice

The objective will be to develop new methods and test the programme and evaluate its effectiveness in the context of practical assessment and progression programmes at the Papworth Trust. Initially, the enhanced approach will be assessed in the context of day-to-day Rehabilitation, assessment and progression activities and the detailed feedback used to modify and improve both the theoretical basis and the practical application. In the longer term, evaluation will be managed using the newly developed approach alongside the existing service and measuring the relative success of the two systems by measuring their effect on a number of previously defined success long-term criteria such as employment rates. The outcomes of the use of the method will be assessed using systematic empirical methodology, such as blind studies.

6.5 Conclusions

We have outlined the cognitive components necessary for a simplistic model to be used to support the assessment of individual assistive technology needs and rehabilitation. The simplistic model has two levels, the overview level gives a framework for embedding detailed models at the second level that can be used to guide the applications of assessment techniques and to evaluate their outcomes and validity. It has been necessary to add; sensory input, perception, input memory, working memory, long tem memory and some kind of central processing resource. All of these factors are well supported by current research and point the way to better ways to carry out assessments for assistive technology for disabled people as well as defining the contents of such assessments. This research can be embedded in the Inclusive context of assessment and holds the potential to provide assessment for computer users that will ultimately empower them both at home and at work with independence and new vocational opportunities. Practitioners and physiotherapists will gain more usable methods and this will enable a better quality of interaction between carers and end users.

6.6 References

Adams RG, Berry C (1981) Cued recall of sentences. Quarterly Journal of Experimental Psychology 33(A): 295-307

Anderson JR (1983) The Architecture of Cognition. Harvard University Press

Argyris C (1991) Teaching smart people how to learn. Harvard Business Review, May-June, pp54-62

Baddeley AD (1996) Your memory: a user' guide. Prion, London

Barnard PJ, May J, Duke D, Duce D (2000) Systems interactions macrotheory. Transactions on Computer Human Interface 7: 222-262

Broadbent DE (1984) The Maltese cross: a new simplistic model or memory. The Behavioural and Brain Sciences 7: 55-94

Broadbent DE, Broadbent MHP (1981) Articulatory suppression and the grouping of successive stimuli. Psychological Research 43: 57-67

Coltheart M (1984) Sensory memory - a tutorial review. Attention and performance X. Lawrence Erlbaum Associates, New Jersey

Cooper CL, Williams S (1994) Creating healthy work organizations. John Wiley, Chichester

Handy TC, Hopfinger JB, Mangan GR (2001) Functional neuroimaging of attention. In: Cabeza R, Kingstone A (eds.) Handbook of Functional Neuroimaging of Cognition. Cambridge, MA, MIT Press

Hartley LR, Adams RG (1974) Effect of noise on the stroop test. Journal of Experimental Psychology 102: 62-66

Keates S, Langdon PM, Clarkson PJ, Robinson P (2001) Towards an Inclusive design approach. In: Proceedings of the 13th International Conference on Engineering Design, Glasgow, UK, pp 355-362

Lee FJ, Anderson JR (2001) Does learning a complex task have to be complex? A study in learning decomposition. Cognitive Psychology 42: 267-316

Marr D (1982) Vision: A computational investigation into the human representation and processing of visual information. San Fransisco: W.H. Freeman

Myers A, Kakabadse A, Gordon C (1995) Effectiveness of French management: Analysis of the behaviour, attitudes and business impact of top managers. The Journal of Management Development 14: 56-72

Rabbitt PMA (1981) Cognitive psychology needs models for changes in performance with old age. In: Long J, Baddeley A (eds.) Attention and performance 1X. New Jersey: Lawrence Erlbaum Associates

Revelle W, Loftus DA (1990) Individual differences and arousal; implications for the study of mood and memory. Cognition and Emotion 4: 161-190

Rumelhart DE, McClelland JL, The PDP Research Group (eds.) (1986) Parallel Distributed Processing. vol 1 - Foundations. Cambridge, MA: MIT Press

Stroop JR (1935) Studies of interferance in serial verbal interactions. Journal of Experimental Psychology 18: 643-662

Treisman AM, Gelade G (1980) A feature integration theory of attention. Cognitive Psychology 12: 97-136

Chapter 7

Control of Virtual Environments for People with Intellectual Disabilities

P.J. Standen, T.L. Lannen and D.J. Brown

7.1 Introduction

Computer-based learning has enjoyed an increasing role in mainstream education with the development of more powerful personal computers available at a lower price. Computer delivered instruction has also started to make a contribution to the education of children with intellectual disabilities (e.g. Dube, Moniz and Gomes, 1995). It enables pupils to take charge of their own learning (Hawkridge and Vincent, 1992). Interactive software encourages active involvement in learning and gives the user the experience of control over the learning process (Pantelidis, 1993) and the learner can work at their own pace, attempting the same task over and over again, making as many mistakes as they like (Salem-Darrow, 1996).

The potential of a specific form of computer software, virtual environments (VEs), for people with intellectual disabilities has been described by Cromby, Standen and Brown (1996). If used on a desktop system the public nature of the display permits interactions between the learner and a tutor or a peer. Cromby *et al.* (1996) noted three characteristics that make VEs particularly appropriate for people with intellectual disabilities. First, VEs create the opportunity for people with intellectual disabilities to learn by making mistakes but not suffering the real, humiliating or dangerous consequences of their errors. Secondly, virtual worlds can be manipulated in ways the real world cannot, perhaps providing less challenging versions of a task for the beginner. Thirdly, in VEs rules and abstract concepts can be conveyed without the use of language or other symbol systems that many people with intellectual disabilities find difficult to use.

Initial work suggests that virtual environments are effective in facilitating the acquisition of living skills for example shopping and navigating new environments (Standen, Cromby and Brown, 1998) and Makaton sign Language (Standen and Low, 1996) by children with severe intellectual disabilities. With the wider availability of computers in both primary and secondary schools for mainstream and special education (Light, 1997) there is a need to investigate a range of questions about this new aid to learning. However, there are adults with intellectual disabilities who may have had little or no computer experience at school but whose continuing educational needs have been recognised by the Tomlinson Report (1997). This highlighted the need to provide courses that teach independent living and communication skills to people with intellectual disabilities.

Around 25 people in every thousand have mild or moderate intellectual disabilities and about four or five per thousand have severe intellectual disabilities (Department of Health, 2001). They are unlikely to enter employment when they leave school or to achieve the level of independence expected by the rest of society. Adults with intellectual disabilities will have the option to attend some form of college or day centre, the role of which is to provide training programmes relating to the development of daily living, social and educational skills.

7.2 The Barriers Created by Current Input Devices

To what extent can the use of VEs help in the development of these skills and through their improvement facilitate community inclusion for adults with intellectual disabilities? Brown *et al.* (1999) have developed a virtual city for people with intellectual disabilities to facilitate the learning of skills like catching a bus, road crossing and buying food in a café. However, in an early evaluation of the city Cobb, Neale and Reynolds (1998) found that to use the virtual city some individuals required considerable support to use the input devices. The joystick was used for navigation tasks and a standard two button mouse for interaction tasks as Hall (1993) had concluded that a joystick limited to two simultaneous degrees of freedom had the greatest utility in navigation. Brown, Kerr and Crosier (1997) evaluating a range of affordable and robust interaction and navigation devices also favoured use of the joystick finding it more suitable for navigation tasks than the keyboard and the mouse. For interaction tasks, the touch-screen and mouse were equally effective although the touch-screen was difficult to calibrate.

Many people with intellectual disabilities have fine motor difficulties as they suffer from conditions where damage has been caused to the central nervous system, such as cerebral palsy, multiple sclerosis, muscular dystrophy and dyspraxia. They therefore find the devices difficult to control. Brown, Kerr and Crosier (1997) concluded that future input device design or modification should ensure that they should be: operable by people with fine motor difficulties; modifiable; robust; easy to calibrate; and affordable. Until this access problem is solved, exploiting the benefits of VEs for this client group will be problematic.

Lannen (1997) reviewed existing computer interface technology, including assistive computer access methods and virtual reality interfaces, to identify any existing devices, which with adaptation could provide a potential solution and to identify technological opportunities for satisfying the design requirements in novel ways. From reviewing assistive technology she identified head-tracking, eye-tracking and the foot mouse as having potential for people with fine-motor difficulties, yet none of these devices met all the requirements suggested by Brown *et al.* (1997). The review of the virtual reality interfaces identified the 'position tracker' and 'motion platform' as having potential and these designs inspired the development of a prototype interactive device, the Mojo interactive seat. It meets some of the requirements suggested by Brown *et al.* (1997) as it is operable by people with fine-motor difficulties, modifiable and affordable, see Figure 7.1.

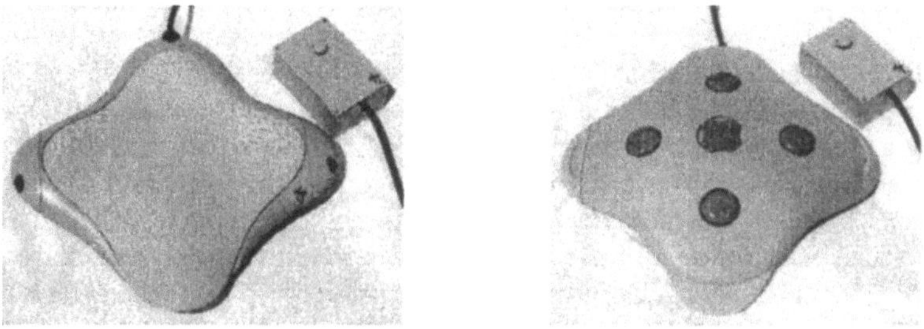

Figure 7.1. Mojo: an interactive seat for VE navigation

Mojo is a navigation device operable with gross motor movement. It consists of an interactive seat that is designed to enable people with intellectual and physical difficulties to explore VEs through movement of the lower body. The user sits on the device, which can be placed on a wheelchair seat, a chair or the floor. The user can rock from side-to-side, forward and back onto the motion sensors, which transfer the movement to the VE. The sensitivity can be adjusted to suit the ability and weight of the user, allowing very slight movements to be detected. Switches on each side of the device can be used to increase its degrees of freedom. Alternatively, external switches can be plugged in to the device. Mojo was compared with a joystick for control of a VE navigation task by students with moderate to severe intellectual disabilities, some of whom were also physically impaired. From the results it was clear that less disorientation occurred when using Mojo than with the joystick, however, it would require considerable further refinement to provide an adequate solution to this human-VE interaction problem.

Soos (1998) developed a device based on a prototype hybrid wheelchair controller. This allowed direct manipulation of VEs by wheelchair users without intellectual disabilities. One of the main findings was that users were already familiar with the operation of their wheelchair controller and it did not impose an extra cognitive load on them when attempting to navigate a VE. This strategy of utilising the characteristics employed in familiar devices has many advantages in the design of input devices for people with intellectual disabilities.

Standen *et al.* (in press) used the virtual city to determine which strategies tutors employ in teaching people with intellectual disabilities to use VEs and how effective these are. Much of the time spent by the tutor in the learner's early sessions was on providing assistance with the input devices. Less time was given to help with the mouse than with the joystick, but the first session had included specific training on using the mouse. Users experienced problems in remembering what tasks were accomplished by each device and in moving from one device to the other as many used the same (dominant) hand for both devices. This suggests that a single device would be easier to use. Whether one or two input devices are needed it may also be the case that the same design may not suit everyone and that different versions of the product need to be produced.

7.3 The Difficulties with Existing Devices

Although several studies have now noted that these users experience difficulties with input devices, which can be both frustrating and ultimately demotivating, the exact nature of the difficulties has not been documented. As a first step to producing a device for school aged students using VEs Lannen, Brown and Powell (in press) carried out a detailed analysis of the difficulties these users experienced using a joystick for navigation and a mouse for interaction. Seven male and seven female students aged between 7 and 19 years formed the user group. Two of the students had mild to moderate intellectual disabilities and the rest had severe intellectual disabilities. All had some degree of co-ordination, gross-motor or fine-motor difficulties. The VEs were displayed on a colour computer monitor and a standard 2-button mouse was used for interaction tasks. Initially, the Axys joystick (Suncom Technologies) was used for navigation tasks. However, as some of the students were experiencing difficulties in gripping the stick on this device, the last 4 students used the Wingman joystick (Logitech). The stick on the Wingman joystick is much taller and wider than the Axys joystick and is shaped to fit the hand, see Figure 7.2.

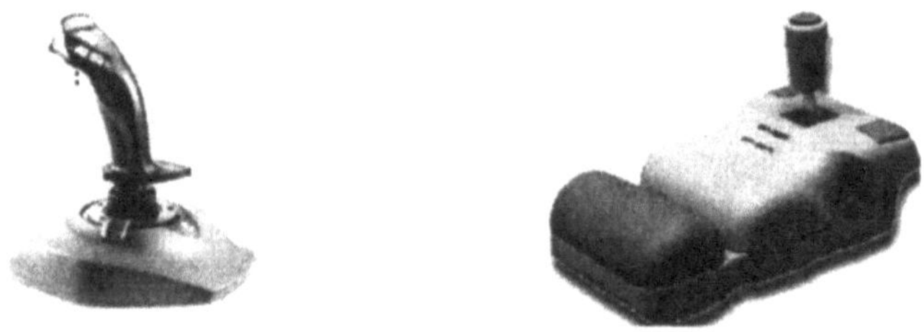

Figure 7.2. The Wingman joystick (Logitech) & the Axys joystick (Suncom Technologies)

The students were asked to complete specified navigation and interaction tasks within the virtual factory, café or supermarket. Demonstrations of the devices and tasks were given before commencing the evaluations. Measures taken included misuse of the device (e.g. non-task related movement, harshness, pressing the wrong buttons); support required (e.g. spoken instruction, physical assistance); physical difficulties (e.g. insufficient strength, inability to grip properly) and user comments and reactions.

Many of the difficulties experienced were due to physical ability and device construction rather than to the user's understanding of how to use each device. For example, when using the joystick users frequently obtained too much left/right rotation, misused the button, had to have the base held still and experienced grip difficulties. The Wingman joystick was easier to grip than the Axys joystick due to its size and shape, highlighting the importance of ergonomic design for usability. Other difficulties appeared to be related to the user's level of understanding of how to use the devices, e.g. occurrence of random movement and frequent pressing of mouse buttons. To overcome these difficulties it may be necessary to gain more knowledge of the users' cognitive and perceptual abilities, so that the devices can be refined to an appropriate level of understanding. Finally, difficulties arose from the design of the VEs which led to 12 students requiring physical help to complete some tasks. This evaluation highlighted the importance of considering the physical and cognitive abilities of the user group, as well as the tasks that the user must complete with the input devices, in order to develop a usable computer interface device. This theory is backed up by contemporary human-computer interaction (HCI) research, which also stresses that you should design for the user, the task and the environment (Faulkner, 1998). This point is also made by Newell and Cairns (1993) who highlight the fact that ergonomics research tends to be focused on ordinary users with average abilities with designers using a single model of the user and making little attempt to specify the actual characteristics of the intended user group. They suggest that some system designers see themselves or their colleagues as archetypes of the system user. The conventional approach for including the consideration of the user, the task and the environment is the user-centred design process.

7.4 User-centred Design

Usability is a crucial factor in the production of a successful interface and is central to the user-centred design process. The usability of a product is defined in ISO 9241, part 11 (1998) (the British Standard giving guidance on usability) as 'the extent to which a product can be used by specified users to achieve specified goals with effectiveness, efficiency and satisfaction in a specified context of use'. According to ISO 13407 (1999) the key activities in user-centred design are:

- understand and specify the context of use;
- specify the user and organisational requirements;
- produce designs and prototypes;
- carry out a user-based assessment.

When the considering people with disabilities in the design process, it is usual to talk about "Design for All", "Universal Usability" or "Equitable Use" implying that the design should be useful and marketable to any group of users. However, Newell and Gregor (2000) consider that this ideal may be very difficult if not impossible to achieve. For example, different user groups may provide very conflicting requirements for a product. As an alternative, they propose a "User Sensitive Inclusive Design" which recognises that inclusivity is more achievable than a universal design. One of their conclusions is that "User Sensitive Inclusive Design needs to be an attitude of mind rather than simply mechanistically applying a set of 'design for all' guidelines."

We are employing a methodology, outlined in Lannen, Brown and Powell (in press) which was determined by combining established guidelines on user-centred design e.g. INUSE (Daly-Jones, Bevan and Thomas, 1999) and USERfit (Poulson, Ashby and Richardson, 1996; Poulson and Richardson, 1998; Poulson and Waddell, 2001) with contemporary human-computer interaction and product design research. This produces a five stage process.

7.4.1 Understand and Specify the Context of Use

This is achieved by conducting a Usability Context Analysis (UCA), which involves a user, task and environmental analysis. In Lannen *et al.* (in press) this involved gathering information about each member of a group of 21 school-aged students with intellectual disabilities, on the attributes that might affect the difficulties they experienced using the input device. This information included their skills and knowledge, their physical, cognitive and perceptual abilities, communication, behaviour and motivations. The next step is a hierarchical task analysis (Dix *et al.*, 1998) which involves breaking down the primary tasks e.g. navigation tasks into subtasks e.g. "use input device to move to position in VE", which are further broken down e.g. "move forward", "move left". This analysis is used to determine the design requirements to carry out each element of the main tasks. Finally the environment analysis involves an analysis of the organisational (e.g. will student be working alone?), technical and physical factors (e.g. level of background noise) of the environment. By gaining an understanding of these factors, an input device can be selected or developed to fit the task environment.

7.4.2 Specify the User and Organisational Requirements

This stage involves the usability team: a multi-disciplinary team which might include project advisors, a design engineer, human-computer interaction and special needs experts, a usability specialist a physiotherapist and an occupational therapist. The team considers the results of the first stage (UCA) translating them into design requirements. A Product Analysis is then conducted in order to describe how the design requirements could be met through specific device attributes. So for example, if the users experience slight hand tremor the device needs to be designed so that it will not detect unintentional movements. The final step in this stage is to collate the device attributes into a design specification that covers such categories as appearance and ergonomic design.

7.4.3 Technology Review

This stage reviews existing technology to identify any computer interface devices that, with adaptation, could provide a potential solution and to identify opportunities for innovation. For the current task the relevant areas would include VR, assistive and general computer interface technology and gaming devices.

7.4.4 Produce Concept Designs and Prototypes

Baxter (1995) described methods for concept and prototype design. Initially, many concepts may be generated with reference to the design specification. Concept selection techniques are then used to select the best concept. Storyboards and sketches can be used to present concepts to the usability team and user group for modification and new idea generation. The selected concept(s) will go through embodiment design, which develops it to the point at which a full working prototype can be made. Finally, engineering drawings, which are the output from embodiment design, will be used to produce the evaluation prototype(s).

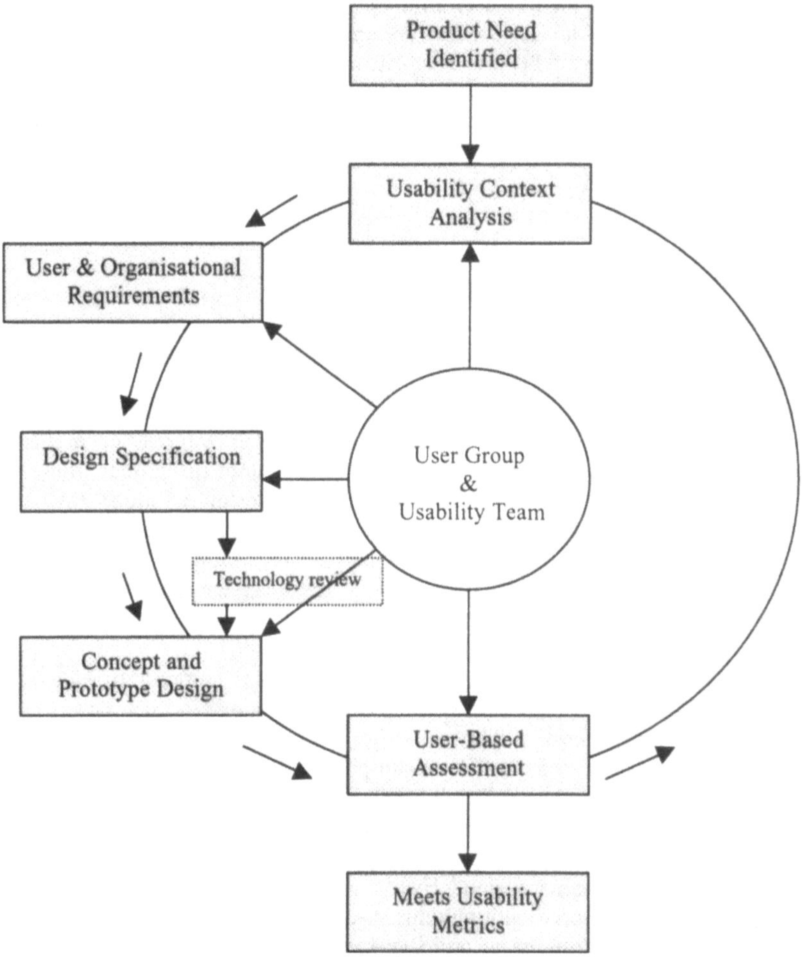

Figure 7.3. The user-centred design cycle

7.4.5 Carry Out a User-based Assessment

The prototype is then taken back to the user group to evaluate the extent to which the user and organisational requirements have been met, and to recommend how the device or devices should be refined (Faulkner, 1998). An evaluation plan will identify the resources required and the intended methodology, which will describe how the data will be collected. In our current study for example, we are using video recordings which are coded using a scheme established in an earlier study (Standen *et al.*, in press) This planning also involves the preparation of a usability specification, which lists the usability attributes and usability metrics. The usability attributes define the success of the prototype(s), i.e. user-satisfaction, misuse of devices. The usability metrics determine how the attributes will be measured for example, frequency of misuse as observed from video recordings. A selected user group then uses the prototype(s) to complete a pre-defined set of tasks within a VE. The results are analysed and recommendations made to refine the prototype(s). A process of evaluation, refinement and re-evaluation is carried out until the usability metrics, outlined in the usability specification have been attained, see Figure 7.3.

7.5 Disability-focused Design

The approach outlined above seeks to solve the problem of design for disability by involving users and specifying in detail their characteristics and the difficulties they experience with existing devices. A danger with this process is that it may reinforce the practice of considering the user population as falling into dichotomous groups: those with disabilities and those without, or in discrete groups: those without disabilities, those with gross motor disabilities, those with sensory impairments, etc. This would suggest that design solutions have to be found for each group in turn and falls back on the solution where systems are designed exclusively for people with disabilities – the "orphan" products referred to by Newell and Gregor (2000). For us, a huge disadvantage of this solution is that the potential market for such a product might be too small to attract a manufacturer.

An alternative way of viewing design for disability is proposed by Newell and Cairns (1993) who believe that considering the needs of extraordinary users can be a spur to a good product or system design for all. Using people with disabilities to evaluate products or systems can also highlight problems that would not have been obvious to those without such disabilities. They see disability as constituting a continuum not a dichotomy. On any given measure of human ability, a range of values will be found in the population, from those who are exceptionally good at this skill, to those who are less good. Everyone will possess this skill to a greater or lesser degree. Even people with obvious disabilities rarely have abilities that are different in quality from those of ordinary users. They are only an exaggeration or lie on a different point on the continuum of ability. These users simply have some functionalities that differ to some degree from the average. So, for example, it is rare for someone to have no motor control, most have more or less motor control relative to one another.

Additionally, Newell and Cairns (1993) remind us that abilities are not static but change with time. Accidents can cause temporary or permanent dysfunction. Disease and age cause substantial changes. In other words, a design solution for the less able will be a design solution for us all. They go on to report an example where technology originally designed to assist people with disabilities became widely used by the general public. Able-bodied people and mainstream researchers have benefited from developments designed for people with disabilities.

Newell and Cairns warned that if users are seen as two distinct groups, mainstream designers might develop too narrow a view of their user population. Presumably, the same argument could be used with designers for disability, especially if the adoption of a user-centred design process involves seeing the users with disabilities as categorically distinct from other users.

7.6 Conclusions

If Newell and Cairns are correct, then a solution to the control of VEs established using people with severe intellectual and physical disabilities, as well as being of benefit to the 3 per cent of the population with intellectual disabilities, may benefit others. Some of these beneficiaries might include those who experience motor difficulties, for example the increasing number of people with neuromuscular disorders, especially those with strokes for whom VEs may have a rehabilitative or therapeutic role (Rose, Attree and Brookes, 1997). Additionally, the elderly who are unfamiliar with computer technology and groups with cognitive impairment might also benefit from a simpler input device. However, just as the remote control is now used by all able-bodied people who wish to change their television channel without leaving their armchair, a VE input device for people with intellectual disabilities may benefit a much wider group of users.

7.7 References

Baxter M (1995) Product design: Practical methods for the systematic development of new products. Chapman and Hall, London

Brown DJ, Kerr SJ, Crosier J (1997) Appropriate input devices for students with learning and motor skills difficulties. Report to National Council for Educational Technology, UK

Brown DJ, Neale H, Cobb SV, Reynolds H (1999) The development and evaluation of the virtual city. International Journal of Virtual Reality 4(1): 28-41

Cobb SVG, Neale HR, Reynolds H (1998) Evaluation of virtual learning environments. In: Sharkey, Rose, Lindström (eds.), Proceedings of the 2nd European Conference on Disability, Virtual Reality and Associated Technologies, pp 17-23

Cromby JJ, Standen PJ, Brown DJ (1996) The potentials of virtual environments in the education and training of people with learning disabilities. Journal of Intellect Disability Research 40(6): 489-501

Daly-Jones O, Bevan N, Thomas C (1999) INUSE: Handbook of User-Centred Design. Serco Usability Services, National Physical Laboratory

Department of Health (2001) Valuing people: A new strategy for learning disability for the 21st century. The Stationery Office

Dix AJ, Finlay JE, Abowd GD, Beale R (1998) Human Computer Interaction. (2nd Edition), Prentice Hall, Europe

Dube WV, Moniz DH, Gomes JF (1995) Use of computer- and teacher delivered prompts in discrimination training with individuals who have mental retardation. American Journal on Retardation 100: 253-261

Faulkner C (1998) The essence of human-computer interaction. Prentice Hall

Hall JD (1993) Explorations of Population Expectations and Stereotypes with Relevance to Design. Undergraduate thesis, Department of Manufacturing Engineering, University of Nottingham

Hawkridge D, Vincent T (1992) Learning Difficulties and Computers. Jessica Kingsley, London

Lannen TL (1997) Mojo: Control of virtual environments for people with physical disabilities. Undergraduate thesis, Department of Industrial Design, Brunel University

Lannen TL, Brown DJ, Powell H (in press) Control of virtual environments for young people with learning difficulties. Disability and Rehabilitation

Light P (1997) Annotation: Computers for learning: psychological perspectives. Journal of Child Psychology and Psychiatry 38: 497-504

Newell AF, Cairns AY (1993) Designing for extraordinary users. Ergonomics in Design, October, pp 10-16

Newell AF, Gregor P (2000) User sensitive inclusive design – in search of a new paradigm. Proceedings of the ACM Conference on Universal Usability, Washington DC. November, pp 39-44

Pantelidis VS (1993) Virtual reality in the classroom. Educational Technology April, pp 23-27

Poulson D, Ashby M, Richardson S (1996) USERFIT: A practical handbook on user-centred design for Assistive Technology. TIDE European Commission, ECSC-EC-EAEC, Brussels-Luxembourg

Poulson DF, Richardson SJ (1998) USERfit - A Framework for User Centred Design in Assistive Technology. Technology and Disability 9: 163-171

Poulson DF, Waddell FN (2001) USERfit: User centred design in assistive technology. In: Nicholle CA, Abascal J (eds.) Inclusive guidelines for HCI, Taylor and Francis

Rose FD, Attree EA, Brooks BM (1997) Virtual environments in neuropsychological assessment and rehabilitation. In: Riva G (ed.) Virtual reality in neuro-psycho-physiology: Cognitive, clinical and methodological issues in assessment and rehabilitation, IOS Press, Amsterdam, pp 147-156

Salem-Darrow M (1996) Virtual reality's increasing potential for meeting needs of person with disabilities: what about cognitive impairments? In: H J Murphy (ed), Proceedings of the 3rd International Conference on Virtual Reality and Persons with Disabilities, California State University Center on Disabilities

Soos R (1998) Unpublished BSc thesis, Computer Studies, Nottingham Trent University

Standen PJ, Brown DJ, Proctor T, Horan M (in press) How tutors assist adults with learning disabilities to use virtual environments Disability and Rehabilitation

Standen PJ, Cromby J, Brown D (1998) Playing for Real. Mental Health Care 1(12): 412-415

Standen PJ, Low HL (1996) Do virtual environments promote self-directed activity? A study of students with severe learning difficulties learning Makaton Sign language. In: Sharkey PM (ed.) Proceedings of the First European Conference on Disability, Virtual Reality and Associated Technologies, Maidenhead, UK, pp 123-127.

Tomlinson J (1997) Inclusive learning: the report of the committee of enquiry into the post-school education of those with learning difficulties and/or disabilities, in England 1996. European Journal of Special Needs Education 12(3): 184-196

Part II

Enabling Computer Access and New Technologies

Chapter 8

Why Are Eye Mice Unpopular? – A Detailed Comparison of Head and Eye Controlled Assistive Technology Pointing Devices

R. Bates and H.O. Istance

8.1 Head Mice and Eye Mice

8.1.1 Introduction

Head-based and eye-based assistive technology pointing devices, or head and eye mice, are used to enable computer control in a similar manner to standard mice, by simply moving the cursor to where a user is pointing either with their head or their eyes. These devices have been in existence for many years within the motor-disabled community and over this time there has been widespread acceptance and adoption of head mice, with many disabled people using these devices to access computers and communication devices. However, anecdotal evidence suggests that eye-based pointing is widely and quickly dismissed as a usable means of pointing in assistive technology due to difficulty of use and inaccuracy, making the potential advantages of eye-based pointing difficult to realise in the face of such quick decisions not to use this approach. It is necessary to understand in detail what the limitations of eye-based pointing are and how these can be overcome. Making relative performance comparisons with head-based pointing can usefully do this, as this is an established technique of assistive technology pointing.

8.1.2 For Eye Pointing

Firstly, eye-gaze has the potential to be a very natural form of pointing, as people tend to look at the object they wish to interact with (Jacob, 1991; Salvucci, 2000). Secondly the speed of eye-gaze to locate a target can be very fast compared with other pointing devices (Ware, 1987; Sibert, 2000). Thirdly, due to the specialised nature of the muscles controlling the eye, natural eye movements exhibit little detectable fatigue and offer near fatigue-free pointing (Saito, 1992). Finally, eye-trackers can be non-encumbering, as they do not require the user to wear anything.

In contrast, head pointing requires conscious movement and steering of the head to point at an object. This form of pointing can be slow due to the high mass of the head restricting rapid movement, it is fatiguing due to the non-specialised nature of the neck muscles, which may tire after repeated head movements and it often requires the user to wear a target or device. Initially it appears that eye-based pointing has considerable advantages over head-based pointing.

8.1.3 Against Eye Pointing

Firstly the eye is not a highly accurate pointing device as it exhibits a positional tolerance (Carpenter, 1991; Jacob, 1995). The fovea of the eye, which gives clear vision, covers a visual angle of $\approx 1°$ arc of the retina, hence when fixating a target the eye only needs to be within $\approx 1°$ of the target position to clearly see the target. This gives an inaccuracy in measured gaze position. Secondly, since eye gaze position cannot easily be consciously controlled or steered, as it is driven by subconscious interest (Yarbus, 1967), the eye tends to fixate briefly on targets of interest before jumping to other points of interest. Thus it requires effort to fixate steadily on a target for any extended period of time. This contrasts sharply with the deliberate, if slow, controlled movement and positional accuracy of head-based pointing. Thirdly the eye is being employed as both an input modality to the user, so the person can see the computer interface, and an output modality from the user to the interface, indicating the pointing intention of the user on the interface. This convergence of interaction point and gaze-point means that the pointing cursor, in contrast to head pointing, cannot be parked or left at a position on the screen whilst the eye momentarily looks away. Such convergence results in unwanted pointing movements at the feedback point on the computer screen as the cursor follows the eye wherever is gazes (Jacob, 1995; Velichkovsky *et al.*, 1997). Finally, unlike head-trackers, eye-trackers are not widely available, and can be expensive.

Clearly, both types of pointing devices have advantages and disadvantages. The question that must be answered is to what extent each of these advantages and disadvantages influence the performance of the devices and lead to the acceptance or rejection of each device by their intended users.

8.2 Assessing the Devices

8.2.1 A 'Real World' Test

A 'real world' experimental test sequence, rather than an abstract target acquisition test, was used to test the performance of the devices. The test consisted of a total of 150 simple tasks across two domains, word-processing with Microsoft Word and web browsing with Internet Explorer, which formed a natural flow of interaction. The proportions of object usage, target sizes and interaction techniques in the two sets of tasks mimicked as closely as possible 'real world' interaction based on previous observation of users. The 150 test task objects that comprised the test, such as a button or menu item, were assigned one of four size categories (0.3°, 0.6°, 0.9°, 1.2°) based on the smallest visual angle subtended by the screen object central to the task at a distance of 60cm from the screen. Typical objects for each category were spin control button or text in the 0.3° category, filenames and scrollbar buttons 0.6°, menu items and toolbar buttons 0.9°, icons and keyboard keys 1.2°. The distribution of object sizes in the test was determined by the nature of the real-world task, with 0.3° objects taking 4%, 0.6° 17%, 0.9° 23% and 1.2° 56% of the total test tasks.

8.2.2 Device Performance

The usability of the two pointing devices was assessed in terms of device *performance* based on the European ESPRIT MUSiC performance metrics method (Macleod *et al.* 1997). Performance was defined as *'The quality of interaction with the device and the time taken to perform that interaction'*. Device performance was calculated by measuring the quality of interaction during the tasks by counting the number of incorrect commands (such as hitting the wrong target), the number of target misses (with no command generated), the number of cursor position corrections (unnecessary position correction cursor movements), and the time taken to complete the tasks (measured from the start of a task until the task was finished or abandoned). Tasks were initially given a quality rating of 5 (perfect) (Szczur, 1994), with subsequent errors reducing the quality until the task was completed or failed, and the next task started. Task performance with each device was calculated by a simple formula (8.1) such that a task that has the highest level of quality and takes no time would give a performance of 100%, with any reduction in quality or increase in time degrading the measured performance:

$$\text{Task performance} = \frac{\text{Quality of interaction (1-5)}}{5 + \text{Time taken for interaction (secs)}} \tag{8.1}$$

8.2.3 Test Participants

Six able-bodied test participants were chosen for the experiment. The participants were selected to give a wide range of experience using the head and eye mice from very experienced users through to novice users with little previous experience of the devices. All participants were experienced hand mouse users. Two participants were categorised as 'low' experience users of both of the devices, two as 'medium' experience users and two as 'high' experience users. (The number of available participants with experience of both test devices was limited and the number of hours experience of using each device to define each category is shown later in Table 8.2).

8.2.4 Experimental Design

The experiment was a within-subjects design, with all six participants completing one session of the 150 test tasks with each of the three devices: hand mouse, head mouse and eye mouse. These sessions were conducted in random order. Prior to these, each participant was given training and practice to become familiar with all of the test tasks. A hand held mouse was used for the practice sessions. Participants were also given the opportunity to practice some of the test tasks with the eye and head mouse until they felt comfortable with the use of these devices.

8.2.5 Test Apparatus

A standard PC was used for the tests. For the eye mouse a Senso-Motoric Instruments infrared video-oculography eye-tracker was used to measure eye-gaze position with a software driver used to move the cursor in response to the eye-gaze of the test participants. A Polhemus ISOTRACK electromagnetic motion tracking system was used to measure the head position of the test participants for the head mouse and a second software driver used to move the cursor in response to head position. Target selection was by a hand held micro-switch and text entry was via a WiViK on-screen keyboard. A standard desktop hand mouse was included in the tests as a baseline for comparison. Participants were seated with a head and eye to monitor screen distance of 60cm on a seat with a backrest and head support to help participants to maintain their head position and to increase seating comfort.

8.2.6 Test Analysis

All data was obtained by capturing the complete contents of the test computer screen during each session, including the cursor position, at a rate of 5 frames per second. The data was analysed by stepping through the video files and recording the quality and time taken to perform each task within a session. In addition, the time taken by any non-productive actions during the task was measured and the nature of the non-productive action was recorded.

8.3 Test Results

8.3.1 Overall Performance

The test showed that there were no overall differences between the word-processing and web-browsing performance for each device, but there were differences in performance between the devices (Figure 8.1). Grouping the word and web results together for each device gave a performance of 65.2% for the head mouse and 51.1% for the eye mouse. This difference was statistically significant

(Mann-Whitney Test, U=301228, n_1=900, n_2=900, p<0.0001), with the head mouse outperforming the eye mouse by 1.28 times. For comparative purposes participants completed the same tasks with a hand-held mouse. The performance for the hand mouse was the same over the two domains, and grouping the data gave a performance of 83.3%, considerably higher than the assistive technology devices.

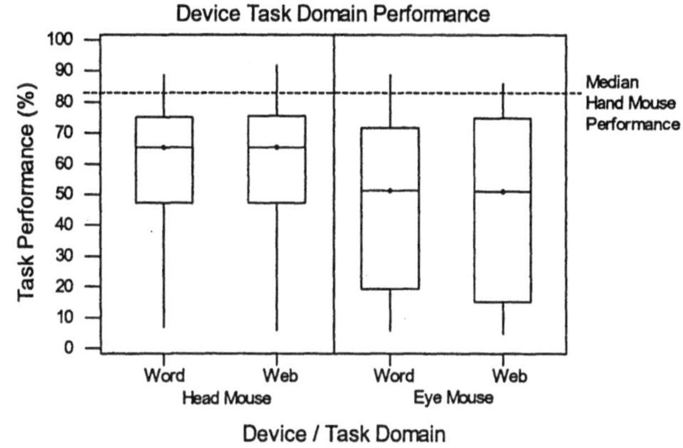

Figure 8.1. Overall device performance

8.3.2 Task Domain Performance

The similarity of device performance between the word and web task domains showed that the context of the tasks had little effect on the performance of the devices. The frequencies of target sizes present in each of the tasks in the domains were similar, which may have accounted for the similarities in measured performance much more than the context of the tasks.

8.3.3 Target Size Performance

Examining the device performance by target size shows a distinct relationship between increasing task performance and increasing target size (Figure 8.2). Here again, the eye mouse was inferior to the head mouse for each of the target sizes. Non-parametric regression was used to determine the relationship of performance to target size (Equations 8.2 and 8.3).

$$\text{Task performance for the head mouse} = 38.9 \times \text{target size} + 21.6 \quad (8.2)$$
$$\text{Task performance for the eye mouse} = 32.2 \times \text{target size} + 16.3 \quad (8.3)$$

Projecting these models to determine at what target sizes the devices have the same performance, or achieve 100% performance, should be treated with caution, as it is probable that device performance will become non-linear as efficiency approaches

100%. Of more use was translating these models into equivalent target sizes for equal device performance over the range of target sizes in the test.

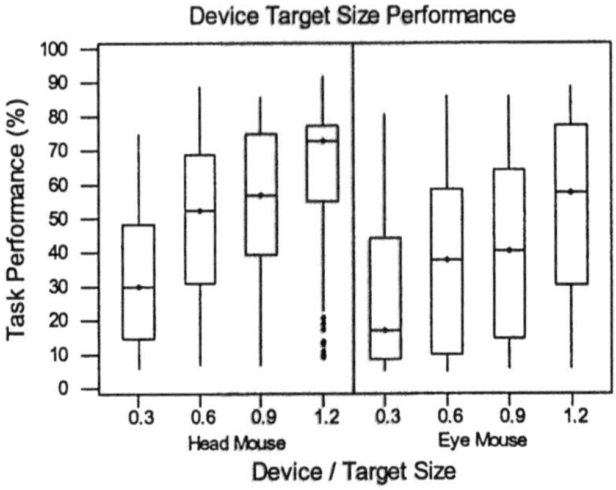

Figure 8.2. Device performance for different target sizes

For example, for the eye mouse to achieve the same efficiency as the head mouse at a target size of 0.3°, the target size for the eye mouse would need to be $((38.9 \times 0.3) + 21.6 - 16.3) / 32.2 = 0.53°$ (Table 8.1).

Table 8.1 Equivalent target sizes for equal performance

Head mouse target size	**Required eye mouse target size**	**Percentage increase in eye mouse target size**
0.3°	0.53°	176%
0.6°	0.89°	148%
0.9°	1.26°	140%
1.2°	1.62°	135%

It is notable that the difference in the required level of target magnification for the eye mouse decreases rapidly with increasing target size, indicating that the eye mouse is capable of performing well on larger target sizes.

Comparing the head mouse target sizes to the required eye mouse target sizes revealed a progression, where for equivalent performance the eye mouse targets must be approximately one size category larger than the head mouse targets. For example, 0.3° head mouse targets gave approximately the same performance as 0.6° eye mouse targets. This strongly suggested that if the target sizes could be increased then the eye mouse could achieve parity with the head mouse. One mechanism to achieve this is to provide the user with an ability to 'zoom in' on an area of the screen (Bates, 1999) which effectively increases target sizes temporarily. The means of controlling this zoom mechanism and the resultant effect on performance are currently being investigated.

8.3.3.1 Elements of Performance and Target Size

The task quality and task time elements that constituted the performance metric showed steady increases in quality and steady reductions in task time with increasing target size. The head mouse was again superior to the eye mouse with the highest quality and lowest times for the target sizes. Of the two elements, the relationship between task time and target size was most interesting (Figure 8.3).

The task time was broken down into six elements: productive time, the time lost generating incorrect commands, misses and cursor control corrections, the time lost whilst the eye mouse cursor was displaced looking at the feedback point on the interface, and finally the time lost during calibrations of the devices. Looking at the individual elements of task time, the most time was lost in cursor control corrections. This was the most detrimental element for both devices, indicating that considerable time was wasted correcting the cursor position onto targets.

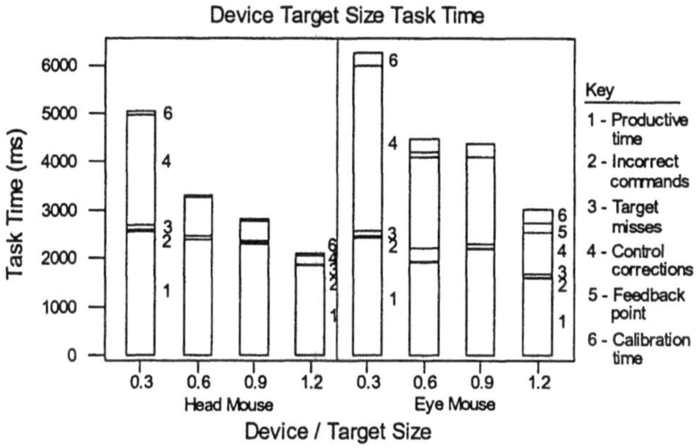

Figure 8.3. Device task time for different target sizes

Most interesting was the similarity in productive time for each of the devices. In particular, the eye mouse had shorter productive times (was more efficient) than the head mouse, indicating that it had the potential to be equal or superior to the head mouse if the non-productive elements could be reduced. The time lost in incorrect commands and misses was not significantly different between the devices.

Looking at elements of the eye mouse task time that could be reduced suggested that if target size continued to increase then the control correction time could be minimised, and the eye mouse would perform as well as the head mouse. It is notable how these results show the performance dependency of the assistive technology devices on the size of the targets present on the computer interface.

8.3.4 Participant Experience and Performance

Table 8.2 shows the numbers of hours of device usage accumulated by participants in each of the three experience categories.

Table 8.2. Participant experience categories and exposure hours

Experience category	Head mouse hours	Eye mouse hours	Numbers of participants
Low	0.25	1 – 2	2
Medium	0.5 – 1	6 – 8	2
High	2 – 3	15 - 30	2

There was a definite relationship between the experience rating of test participants with the devices and their performance, with increasing experience resulting in increasing task performance (Figure 8.4).

Here again, the eye mouse was inferior to the head mouse for the low and medium experienced participants. However, the two devices achieved parity of performance, at 73.0% for the head mouse and 73.5% for the eye mouse in the high experience participants. While the number of hours device experience for these participants is very different between devices, the data suggests that the eye mouse could approach the performance levels of the head mouse if participants are sufficiently practised. In steady-state, performance with neither device is likely to exceed the 83% performance baseline obtained from the hand mouse.

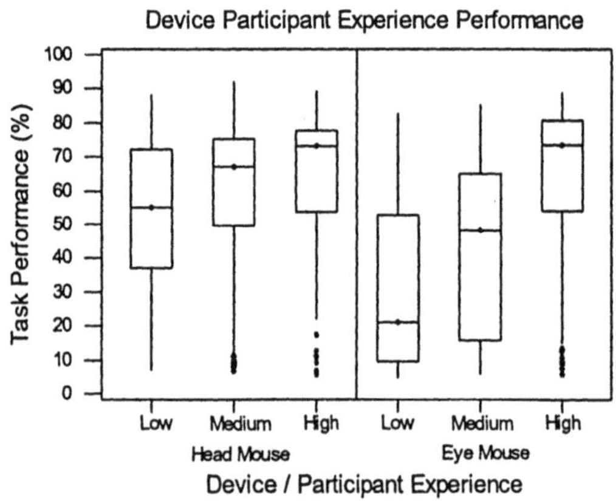

Figure 8.4. Device performance for different participant experience

The performance of the medium group of head mouse users after 0.5 to 1 hour experience is far higher than the low experience eye mouse group with 1 to 2 hours experience. The learning times coupled with the poor performance results for low and medium experienced participants for the eye mouse strongly suggested that considerable effort and dedication would be required to obtain even a moderate level of performance with the eye mouse. This was a strong indicator as to why eye mice appeared to be rarely used, and suggested that more work is needed to investigate the most efficient means of training participants to use the eye mouse in order to reduce the time needed to achieve these levels of performance.

8.3.4.1 Elements of Performance and Experience

Examining the task quality and task time elements that constituted the performance metric showed steady increases in quality and steady reductions in task time with increasing participant experience. The head mouse was superior to the eye mouse with the highest quality and lowest times for the low and medium experience participants, with the eye mouse achieving parity for the highly experienced participants. Again, of the two elements, the relationship between task time and experience was most interesting (Figure 8.5).

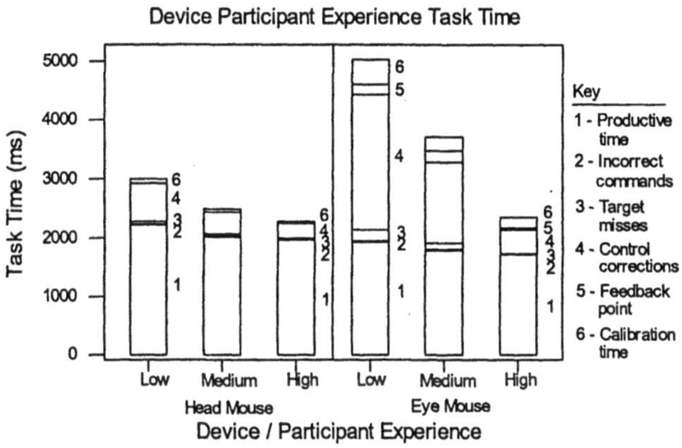

Figure 8.5. Device task time for different participant experience

Here we see dramatic reductions in the non-productive elements of the eye mouse task time for highly experienced participants. Calibration time and time spent at the feedback point has been cut significantly and the time lost in cursor control corrections reduced to near parity with the head mouse. Both sets of data show a levelling out of the productive time component with increasing experience. This suggests that it is possible with much practice to overcome the weaknesses of the eye mouse and use the strengths of the device to match the performance of the head mouse.

8.3.5 How Good Can an Eye Mouse Get?

To investigate just how good the performance of the eye mouse could be, the target size performance of the highly experienced participants was separated from the data for all of the devices, including the baseline hand mouse, and compared (Figure 8.6). Here we see that the hand mouse was superior to the assistive technology devices, even when experienced participants use these devices. However as the target size increased, so the performance of the head and eye mice approached that of the hand mouse. Examining the largest target size, the hand mouse had a performance of 83.3% compared to the head mouse at 75.2% and the eye mouse at 78.1%. At this point the eye mouse exceeds the performance of the head mouse, this difference was statistically significant (Mann-Whitney Test, $U=10906$, $n_1=168$, $n_2=168$, $p=0.0003$), and reaches to within a few percentage points of the hand mouse. This showed that if target sizes were larger and users experienced then the performance of an eye mouse might exceed a head mouse, and approach that of a hand mouse.

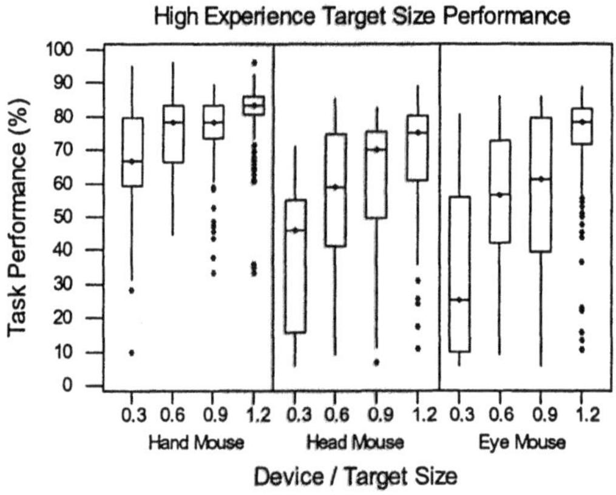

Figure 8.6. High experience participant device performance for different target sizes

8.4 Summary

The question this chapter raised was why are eye mice dismissed as unusable when head mice are widely accepted, particularly in view of the advantages of eye mice in terms of speed and ease of use?

There were no differences in task domain performance for a given device, so the nature of the tasks did not distract or influence the performance of the participants with the eye mouse. The overall performance of the eye mouse was found to be poor.

Breaking down the tasks by target size revealed a trend of increasing performance with target size and showed that the eye mouse performance approached the head mouse for larger sizes, as the non-productive elements of pointing were reduced. It also showed that the actual productive time for the eye mouse was shorter than the head mouse.

Looking at participant experience it was found that highly experienced eye mouse users could exceed their performance with the head mouse in the test as they had learnt how to minimise the non-productive elements of eye mouse pointing. However, this came at a cost of a much longer learning time with the eye mouse compared with the head mouse. It should be noted that it is possible that the performance of the head mouse could improve further than that found in the test if a user had extended head mouse experience up to the 30 hours of the experienced eye mouse users. However, it was observed that the head mouse was extremely quick to learn, as evidenced by performance improvements over time. From this rapid learning time, it was expected that head mouse performance would not improve significantly with extended experience.

Finally, it was shown that an eye mouse could exceed the performance of a head mouse and approach that of a hand mouse if target sizes were large and users sufficiently well practised.

This experiment used able-bodied participants. It is interesting to speculate as to how the results would change if disabled participants had been used. For example, the range of neck motion and the potential for fatigue may reduce the performance of the head mouse and favour the eye mouse. Conversely any reduction in the gaze performance of the participants, due to nystigmus for example, will degrade eye mouse performance in favour of the head mouse.

To answer the question, why have eye mice not been adopted, is that they require slightly larger target sizes and higher user experience to perform well. For novice users the eye mouse would manifest itself as unusable and the system would be quickly rejected, despite its potential benefits. In comparison, the head mouse has moderate performance on smaller targets and a short learning time, so a new user would be able to use the system to some extent on their first attempt, making the system much more attractive. Methods to allow users to control target sizes through 'zooming in' on the screen can overcome this and are already being investigated. This could be coupled with training for users to reach an experienced level quickly. Users should be encouraged to have patience with the eye mouse until they become experienced.

With sufficient control over target size, and sufficient experience, eye mice can be used effectively. For people with motor disabilities who dislike or have difficulties using a head mouse, or cannot use a head mouse, the option to use an eye mouse at least as effectively as a head mouse would greatly enable them to operate the computers and environmental controls around them.

8.5 References

Bates R (1999) Multimodal Eye-based Interaction for Zoomed Target Selection on a Standard Graphical User Interface. In: Proceedings of Interact'99, British Computer Society, vol. II, pp7-8

Carpenter RHS (1991) Eye movements, MacMillan

Jacob RJK (1991) The Use of Eye Movements in Human-Computer Interaction Techniques: What You Look At is What You Get. ACM Transactions on Information Systems 9(3): 152-169

Jacob RJK (1995) Eye Tracking in Advanced Interface Design. In: Barfield W, Furness T (eds.) Advanced Interface Design and Virtual Environments, Oxford University Press, 258-288

Macleod M, Bowden R, Bevan N, Curson I (1997) The MUSiC performance measurement method. Behaviour and Information Technology 16(4-5): 279-293

Saito S (1992) Does Fatigue Exist in a Quantitative Measurement of Eye Movements? Ergonomics 35(5-6): 607-615

Salvucci DD, Anderson JR (2000) Intelligent gaze-added interfaces. In: Proceedings of CHI 2000, ACM Press, vol. 2, pp 273-280

Sibert LE, Jacob RJK (2000) Evaluation of eye gaze interaction In: Proceedings of CHI 2000, ACM Press, vol. 2, pp 281-288

Szczur M (1994) Usability testing - on a budget: a NASA usability test case study. Behaviour and Information Technology 13(1-2): 106-118

Velichkovsky B, Sprenger A, Unema P (1997) Towards Gaze Mediated Interaction: Collecting Solutions of the "Midas Touch" Problem. In: Howard S, Hammond J, Lindgaard G (eds.) Proceedings of Human-Computer Interaction, Chapman & Hall

Ware C, Mikaelian HH (1987) An Evaluation of an Eye Tracker as a Device for Computer Input. In: Proceedings of CHI 1987, ACM Press

Yarbus AL (1967) Eye Movements and Vision. Plenum, New York

Chapter 9

Cursor Characterisation and Haptic Interfaces for Motion-impaired Users

F. Hwang, P. Langdon, S. Keates, P.J. Clarkson and P. Robinson

9.1 Introduction

For people with functional impairments, independent control of a computer is often an important part of everyday life. However, in order to be of benefit, computer systems must be accessible. For people with motion-impairments, the keyboard, mouse and monitor arrangement can be difficult, if not impossible, to use. Symptoms such as tremor, spasm, restricted range of motion, and reduced strength can often restrict the extent to which a keyboard and mouse are useful.

This chapter describes research in developing more effective means of computer access for people with motion-impairments. The objective is to gain an understanding of the nature of computer interaction, and to use this understanding as a basis for developing methods of improving computer accessibility. This work focuses on the study of cursor trajectories during "point and click" interactions using a mouse. Seven measures are proposed as ways of characterising a user's cursor control. The measures are applied to the cursor paths of users with motion-impairments to illustrate their ability to capture differences among people with varying severities and types of impairments. The measures are also useful in identifying some of the difficulties experienced by the users. The cursor characterisation then forms the basis for the development of assistive techniques involving haptic feedback.

9.2 Characterisation of Cursor Movements

Analyses of "point and click" interactions are common in the literature (e.g. Douglas *et al.*, 1999), but have tended to focus on gross measures such as movement time and error rate. Although these measures may adequately establish that differences exist, for example among people or among devices, establishing *why* they exist is more likely accomplished by studying cursor trajectories throughout a target selection task (MacKenzie *et al.*, 2001).

9.2.1 Related Work

In the past, studies of cursor movements have examined a variety of characteristics. Mithal and Douglas (1996) studied cursor velocity throughout a movement to elicit and provide an explanation for performance differences between mouse users and joystick users. Munch and Dillman (1997) reported that certain features of cursor trajectories could help predict a user's actions. The features included smoothed acceleration, velocity, curvature, stopping distance, and overall distance. Keuning-Van Oirschot and Houtsma (2001) found that studies of mean path curvatures, the variability around the mean path, and velocity profiles appeared to be helpful in creating a useful prediction algorithm. MacKenzie *et al.* (2001) proposed seven accuracy measures intended to elicit subtle differences among devices through an analysis of the cursor movement along the cursor path.

9.2.2 Characteristics of Cursor Movements

In the above studies, the focus was on the cursor movements of able-bodied individuals. However, characteristics derived with able-bodied people in mind are not necessarily suitable for people with motion-impairments, and do not preclude examination of new characteristics that may be more appropriate. Seven characteristics, proposed to capture a variety of features of cursor movements of people with motion-impairments, are described in this section. Cursor movements are studied in terms of the path taken by the cursor between the start point and the point where the target is successfully selected.

9.2.2.1 Target Re-entry

A target re-entry occurs when the cursor enters the target, leaves, then re-enters the target (MacKenzie *et al.*, 2001). This characteristic is intended to capture the ease with which an individual is able to hold the cursor inside a target while selecting it.

9.2.2.2 Distance Travelled Relative to Cursor Displacement

This characteristic is defined as $D1/D2$ where $D1$ is the distance travelled by the cursor and $D2$ is the magnitude of the cursor's displacement. This characteristic is intended to capture how closely the cursor path follows a straight line. A value of 1 indicates motion directly towards the target, and larger values indicate deviations.

9.2.2.3 Distribution of Distance Travelled for a Range of Cursor Speeds

This characteristic is a *distribution* that indicates how far the cursor travelled while moving at a particular speed. This characteristic may be particularly effective at capturing the occurrence of spasms that often result in high-speed movements.

9.2.2.4 Submovements
A submovement is one cycle of cursor acceleration and deceleration. A large number of submovements within a trial indicates difficulties in making fluid cursor movements - the cursor frequently "stops and starts" on the way to the target.

9.2.2.5 Cursor Distance Travelled Away from the Target
This characteristic is the total distance travelled by the cursor in a direction that takes it farther away from the target. It is intended to capture how well the user is able to move the cursor toward the target.

9.2.2.6 Distribution of Distance Travelled for a Range of Curvatures
A curved path can be represented as a series of arc segments, each formed from the arc of an associated circle having a particular radius of curvature. This distribution indicates how far the cursor travelled at a particular radius of curvature, thereby capturing "twists and turns" in the path. For example, a straight path will have 100% of the distance travelled at a radius of curvature of infinity.

9.2.2.7 Distribution of Distance Travelled for a Range of Radii from Target
This distribution indicates how far the cursor travelled while at a particular radius from the target's centre. For a straight path, the distribution will be uniform across all radii up to the cursor's initial distance from the target. This characteristic is intended to capture the "spatial spread" of the cursor movement about the target, and can reveal where along the path difficulties with cursor control occur.

9.3 A Study of Cursor Movements

The seven cursor measures were applied to the cursor movements of motion-impaired users (Table 9.1) from the Papworth Trust and, for comparison, three users without motion-impairments (CU1-3).

Table 9.1. Study participants from the Papworth Trust

User	Condition
PI3	Athetoid Cerebral Palsy, spasm, wheelchair user
PI5	Athetoid Cerebral Palsy, deaf, non-speaking
PI6	Athetoid Cerebral Palsy
PI7	Friedrich's Ataxia, tremor, wheelchair user

A Logitech Wingman force-feedback mouse with the force-feedback turned off was used as an input device. The task was a Fitts' Law task, involving point-select interactions. 16 "target" circles (diameter = 40 pixels) were arranged in a circular layout (diameter = 574 pixels) around a central "home" circle at a screen resolution of 1024 by 768 pixels. A sequence of trials began when a participant clicked in the "home" circle. The next selection was a "target" circle randomly selected by the software. The "home" circle had to be selected again before the next "target" was activated. The circle to be selected was always filled in red. Each sequence comprised 16 "target" selections and 17 "home" selections, and data collection began after the first "home" selection.

9.3.1 Results

9.3.1.1 Target Re-entry

Figure 9.1 shows the distributions of the number of target re-entries for each user. The boxes have lines at the lower quartile, median, and upper quartile values of the distribution, and values outside the interquartile range are indicated by a '+'. For CU1-3, PI5, and PI6, fewer than 5% of the trials had more than one target re-entry. PI3 and PI7, however, were less consistent. The number of target re-entries ranged from 0 to 7, and was as high as 12 for PI7. For PI3, many of the target re-entries resulted from spasms that occurred when the cursor was in the vicinity of the target. Target re-entries for PI7 were often the result of difficulties in keeping the mouse stationary while clicking. PI7 operated the mouse using two hands, and an attempt to click the mouse button would often drive the cursor outside the target.

9.3.1.2 Distance Travelled Relative to Cursor Displacement

Figure 9.2 shows the distributions of the distance travelled relative to cursor displacement for each user. The dashed line indicates perfectly straight motion. Spasms often make the cursor deviate widely from the intended path, giving large values of *D1/D2* for PI3, particularly when multiple spasms are experienced during a trial. For PI7, a constant tremor often results in a path with many "twists and turns" which increases *D1/D2*. Very high values can also occur when there is a lot of movement in the vicinity of the target while attempting to click on it. In contrast, CU1 moves in almost perfectly straight lines with few occurrences of overshoot, giving values clustered about 1.

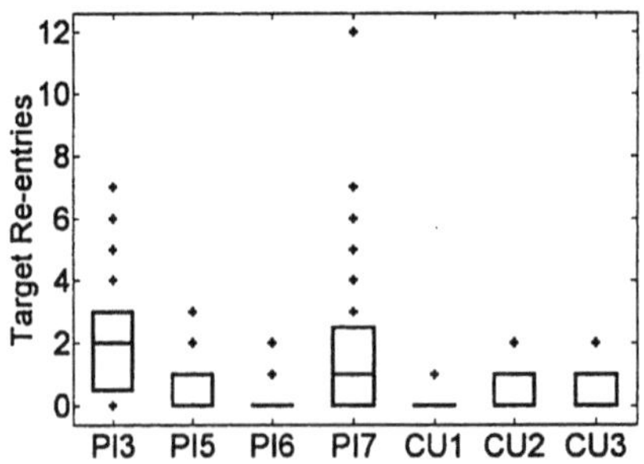

Figure 9.1. Number of target re-entries

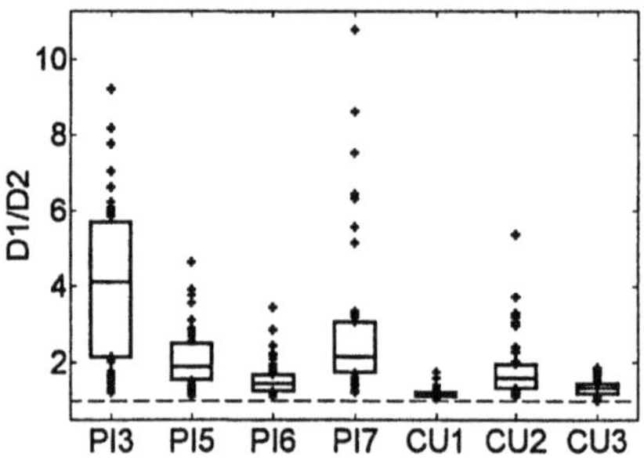

Figure 9.2. Distance travelled relative to cursor displacement

9.3.1.3 Distribution of Distance Travelled for a Range of Cursor Speeds

The distributions for this characteristic showed that for all users except PI3 and CU2, few samples were found at speeds higher than 4 pixels/ms. For PI3 and CU2, however, speeds greater than 10 pixels/ms were frequently observed. For comparison, Figure 9.3a shows the complete distributions for PI3 and CU1, and Figure 9.3b provides a closer look at the values for high speeds. A direct comparison of the magnitudes in each bin is not appropriate since they must be related to the total distance travelled to be meaningful. Of interest, however, is the presence of high-speed samples for PI3 where they are completely absent for CU1. The high-speed movements for PI3 are most likely to have been caused by spasms. High speeds for CU2 can be attributed to "ballistic" motions at the start of a trial.

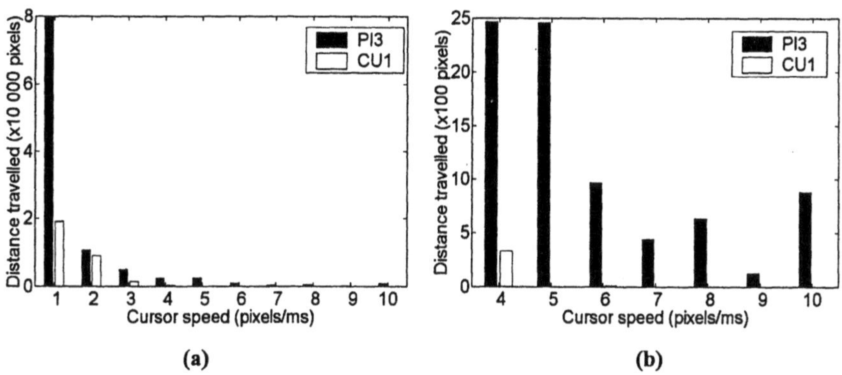

Figure 9.3. Distribution of distance travelled for a range of cursor speeds

9.3.1.4 Submovements

The number of submovements was estimated by counting the number of times that the cursor speed rose above a 0.5 pixels/ms empirically determined threshold. Figure 9.4 shows that for CU1-3 and PI6, tasks are usually completed in 1-3 submovements, and in 2-5 submovements for PI5. The motions of PI3 and PI7, however, are far less fluid. For PI3, cursor motion stops momentarily after a spasm as the user regains control of the mouse. PI7 often navigates by a series of small movements, rather than attempting to reach the target using large motions.

9.3.1.5 Cursor Distance Travelled Away from the Target Centre

Figure 9.5 shows the distributions of the cursor distance travelled while moving in directions that take the cursor farther away from the target's centre. Ideally, the cursor would always move *toward* the target, as exhibited by CU1 with a cluster of values near zero. By contrast, the cursor movements of PI3 often move large distances in directions away from the target. These distances can be greater than 700 pixels – more than twice that required to reach the target (= 287 pixels).

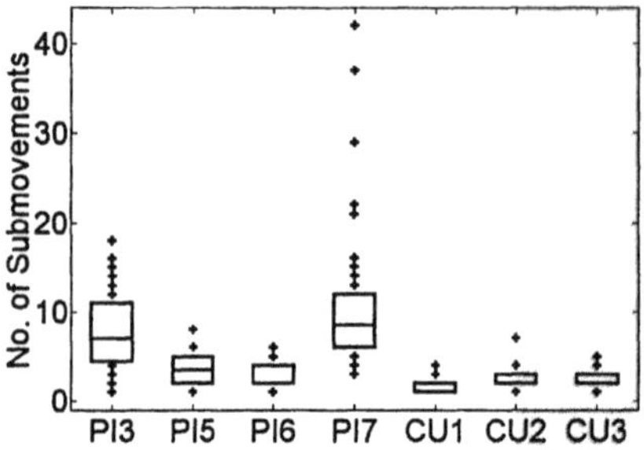

Figure 9.4. Number of submovements

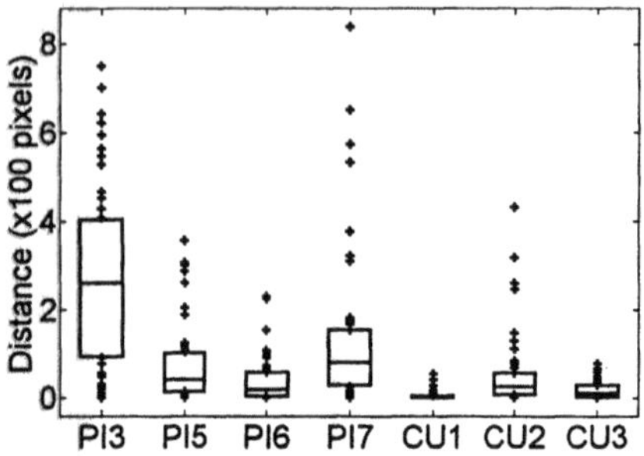

Figure 9.5. Distance travelled away from the target centre

9.3.1.6 Distribution of Distance Travelled for a Range of Curvatures

This characteristic showed that PI3 and PI7 were notably different from the others in that the distribution failed to tail off for bins of high curvature. Figure 9.6 compares PI7 and CU1. Negative radii indicate curved motion in an anti-clockwise direction. Of interest is the presence of high curvature movements for PI7 where they are almost absent for CU1. These distributions are capable of capturing the difference between the cursor paths of PI7 which contain many "twists and turns" and those of CU1 which are relatively straight. For PI5-6 and CU2-3, some high curvature movement was also observed, mostly attributed to overshoot.

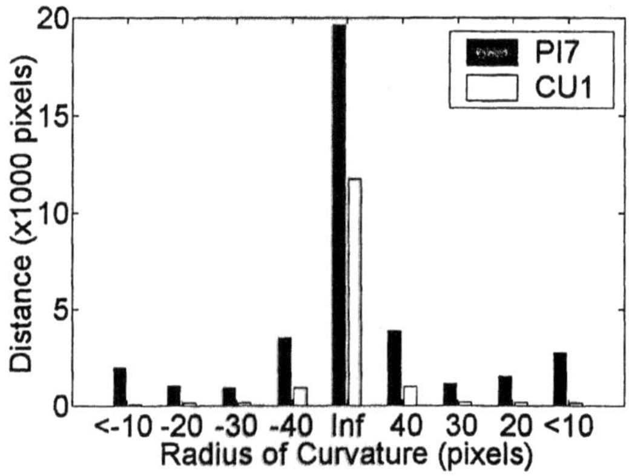

Figure 9.6. Distribution of distance travelled over curvature

9.3.1.7 Distribution of Distance Travelled for a Range of Radii from Target

Figure 9.7 shows this characteristic for PI7 and CU1. For CU1, the cursor travels in straight paths to the target, shown by the uniform nature of the distribution. In contrast, PI7 has difficulty clicking on the target and there is a lot of cursor movement near the target, reflected in the peak in the low end of the distribution.

Distributions for PI3 exhibit a similar peak. For PI5-6 and CU2-3, a smaller peak in the low end of the distribution was observed.

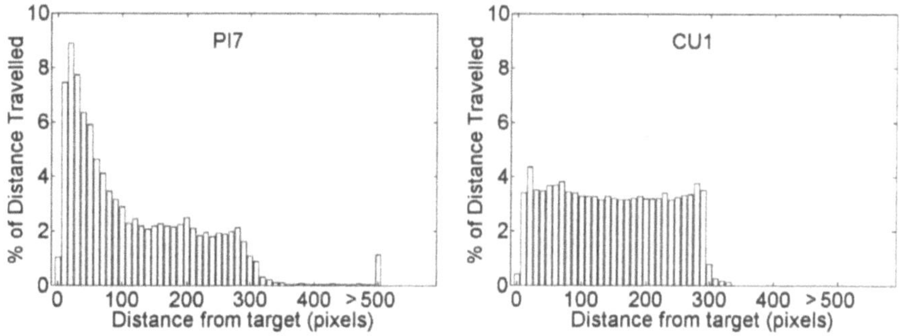

(a) (b)

Figure 9.7. Distribution of distance travelled over distance from target

9.3.2 Discussion

Seven cursor characteristics have been proposed as potential ways to capture important features of the cursor movements of people with motion-impairments. These characteristics appear promising in their ability to represent cursor behaviour as it varies both in space and time. The outcome of research in cursor movement characterisation may be applied in several contexts. These characteristics can form the basis of new user models, or may be developed into new performance measures. Also, these characteristics may give insight into where difficulties may lie. These difficulties in turn can suggest which methods of assistance may be of most benefit. The remainder of this chapter explores this last point further. Some of the characteristics are discussed in terms of how they highlight difficulties experienced by the users. The nature of the difficulties suggests forms of haptic assistance that may be effective.

9.4 Design of Assistive Haptic Interfaces

Force-feedback has been shown to improve the performance of motion-impaired users in computer interaction tasks (Hwang *et al.*, 2001; Langdon *et al.*, 2001; Keates *et al.*, 2000). However, the implementation of haptic feedback requires careful consideration. If implemented inappropriately, haptic effects are not only non-effective but also can be detrimental to performance (Langdon *et al.*, 2001) and increase fatigue (Oakley *et al.*, 2000). To facilitate the design of effective haptic interfaces to assist computer interaction for motion-impaired users, a systematic approach is proposed whereby cursor movements are first studied to identify the nature of the difficulties experienced by a user. The needs of each user may vary. The haptic effects are then designed specifically to address these needs.

9.5 Investigating Forms of Haptic Assistance

The characteristics of cursor paths revealed several aspects of "point and click" tasks that presented difficulties to certain users. Three are addressed in this section: (1) entering a target and remaining inside it while selecting it, (2) controlling high speed cursor movements, and (3) moving the cursor in a straight line. The nature of these difficulties suggest assistive haptic techniques. A series of experiments, involving the same people and based on the same task, was carried out to investigate the effectiveness of three forms of haptic assistance to address the three areas of difficulty: (1) a gravity well around targets, (2) non-directional viscous damping throughout the workspace, and (3) haptic "tunnels" to targets. Haptic feedback was provided through the Logitech Wingman force-feedback mouse.

9.5.1 Gravity Wells

The number of target re-entries and the distribution of distance travelled over distance from the target indicated that both PI3 and PI7 experienced difficulties in entering a target and remaining inside it while selecting it. To assist the users in this, a gravity well surrounding the target was implemented. In the first study, the task was performed under two conditions – *None* and *Gravity Well*. In *None*, no force-feedback is applied. In *Gravity Well*, the desired target sits at the centre of a circular gravity well. When the cursor enters the gravity well, a spring force pulls the mouse toward the centre of the target.

The use of a gravity well around a target appears to give a considerable improvement in times to target. The times averaged over all users were reduced by over 40% (3.9s compared with 2.3s). The most dramatic improvements were seen for PI3 and PI7 where times were reduced by 52% and 48% respectively. This result is in accordance with that expected based on the observed characteristics. The characteristics of cursor movement indicated that PI3 and PI7 experienced greater difficulty than PI5 and PI6 in entering a target and remaining inside it. Accordingly, when gravity wells were used, the improvement in performance for PI3 and PI7 was greater than that for PI5 and PI6.

9.5.2 Non-Directional Damping

The distribution of distance travelled over cursor speeds indicated that PI3 experienced many high-speed movements. Empirical observations indicated that many of these movements were the result of spasms, and were detrimental to performance. To reduce the effects of the spasms, non-directional viscous damping was investigated. In the second study, the task was performed under 4 damping conditions – *None, Acceleration Damping, Velocity Damping,* and *Combined Damping*. Non-directional damping was implemented as a viscous force that increases linearly with mouse acceleration (*Acceleration Damping*), mouse velocity (*Velocity Damping*), and a combination of the two (*Combined Damping*).

The results indicated that all forms of damping have a favourable effect for PI3, reducing times to target by over 50%. The damping does not appear to have a great effect on times for the other participants. Again, these results are in accordance with those expected based on the observed characteristics, which indicated that PI3 exhibited high-speed movements where the others did not. However, it is also possible that the force-feedback from the Wingman mouse, a limited-power device, was not strong enough to have a significant effect for the others.

9.5.3 Haptic Tunnels to Target

The distance travelled relative to cursor displacement, the distribution of distance travelled over curvature, and the cursor distance travelled away from the target centre indicated that PI3 and PI7 had difficulties moving the cursor in a straight line to the target. To assist the users, haptic tunnels to the targets were investigated. In the third study, the task was performed under 5 conditions – one with no haptic feedback (*None*), and four with haptic tunnels to the target (*T1 to T4*). Haptic tunnels have a tunnel width (i.e. distance between the tunnel's inside walls) and a wall thickness. When the cursor passes over a tunnel wall, a spring force pulls the cursor to the inside wall. The four implementations of haptic tunnels used are described in Table 9.2. An infinite wall thickness effectively means that users can never move outside the tunnel. The tunnels extended to the edge of the screen.

Table 9.2. Haptic tunnel descriptions

Tunnel Type	Tunnel Width (pixels)	Wall Thickness (pixels)
T1	0	20
T2	20	20
T3	0	Infinite
T4	20	Infinite

In terms of average times to target, the haptic tunnels do not appear to be of any benefit to PI5 and PI6. This may be because they do not experience great difficulty in moving in straight paths. For PI3 and PI7 however, the haptic tunnels appear to be beneficial, with *T1* reducing times to target by approximately 25% and 35% respectively. Surprisingly, *T3* did not appear as effective for PI7 as did *T1* despite the fact that both conditions effectively constrained the cursor to linear motion. It is possible that this may be due to differences in the software implementation of the two haptic effects. Finally, the width of the tunnel wall does not appear to affect performance for PI3, and for PI7, infinite wall widths appear less effective than finite wall widths. Again, this may be due to implementation differences, and requires further study.

9.6 Conclusion

This chapter has described research that aims to provide insight into the nature of computer interactions of motion-impaired users, and to use this understanding as a basis for developing methods of improving computer accessibility. Seven characteristics have been proposed to elicit information about a cursor's path of movement. The characteristics are promising in their ability to capture features of cursor behaviour as it varies both in space and time. The characteristic profiles of cursor movements highlighted three areas of difficulty experienced by motion-impaired users: (1) entering a target and remaining inside it while selecting it, (2) controlling high speed cursor movements, and (3) moving the cursor in a straight line. Three forms of haptic assistance were investigated to address these difficulties: (1) gravity wells, (2) damping, and (3) haptic tunnels to targets. Results indicated that haptic force-feedback can improve performance, particularly when matched to a user's need as indicated by the characteristic profile.

9.7 Acknowledgements

The authors would like to thank the volunteers and staff of the Papworth Trust. This research is funded by the Canadian Cambridge Trust, NSERC, and EPSRC.

9.8 References

Douglas SA, Kirkpatrick AE, MacKenzie IS (1999) Testing pointing device performance and user assessment with the ISO 9241, part 9 standard. In: Proceedings of CHI'99, ACM Press, pp 215-222

Hwang F, Keates S, Langdon P, Clarkson PJ, Robinson P (2001) Perception and haptics: towards more accessible computers for motion-impaired users. In: Proceedings of PUI 2001, ACM Press

Keates S, Langdon P, Clarkson J, Robinson P (2000) Investigating the use of force feedback for motion-impaired users. In: Proceedings of the 6th ERCIM Workshop, pp 207-212

Keuning-Van Oirschot H, Houtsma A (2001) Cursor displacement and velocity profiles for targets in various locations. In: Proceedings of Eurohaptics 2001, pp 108-112

Langdon P, Keates S, Clarkson J, Robinson P (2001) Investigating the cursor movement parameters for haptic assistance of motion-impaired users. In: Mokhtari M (ed.) Integration of Assistive Technology in the Information Age. IOS Press, Evry, France, pp 237-242

MacKenzie IS, Kauppinen T, Silfverberg M (2001) Accuracy measures for evaluating computer pointing devices. In: Proceedings of CHI'01, ACM Press, pp 9-15

Mithal AK, Douglas SA (1996) Differences in movement microstructure of the mouse and the finger-controlled isometric joystick. In: Proceedings of CHI'96, ACM Press, pp 300-307

Munch S, Dillman R (1997) Haptic output in multimodal user interfaces. In: Proceedings of IUI'97, ACM Press, pp 105-112

Oakley I, McGee MR, Brewster S, Gray P (2000) Putting the feel in 'look and feel.' In: Proceedings of CHI 2000, ACM Press, pp 415-422

Chapter 10

Web-based Multimodal Graphs for Visually Impaired People

W. Yu, D. Reid and S. Brewster

10.0 Abstract

This chapter describes the development and evaluation of Web-based multimodal graphs designed for visually impaired and blind people. The information in the graphs is conveyed to visually impaired people through haptic and audio channels. The motivation of this work is to address problems faced by visually impaired people in accessing graphical information on the Internet, particularly the common types of graphs for data visualisation. In our work, line graphs, bar charts and pie charts are accessible through a force feedback device, the Logitech WingMan Force Feedback Mouse. Pre-recorded sound files are used to represent graph contents to users. In order to test the usability of the developed Web graphs, an evaluation was conducted with bar charts as the experimental platform. The results showed that the participants could successfully use the haptic and audio features to extract information from the Web graphs.

10.1 Introduction

The work described in this chapter is part of an ongoing research project 'Multivis' which aims to develop a multimodal data visualisation system for visually impaired and blind people. Common data visualisations such as line graphs, bar charts and pie charts, etc, are presented to users through haptic and audio channels. To achieve this multimodal representation, we use force feedback devices, spatialised non-speech sound and synthesised speech. This work introduces our attempt at rendering various graph types on the World Wide Web with the aim of providing universal access.

The advent of World Wide Web (WWW) has changed many people's way of life. Not only do sighted people benefit from the growth of the Web but so do visually impaired people. With the help of synthesised speech and Braille display technology, visually impaired people can access a wealth of information and services such as news, travel timetables, online shopping and banking, etc. (RNIB, 2001). However, for these assistive technologies to work properly, Web pages must be appropriately designed and written in valid HyperText Mark-up Language (HTML). Moreover, due to the Graphical User Interface (GUI) orientated design, Web pages often contain invisible tables, columnar text and graphical icons which are potential barriers to the assistive technologies mentioned above (Nguyen, 2001). Furthermore, pictures, diagrams and graphs, which are often found on Web pages, cannot be represented easily by synthesised speech or Braille. It is desirable to provide means for visually impaired people to access these kinds of information on the Web.

To address the inaccessibility of the GUI for visually impaired people, force feedback devices have been developed (Mynatt and Weber, 1994; Ramestein *et al.*, 1996). Therefore, icons, window frames and other standard GUI features can be felt by visually impaired people through the device. Besides tackling GUI problems, other research has been done in the haptic representation of graphical contents on Web pages. Blind people's perception of virtual 3D objects and ability of using online education tools have been investigated (Hardwick *et al.*, 1998; Wies *et al.*, 2001). The commonly used force feedback devices are expensive 3D position input and force output devices. Our approach is to use a low-cost (~£60) Logitech WingMan Force Feedback Mouse (Figure 10.1) to relay information. The aim of this work is to create universal accessible Web pages which contain various types of graphs.

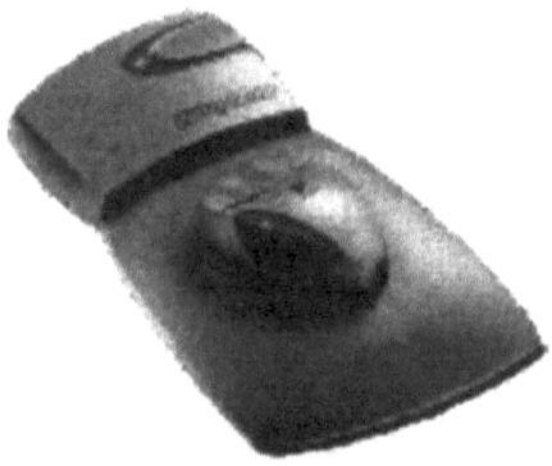

Figure 10.1. Logitech WingMan Force Feedback Mouse

This chapter describes the design and implementation of the Web-based graphs. Most effort has been put into the making of haptic and audio features in order to meet the needs of visually impaired people. Details of the evaluation, which has been conducted to assess the usability of Web graphs, are also given in this chapter.

10.2 Web Graphs Development

Multiple senses modalities were used to present Web graphs. Besides the graphical display, haptic effects and audio feedback are incorporated into the Web pages.

The haptic effect enables users to touch and interact with the graphical objects whereas audio provides additional information about the graphs. JavaScript is used for inserting the haptic effects into the Web pages as well as triggering the audio feedback based on users' mouse activities. The format of the Web pages and co-ordination of haptic and audio features are controlled in Cascading Style Sheets.

10.2.1 Web Page Format

Cascading Style Sheets (CSS) have been proposed by the World Wide Web Consortium (W3C) to control the style of appearance of a Web page (W3C, 2001). In this approach, the content of a Web page can be separated from its presentation. It is a simple, declarative language that allows Web developers to control the style and structure of documents written in HTML or XML (Extensible Mark-up Language). Values such as font, size, colour and positioning can be assigned to a document tag. The word 'cascading' in CSS refers to what occurs when several sources of style information are available for control of the elements on a page. Style information is passed down from a higher level style sheet until it is over-ridden by a style command with more weight. The CSS language is simple and easy to implement, and most importantly using it fulfils the requirements stated in the W3C Web page design guidelines (W3C, 1999).

Using CSS also has advantages when assistive technologies, i.e. screen readers, refreshable Braille displays, are used. The content can be accessed directly without confusions from style controls embedded in HTML. CSS also gives the flexibility required for multimodal Web pages. Due to the architecture of integrating multiple modalities into one Web page, two layers of images are needed. They can be implemented and controlled easily in style sheets. Flexible control and consistent appearance of the Web pages have been achieved.

10.2.2 Haptic Graph Implementation

The haptic effect, which makes the Web graphs tangible, is constructed by using the Immersion Web ActiveX control and Web Plug-in. These allow the communication between JavaScript within the source script of a Web page and a force feedback device to produce the desired sensations on the page. The plug-ins need to be installed on a user's computer for the force effect to be activated. The force feedback device used in this work is the Logitech WingMan Force Feedback mouse. It is an absolute positioning device and provides 2-degree-of-freedom force feedback. The amount of force and the size of the workspace provided by the mouse are limited, but it is affordable to most blind individuals.

The haptic features of the Web graphs are constructed by integrating appropriate primitive haptic objects supported by the Immersion Web Plug-in. The general procedure to create the haptic effect involves three basic steps. Firstly, the appropriate type of haptic effect has to be decided. Secondly, parameters of the haptic effect such as location, size and force response have to be set to match with the modelling object. Finally, the events that control the start and stop of the haptic effect have to be defined. In general, these events are based on mouse movements.

To render different types of graphs which are commonly used, such as line graphs, bar charts and pie charts, dissimilar implementation is required. The methods that we used in this work are based on the primitive haptic objects supported by the Immersion Web Plug-in. The most used effect is enclosure which constrains the mouse movements in a pre-defined area (both rectangular and elliptical). If users wish to exit from the enclosed area, they just need to push the mouse harder against the resisting force. The rectangle effect is used to construct the bar charts and line graphs whilst combination of ellipse and rectangle effects is used for pie charts.

A bar chart is relatively easy to implement due to its regularity. A rectangular enclosure effect is used to model the bars. The co-ordinates of each bar on the graph are measured and subsequently used to define the location and size of the effects. Both the inside and outside walls of the effect are set as 'touchable' so that users can feel the boundary of the bar. If only one side of the wall is enabled, force feedback only applies to the mouse when it travels towards the same side of the wall (Figure 10.2). Therefore, both sides of the wall are enabled to give a realistic wall simulation.

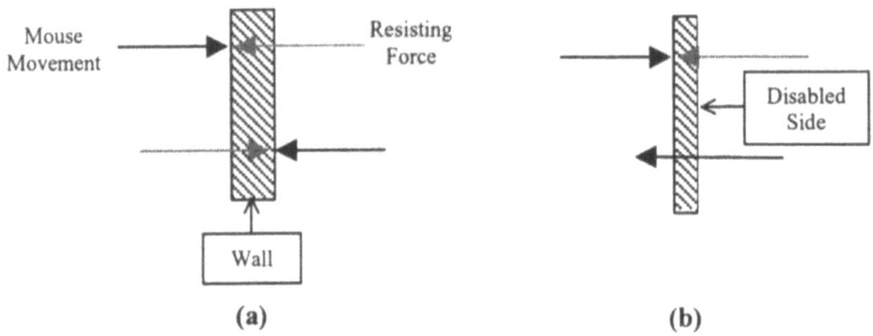

Figure 10.2. (a) A virtual wall with both sides enabled, (b) one side of the wall is disabled and the mouse can move across without any restrictions

To render pie charts, both rectangular and elliptical enclosure effects have to be used. The ellipse effect is used to form the circumference of the pie. Only the inner wall of the ellipse is enabled so that users can feel the internal area of the pie. This is because the most interesting part of pie charts is the divisions of the pie rather than its overall size. The boundary of different portions of the pie is represented by a very narrow rectangular enclosure effect. Only the top and bottom walls of the rectangular effect are active and the gap between them is kept to a minimum distance. Therefore, moving between the top and bottom walls is like following a straight line. The position of the rectangular effect has to be precisely positioned so that the line effect starts from the centre of the pie to the edge. Figure 10.3a shows this transition, a rectangle enclosure is rotated and translated into the desired position. The number of rectangular effects required depends on the number of pie divisions.

Line graphs are more difficult to model using the primitive haptic objects. This is due to the potential complexity of the line or curve shapes. In order to construct a smooth curved line, techniques proposed by Fritz and Barner (1999) are more appropriate. However, it is not feasible to implement those techniques based on the functions provided in the plug-ins. Therefore, the rectangular enclosure effect is used to simulate simple straight-line approximations. The same technique used in the pie charts to form pie divisions is used here to represent line segments. Multiple straight lines are rotated and positioned on the graph so that the end points of each line segments are jointed together (Figure 10.3b). The problem with this kind of formation is that smooth transition cannot be achieved when the line changes direction sharply.

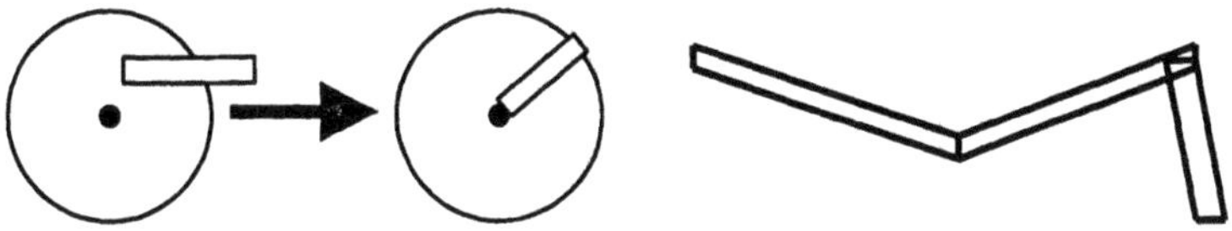

(a) **(b)**

Figure 10.3. (a) Pie chart arrangement, (b) Line graph arrangement.

10.2.3 Audio Implementation

Web-based graphs have an advantage over their traditional paper-based counterparts in that they have the capacity to include interactive sound to relay further information to the user. Our previous work has shown that users' performance has significantly improved when audio is introduced into a haptic graph (Yu and Brewster, 2002). In this work, redundant sounds were added to give additional feedback on the numerical information presented on these graphs.

Different forms of audio exist on the Internet including Wave, Musical Instrument Digital Interface (MIDI), Real Audio, MP3, etc. Each audio format has its own advantages and disadvantages. The criteria for choosing suitable audio format in this work are based on the popularity and bandwidth requirements. Popularity means whether the audio format has universal support so that it can be accessed in any Web browser. Not all Web users have the capacity or the desire to download and use plug-ins. Moreover, the downloading and installation of an audio plug-in can be a fairly daunting task even for the computer literate (RNIB, 2001; WCAG, 2001).

The limited bandwidth of standard analogue modems means Web developers can barely afford a fully featured graphical interface, even before audio content is considered (Beggs and Thede, 2001). The combination of intensive visual/audio pages, and slow modem speeds can result in slow loading of images, and audio frequency dropping or skipping ahead. Bandwidth limitations can also reduce the quality of the sound.

The suitable candidates for the audio feedback are MIDI and Wave. MIDI offers the smallest file size per minute of any audio format as a MIDI file only contains a simple set of instructions to how a synthesiser or sound engine should play back the file. Therefore, the download time is short and it is platform independent. However, the sound quality depends on the sound card installed on users' computer. The playback sound may sound different as each manufacturer may use a slightly different technique to sample and reproduce sounds.

Wave is a common sound format. It has an excellent browser compatibility rating with most browsers carrying a ready installed plug-in to play Wave files. The format is also easy to place onto a standard Web server for downloading, and is ideally suited for simple Web sound effects such as button rollovers. The sound reproduced on users' computer will be more or less the same as the sound recorded on the developer's computer. However, Wave does not offer elegant compression and is therefore not suited for playback over limited bandwidth conditions. As the number of audio notes that playback on the Web graphs is fairly small, the limitation of Wave is not really a problem in the audio representation. Therefore, Wave format is used in the current development to present audio feedback.

Currently, audio feedback is only implemented on bar charts. Audio notes are played when the mouse cursor moves over a bar. A JavaScript method is used to perform this task. As the 'mouse over' event that triggers a JavaScript function is linked to one image only, multiple images have to be included on a Web page for a series of audio notes to be playback interactively. A separate layer of image is therefore implemented on top the haptic image. The arrangement of different layers of images is managed in the style sheet. The audio images are slightly smaller than the haptic images and overlay them. Sound used on the haptic graphs is recorded from a MIDI synthesiser. The height of the bars is mapped proportionally to the MIDI notes. Therefore, a tall bar will generate a high note and vice versa. By moving the mouse cursor across all the bars, the changing pitches will give users an idea about the bar values (Ramloll *et al.*, 2001).

10.3 Evaluation

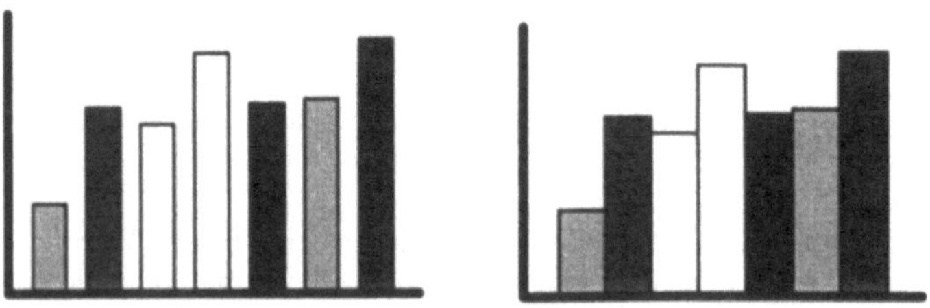

(a) (b)

Figure 10.4. Two sample graphs used in the experiment: (a) Condition 1, (b) Condition 2.

An evaluation was conducted to assess how the Web-based graphs could be used. Bar charts were selected for the evaluation as they have been developed further in terms of haptic and audio features. In the experiment, the effect of two different bar chart arrangements was also investigated. In the first condition, bars have a gap between them (Figure 10.4a). In the second condition, all the bars are flush together (Figure 10.4b). The main testing purpose is to see which one is easier for users to navigate and understand the graph content. Therefore, the experiment was designed to compare their individual effectiveness in transmitting information to the user. The major investigation issues include how the different graph arrangements affect users' navigation through the graphs, how the individual bars were compared against each other, and how much workload they placed on the users.

10.3.1 Experiment Setup

This experiment consisted of a two condition within subjects counter-balanced design. Six bar charts were constructed for each experiment condition. The data used to generate the bar charts were taken from the web-site of the UK Department of Health (DOH, 2001). They were the statistics of hospitals in England from 1993 to 2000. There were seven bars on each chart and arranged according to the condition, either having a gap in between (Condition 1) or flush together (Condition 2).

Twelve sighted people took part in our experiment and they were students of the Department of Computing Science at the University of Glasgow. We did not use blind people in the experiment because our previous experimental results as well as other researchers' work indicate that there is no significant difference between blind and sighted people's performance in using the novel haptic interface (Ramstein *et al.*, 1996; Yu *et al.*, 2001). During the experiment, participants did not have any visual feedback on the graphs and had to work on the Logitech WingMan Force Feedback mouse and wore a pair of headphones.

In order to test whether participants could successfully use the haptic and audio features on the bar charts to extract useful information, four questions were asked:

Q 1. What is the general trend of the graph?
Q 2. Which bar represents the lowest value?
Q 3. Which bar represents the highest value?
Q 4. Which two bars are the closest in value?

A four minute time limit was placed on each graph. The participants were instructed to answer the questions as quickly as possible but keep a high accuracy. The time taken by the participants to answer all four questions was noted. Before the experiment started, four practice graphs were given to the participants for training purposes. In the experiment, the sequence of which condition came first was randomised in order to counter-balance the effect of learning. After the experiment, each participant was asked to fill in a questionnaire regarding the workload they experienced in the experiment. The screen activity, which shows the users' cursor movement, was recorded on video tapes.

10.3.2 Experiment Results

Three major measurements were taken in the evaluation process: number of correct answers, time taken to answer all questions, and the NASA task load index. The task load index is designed to assess the workload placed on a user based on his/her subjective responses on the contributing factors (Harts and Wicken, 1990). There are six factors including mental demand, physical demand, temporal demand, effort, performance and frustration.

Figure 10.5a shows the results of the average number of correct answers per question across all 6 bar charts. The results of the first three questions in both conditions are very similar. Participants were able to obtain a large percentage of correct answers. A significant drop in accuracy occurs in Question 4. Only 29.17% correct answers was obtained in Condition 1. Situation in Condition 2 is better with 40.28% accuracy. The t-test revealed a significant difference between them (T_{11}=2.345, p=0.0388). The overall accuracy in conditions 1 and 2 is 77.78% and 80.21% respectively. However, no significance has been found (T_{11}=1.865, p=0.0891).

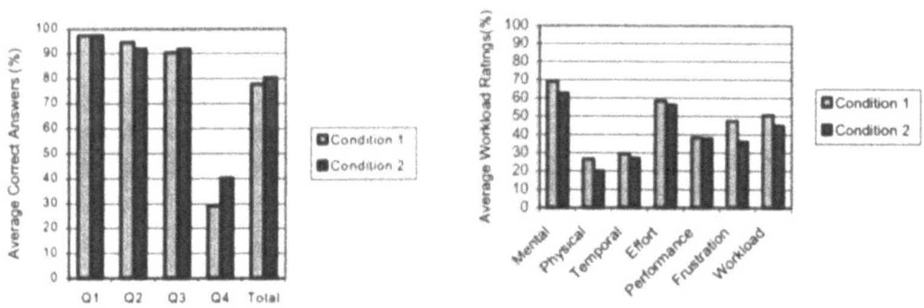

(a) (b)

Figure 10.5. (a) Average correct answers, (b) Average workload index (Condition 1 – bars separated, Condition 2 – bars close together)

The task completion time recorded varies between participants. The average time taken by the participants in condition 1 is 2 minutes and 7 seconds which was longer than the time required in condition 2, 1 minute and 49 seconds. The difference between them was not significant as the t-test only shows T_{11}=1.985 and p=0.0727.

A similar situation happens to the workload index. The participants perceived lower workload in condition 2 and thus gave a workload index 44.9%. The workload index of condition 1 was rated 50.7%. Again no significant difference was found (T_{11}=0.975, p=0.351). The average distributions of participants' ratings on the six contribution factors are plotted in Figure 10.5b.

10.3.3 Discussion

According to participants' performance, the first three questions are easier to answer than the last question. The accuracy of the answers to the last question dropped significantly which means that it is difficult to compare the height of different bars. The two different arrangements of the bars had very little effect on participants' answers to the first three questions due to the ceiling effect. High accuracy is maintained in both conditions. The difference between two conditions shows in the answer to the last question (the comparison). Condition 2 received slightly more correct answers (40.28%) than condition 1 (29.17%). This implies that arranging bars close together helps participants to compare different bar heights more than separating bars by a gap. However, the overall correct answers did not show a significant difference between two conditions.

Task completion time varies between individuals, some participants needed more time, the other did not. The average task completion time in condition 2 is shorter than the one in condition 1. However, a t-test did not reveal a significant difference between them.

In the workload index assessment, the overall workload index in condition 2 is again less than the one in condition 1. However, t-test did not produce a significant result. On the other hand, the variance of the participants' ratings showed a significant difference between two conditions ($F_{11}>2.82$, $p=0.024$). The variances in condition 1 and 2 are 18.07 and 5.13 respectively. This indicates that the workload perceived by participants in condition 2 is more consistent.

Mental demand and effort received much higher ratings from participants than other factors. Obviously, to perceive information through haptic and audio channels is much harder than using vision. The narrower bandwidth of these two channels has placed a heavy burden on the participants when they were trying to assemble pieces of information picked up through the interface into a complete picture. Moreover, all participants are sighted people, it is very unusual for them to ignore vision and use senses of touch and hearing alone.

Participants' ways of exploring the graphs during the experiment were observed. The common technique adopted by most participants is to move the mouse cursor across the bars. Based on this pattern of cursor movement, it can be seen that most of the participants were using the haptic feedback as a navigation guide rather than a tool to extract information about the bars, i.e. bar height. The haptic feedback informs the participants when they were entering the graph or moving into a new bar. Participants relied on the audio feedback on the bars to determine their value. Force feedback was rarely used for this purpose, or as a backup to the audio interpretations. This may explain why participants' answers to the last question were so inaccurate. The nature of the graph representation might affect users' way of using haptics. As detecting the height of the bars by haptics is an indirect and time-consuming process in comparison with the audio representation. Users would not bother to move the mouse up and down on the bars to find the answers, instead they would use the audio provided by the interface. On the other hand, a MIDI note stored in a Wave file is an abstract form of information. It is very difficult to make comparisons based on the MIDI notes alone. Moreover, very few people have perfect pitch. More precise forms of data representation are required for comparison. At the moment, while this kind of information cue is not available at the interface, users should be encouraged to use haptic features on the graph to assist their exploration. Hopefully, the performance of people who can successfully use both haptic and audio features can be improved.

Based on the overall number of correct answers, task completion time and workload index, both experiment conditions provided participants with similar performance. Participants' comments were also noted. In condition 1, a user commentated that the graph was "tough to navigate" in comparison to condition 2. Participants often seemed to get slightly more disorientated on condition 1 graphs, especially where there were dramatic changes in bar height. The fact that condition 2 bars led onto each other was preferred by some of the participants. To them, the feeling of empty space between the bars with no haptic or audio feedback was disconcerting and perhaps putting a slightly greater demand. This has coincided with the design guidelines for tactile display proposed by Challis and Edwards (2001). Space between the bars can be confusing and cause disorientation to users.

On the other hand, some participants preferred having a gap between bars. With bars close together, some users felt there was no definite distinction between the bars, with the possibility arising of mistaking one bar for another. In summary, although the bars arranged close together has little effect on the participants' performance except in the data comparison, majority of participants would prefer this layout.

10.4 Conclusions

Web-based multimodal graphs have been developed. Three types of graphs have been implemented including bar charts, pie charts and line graphs. They were designed to address problems faced by visually impaired people in accessing graphical contents on Web pages. The Web graphs are presented to users in visual, haptic and audio forms. At the current stage, audio feedback is available on the bar charts. Haptic features can be explored by using a Logitech WingMan Force Feedback mouse.

An evaluation, which was conducted to test the effectiveness of using haptic and audio effects in conveying information the users, has shown that participants are able to use the features after a very short training. A high accuracy of participants' answers has revealed the successful use of the Web pages. It has been observed that most participants use haptic features for navigation. They were guided to explore the bar charts and able to discover their position on the graph. Audio features were used to access the information presented on the bars. This works well with locating general and approximate information from the graph. A problem arises when precise information is required for data comparison. It shows that non-speech audio alone cannot give participants a very good indication of the data value therefore a low accuracy is obtained in the last question. The audio used in this implementation is hence regarded as useful in trend detection but not in detailed information representation. However, when synthesised speech is introduced, the amount of information that can be presented will be increased.

The experiment only gives inconclusive results on the difference between two types of bar charts. There are not significant differences with respect to the overall number of correct answers, task completion time and overall workload index. In general, very few differences exist whether the bars are arranged close together or having a gap in between. However, a difference exists in the accuracy of the answers to the last question. Participants did better in finding out two similar bars in height in condition 2 and gave more consistent ratings to the workload index which is slightly lower than in condition 1. Moreover, based on the feedback from participants, most of them prefer to have the bars closely arranged together to minimise the chance of disorientation in the empty space. Therefore, to render an effective haptic bar chart, it is recommended to have bars placed next to each other closely.

10.5 Future Work

Constructing the Web-based graphs is a very tedious process. The implementation of the graphics and audio clips, as well as the positioning of these components is very laborious. The next stage of development will be to produce a system by which online haptic graphs can be produced automatically from raw data. We are currently looking at the possibility of using Java Applets in conjunction with JavaScript to make the graph production easier and more flexible. Moreover, we will conduct case studies on the new system with blind people.

10.6 Acknowledgements

Multivis project is funded by EPSRC Grant GR/M44866, ONCE (Spain) and Virtual Presence Ltd.

10.7 References

Beggs J, Thede D (2001) Designing Web Audio – RealAudio, MP3, Flash and Beatnik. O'Reilly

Challis BP and Edwards ADN (2001) Design Principles for Tactile Interaction. In: Proceedings of Haptic Human-Computer Interaction, Springer, pp 17-24

Department of Health, Hospital Activity Statistics (2001) Available at: http://www.doh.gov.uk/hospitalactivity/index.htm

Fritz JP, Barner KE (1999) Design of a haptic data visualisation system for people with visual impairments. IEEE Transactions on Rehabilitation Engineering 7(3): 372-384

Hardwick A, Furner S, Rush J (1998) Tactile display of virtual reality from the World Wide Web - a potential access method for blind people. Displays (18): 153-161

Hart SG, Wickens C (1990) Workload assessment and predication. In: MANPRINT, an approach to systems integration, Van Nostrand Reinhold, New York
Mynatt ED, Weber G (1994) Nonvisual presentation of Graphical User Interfaces: Contrasting two approaches. In: Proceedings of ACM CHI 94, ACM Press, New York, pp 166-172
Nguyen K (1996) The accessible web: Web access through adaptive technology. Available at: http://www.utoronto.ca/atrc/rd/library/papers/WebAccess.html
Ramloll R, Yu W, Riedel B, Brewster SA (2001) Using non-speech sounds to improve access to 2D tabular numerical information for visually impaired users. In: Proceedings of BCS IHM-HCI 2001, Lille, France, Springer, pp 515-530
Ramstein C, Martial O, Dufresne A, Carignan M, Chasse P, Mabilleau P (1996) Touching and hearing GUI's: Design issues for the PC-access system. In: Proceedings of ACM ASSETS 96, ACM Press, New York, NY, pp 2-9
Royal National Institute for the Blind (RNIB) (2001) Accessible web design. Available at: http://www.rnib.org.uk/digital/hints.htm
Web Content Accessibility Guidelines (W3C Recommendation 5-May-1999). Available at: http://www.w3.org/TR/1999/WAI-WEBCONTENT-19990505
Web Content Accessibility Guidelines 1.0 (W3C) (2001). Available at: http://www.w3.org/TR/WCAG10/
Wies EF, Gardner JA, Sile O'Modhrain M, Hasser CJ, Bulatov VL (2001) Web-based touch display for accessible science education. Haptic Human-Computer Interaction, LNCS 2058, Springer, pp 52-60
World Wide Web Consortium (W3C) (2001) Style sheet activity statement. Available at: http://www.w3.org/Style/Activity
Yu W, Ramloll R, Brewster S, Ridel B (2001) Exploring computer-generated line graphs through virtual touch. In: Proceedings of the 6th International Symposium on Signal Processing and Its Applications, IEEE, vol. 1, pp 72-75
Yu W, Brewster S (2002) Comparing two haptic interfaces for multimodal graph rendering, Accepted by IEEE VR2002, 10th Symposium on Haptic Interfaces for Virtual Environment and Teleoperator Systems (Haptics 2002), in Orlando Florida, 2002, IEEE

Chapter 11

Automatically Rearranging Structured Data for Customised Special-Needs Presentations

S.S. Brown and P. Robinson

11.1 Introduction

Computers are most frequently used for processing text, or for processing signal-based data such as graphics, audio and video. However, there is also a significant amount of non-textual symbol-based data, such as musical scores, mathematics, schematics, and scientific models, that are encoded in such a way that they can be manipulated by algorithms at a higher level than simply processing the signal. Such data can be used for complex search queries, for example.

In order to present such data to people, it must be sent to an output device, such as a screen, a printer, a Braille embosser, or a speech synthesiser. This usually involves one or more *transformations*, in which the data is changed by an algorithm. If an alternative form of presentation is required, perhaps for a special need, then this algorithm often needs to be customised, modified, or re-written altogether. Such modifications can be beyond a developer's resources, and this limits the ability of software to adapt the presentation to the needs of a diverse range of people. It also limits the extent to which end-users can customise the presentation to their own individual needs.

This chapter proposes a different paradigm for representing and transforming structured data, which can help developers (particularly print-disabled developers) to build systems that automatically transcribe data into different formats. This benefits universal access because the methods of presenting data to print-disabled people are far more diverse than one might think, and the need cannot be completely addressed simply by writing a limited number of conversion programs or by adopting a standard "accessible" presentation.

11.2 Related Work

11.2.1 Diversity of Special Needs

Special needs are diverse and can be difficult to anticipate. A person's ability to use data in printed form may be hampered by a print disability, such as blindness, low vision, or dyslexia. It may also be hampered by educational and cultural differences — the person may have learned a notation system that is different from the one being used in the presentation.

The diversity of print disabilities is rarely acknowledged in the literature. Many papers use the phrase "blind and visually impaired" when discussing designs for blind people, implying that people with low vision work in the same way; in fact, many with low vision use their residual sight as much as they can. Other papers (such as Hermsdorf *et al.*, 1998) assume that the needs of all partially-sighted people are much the same. Jacko *et al.* (1998, 1999) show that this is not true, and suggest that a user's needs can be determined by clinical assessment. Even this can be difficult in the case of some eye conditions, such as nystagmus, which can vary over time and can produce different perceptual results for different people (Taylor and Harris, 1999). Some users need to be given control over the presentation themselves, as Gregor and Newell (2000) explain for some cases of dyslexia.

Many industry-standard applications already allow the customisation of fonts, sizes and colours, although it can be difficult and is not always reliable. Not all of these applications allow the layout of structured data to be changed to compensate for the reduced viewing area to text size ratio (a problem that is also prevalent in the mobile telephone industry). Also, people who have difficulty fixing their gaze can sometimes be helped by different layouts, and this requires even more customisation.

Educational background can also contribute to the requirement for an alternative presentation. A good example of this is in music — besides Western staff notation, musicians use various tablature and instrument-specific notations, as well as *sol-fa*, Chinese *Jianpu*, and others, and it is often possible to transcribe a piece of music from one notation into another in order to make it accessible to a greater number of musicians. Braille music also has numerous different versions across the world, and most existing transcription software, such as Goodfeel (McCann), cannot generate all of them. And sometimes an educational establishment will customise a notation for pedagogical purposes — while students are learning a complex notation, they need documents that only use the subset of it that they already know (Ofsted, 2000).

Although it is common practice to focus on one need at a time, it is possible to envisage individuals who have a combination of several of the above-mentioned special needs, and this gives rise to even more diversity.

11.2.2 Existing Transformation Systems

There is no shortage of books and web-sites on XML (W3C, 2000), and on related tools for presenting it (such as the Apache Cocoon project), many of which make use of the XSLT transformation language (W3C, 1999). It is often claimed that this language is Turing-powerful and is therefore adequate for any transformation task.

However, some common transformation tasks are relatively difficult to achieve in XSLT, particularly for people with print disabilities, because so much code needs to be written. Consider, for example, matrix transposition. This is frequently encountered when processing musical scores, which can be structured either with many bars (measures) within each part or with many parts within each bar:

```
<SCORE>                          <SCORE>
 <PART>                           <BAR>
 <BAR> a </BAR>                   <PART> a </PART>
 <BAR> b </BAR>                   <PART> c </PART>
 </PART>                          </BAR>
 <PART>               ↔           <BAR>
 <BAR> c </BAR>                   <PART> b </PART>
 <BAR> d </BAR>                   <PART> d </PART>
 </PART>                          </BAR>
</SCORE>                         </SCORE>
```

While this transformation can be done in XSLT, the resulting code is long and complex.

In an earlier project (Brown, 2000), the first author represented musical scores in an unstructured tuple space. Each tuple was a list of attribute/value pairs that represented an isolated event in the music, such as:

```
(type=note, letter=c, octave=2, barNumber=5,
part=1, time=5, notatedLength=2, realLength=1/2,
accidental=sharp, staccato=1)
```

A scripting language was developed for transforming this into the output; it contained a construct called `foreach`, which sorted the tuple space using a given attribute as the sort key, divided the result into subspaces (one for each unique value of the given attribute), and executed the enclosed code on each of these subspaces. Thus it was easy to write code that structured the output without having to consider how the input was structured, such as:

```
foreach bar
 foreach part
 foreach time
 ...
 end foreach time
 end foreach part
end foreach bar
```

However, this model does not adequately deal with cases where the original hierarchy *does* need to be preserved, such as mathematical expressions (which are recursive). For these, XSLT is much simpler. A general system must be able to deal with documents that contain a mixture of text, music, mathematics and other notations (consider an encyclopaedia for example), which suggests that some sort of hybrid system is needed, which gives the benefits of both XSLT and the tuple space paradigm.

11.3 A Four-Dimensional Mark-up Language

Mark-up languages, such as XML, can be used for describing hierarchical structures over documents and data. A piece of data can be enclosed within an "element," which can in turn be a member of a higher-level element, and so on. As described above, this model becomes more difficult to work with when the data can be divided in more than one manner.

The proposed four-dimensional mark-up language (4DML) allows the scope of an element to be non-contiguous; this makes it easier to represent and address multiple, overlapping sets of mark-up. The document is represented as a set of points in a discrete four-dimensional space (fourspace) with the following dimensions:

- Element name;
- Element position (it is possible for elements of different names to share the same position);
- Element 'depth,' indicating how deeply nested the element is in the tree (this is required for disambiguating between identical elements at different levels of a recursive structure);
- Scope. Each value on this axis corresponds to a unique instance of a symbol (a string of any length) in the document. No ordering is implied — that is defined by element positions. Symbols can be empty placeholders to represent elements that have no data.

An element has one point for each symbol in its scope (including those in the scope of its children). Thus there are many points for each symbol. To identify an element in the fourspace, it is sufficient to specify any one of that element's points.

It is not intended for the fourspace to be directly visible to the user; it is interacted with by converting to and from XML or another language (this chapter uses XML without trailing closing tags). When representing XML, elements with empty names are added around XML cdata (to preserve the position information when mixing cdata with other child elements), and XML attributes are represented as children of a child element named `!attributes` (not valid in XML) which does not disturb the position numbers of the other children.

11.3.1 Transformation by Model

This operation takes as inputs two fourspaces — the input and the model (or template). The return value is the result of transforming the structure of the input to match that of the model. For example, the model to effect the transformation in the example above is `<SCORE> <BAR> <PART>`. Note that the models are written using the structure of the output only — the user does not have to know what (if any) transpositions should occur to achieve the desired structure.

The model fourspace is recursively traversed top-down (if two or more elements share the same position number then they are processed in an undefined order). For each element *e* in the model, the *input* fourspace is searched for elements with the same name as *e*, and only the least deeply-nested of those elements are considered. The input is divided into subspaces, one for each of these elements, with the elements themselves removed. The part of the model enclosed within *e* is then applied to each of these subspaces, and each result is "covered" with an element named after *e*. If *e* is a leaf node in the model, then each result is a symbol representing all the data in that subspace, in the order given by top-down traversal.

Reporting lost data. If the model does not specify every element, it is possible that some data will be lost. The algorithm can return this data, as a fourspace containing points that were in the input fourspace but were not used in generating the output. This will contain just enough of the input's structure to show where the lost data was. If this is presented to the user in some way, it can be used for debugging the model, or at least for summarising what had to be lost in the conversion.

11.3.1.1 Parameters in the Model

Parameters to the model's elements are stored in the same way as XML attributes. The following parameters are defined, and the design is extensible with new parameters. When doing this, one should not be afraid of redundancy, because different users approach tasks in different ways.

rename and nomarkup. `rename` specifies a new name for the element, to be used in the output. This is useful if the nomenclature is different (e.g. `<BAR rename="MEASURE">`). Element names that are empty (`rename=""`) are accepted; when converting to XML, no mark-up is outputted around such elements. For convenience, the parameter `nomarkup`, if present, is equivalent to setting `rename=""` for this and all child elements.

before, after, between, begin, end, and arbitrary text. `<TD before="a" after="b" between="c"/>` specifies that, if there are any `TD` elements at all, then *a* should be added as cdata *before* the first element, *b* *after* the last element, and *c* *between* each. Parameters `begin` and `end` are also provided for adding cdata *within* each element (at its beginning and end respectively). Additionally, any text in the model is copied to the output whenever it is encountered. Thus the model:

```
<TABLE> begin table
 <TR> <TD/> end tr </TR>
end table
```

will insert the text "begin table," "end table" and "end tr" at the appropriate places in the output; this could be used to output a structure in a non-XML language, particularly if nomarkup is used. However, the effect of <TD> text </TD> may not be obvious – the TD is no longer a leaf node in the model, so its contents are completely replaced by "text." The use of parameters begin and end is recommended instead.

In all cases, if XML is used to enter the model then there should be some means of representing characters like < or " in the text. This could be done by expanding XML entities (such as <).

start-at, end-at and number. start-at and end-at can be used to restrict which elements are processed. For example, start-at="4" end-at="5" causes only the 4th and 5th elements that are found to be processed. For convenience, number="*n*" sets both values to *n*.

Reserved element names and wildcard. It is sometimes necessary to combine the above with a way of matching any element name; for example, the two parameters of a MathML msub element may need to be treated differently (number required) but each can be one of a number of possible element types. It would be useful to reserve a "wildcard" element name that, when encountered in the model, causes that model element to match on all top-level input elements, and not to remove the said input elements from the subsets it generates.

However, reserving special element names introduces complications when an element in the input has the reserved name. One way around this is to make the reserved name customisable (with no default). This can be done in the model — the wildcard parameter specifies the name of the wildcard elements, and applies within the scope of the current model element (perhaps the top-level element).

Namespaces. XML namespaces are a useful alternative to reserved words, and namespaces can also be defined which are equivalent to setting certain attributes in a model element. This can lead to more concise models; for example, if the namespace seq pointed to http://ssb22.cam.ac.uk/set/sequential/1, then <seq:P> would be equivalent to <P sequential="1">. However, the use of namespaces should not be enforced, since not all editors support them, and they can detract from the conciseness of small models.

children-only and sequential. The children-only parameter, if present, causes only elements that are (direct or indirect) children of the given element to be considered. For example, consider the effect of the model <B><A> on the input <A_1><B><A_2/><A_3/> (the subscripts are added for annotation). As it is, the model's <A/> will apply to the input's A_1, but if <B children-only="1"> were used, it would instead apply to A_2 and A_3 (A_1 would be ignored).

sequential causes each input element's immediate children to be processed sequentially, rather than being grouped by element name as would normally happen. This will often be used when processing documents that contain a mixture of different types of object in any order (as is the case with XHTML). `sequential` implies `children-only`, and also that only an element's *immediate* children are considered by the next level of the model. As a special case, `sequential="cdata"` additionally causes any cdata elements (at that level) to be copied from input to output.

call. This is a means of adding recursion to the model. For example, in:

```
<math>
 <mrow call="math"/>
 <mi>...</mi>
 ...
```

each `mrow` element is treated as though it were another `math` element. It is also possible to call elements non-recursively, as in:

```
<math>...</math>
<p sequential="1">
 <math call="math"/>
 ...
```

external. Consider the effect of the model `<SCORE><PART><TITLE/>` ... on the input:

```
<SCORE>
 <TITLE> ... </TITLE>
 <PART> ... <PART>
 ...
```

The intention here is that each `PART` bears the `TITLE` of the `SCORE`. However, `TITLE`'s data is outside the scope of the `PART` element and will therefore not be present in the corresponding subset of the input when `PART` is processed. It can be reached by searching a display stack of fourspaces that contain all points not present in any of the subspaces generated by the model. Hence, if no `TITLE`s are found in the `PART`, then the `SCORE` will be searched (this search excluding all of the `PART`s); if no `TITLE`s are found there then the next level up will be searched and so on.

This behaviour can be overridden with the `external` parameter; `external="never"` would cause only the `PART` to be searched; `external="always"` would cause only the `SCORE` and higher-level elements to be searched.

11.4 Evaluation

The transformation by model algorithm has been implemented in Python. The model and input are read from XML files, and the output is generated as XML (or as plain text if `nomarkup` is used at the top level).

The prototype can be used from the command line or as a filter in a pipe. Additionally, a graphical user interface was constructed that displays the model, output, and lost data as tree controls (similar to those used in Windows Explorer), and allows the user to edit the model tree while observing the effects of these changes on the other two trees.

Test cases. The British Broadcasting Corporation (BBC) has a web-site that publishes local weather forecasts; each forecast is some 30Kb of HTML. After this was converted to XHTML, the prototype was used to transform it into a one-line textual summary suitable for being read by a speech synthesiser, sent as an SMS message, or being displayed in a login script or similar (Figure 11.1).

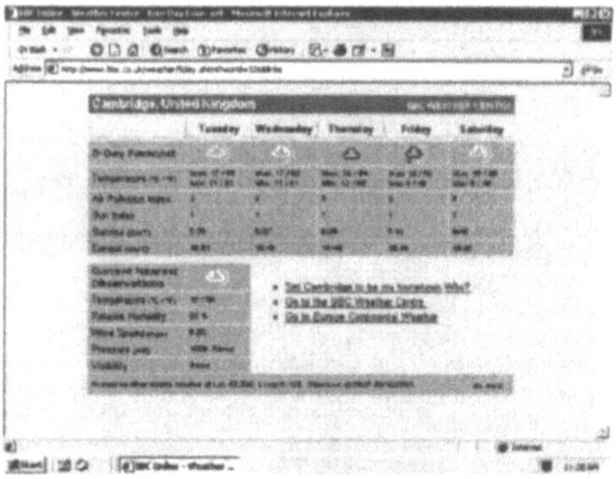

→

BBC Weather Centre. Tuesday: Sunny Intervals. Wednesday: Sunny Intervals. Thursday: Cloudy. Friday: Light Showers. Saturday: Sunny Intervals

Figure 11.1. The BBC Weather Cantre

Although the transformation is easily invalidated by changes in the BBC's house style, it does demonstrate the relative simplicity of the prototype's models:

```
<TABLE nomarkup="1">
 <TABLE children-only="1">
 <TD start-at="4">
 <TR start-at="2" end-at="7">
 <B before=". " after=": "/>
 <ALT/>
```

The prototype was also used to parse a MathML document (which was generated from LaTeX by the utility **tex4ht**), and to output it as English text. For example, the expression:

$$\sum_{n=0}^{k} \frac{f^n a}{n} \tag{11.1}$$

became "sigma from n equals 0 to k of f to the n a over n". Since **tex4ht** outputs MathML in "presentation" format and uses Unicode entities for such things as Σ, it was necessary to extend the model language with a `value` attribute, so that entries like `<mo value="∑"> sigma </mo>` could be used to translate the symbols.

11.5 Conclusion

A system was developed that allows the user to specify the structure of the desired output in a relatively concise manner. The concept described can be used to prototype more quickly systems for presenting structured data in alternative formats for people with special needs. The system can be extended for use with a wider range of transformation tasks. It will probably be more useful when dealing with multi-dimensional data such as musical scores.

The method of inputting the desired structure is left open; it need not be XML. Future work may include allowing the user to describe the desired structure by creating an annotated example document. It might also be possible to develop a parser generator that takes similar specifications, so that there is greater conceptual similarity between parsing data and formatting it.

The prototype tends to generate large numbers of points in the fourspace, and this is not efficient in space or time, even though the points are stored in a data structure that allows for faster queries. There is scope for developing a more efficient model for use in real-time or embedded applications.

11.6 Acknowledgements

The first author is supported by a studentship from the UK Engineering and Physical Sciences Research Council.

11.7 References

Brown S (2000) An extensible system for conversion of musical-notation data to braille musical notation. Computing in Musicology 12: 45-74, 2001. The original was an undergraduate dissertation entitled A Representation and Conversion System for Musical Notation, Cambridge University Computer Laboratory

World Wide Web Consortium (1999) XSL Transformations (XSLT) Version 1.0, W3C Recommendation, Nov 1999. Available at: http://www.w3.org/TR/1999/REC-xslt-19991116

World Wide Web Consortium (2000) Extensible Markup Language (XML) Version 1.0 (Second Edition), Oct 2000. Available at: http://www.w3c.org/TR/2000/REC-xml-20001006

Office for Standards in Education (2000) Inspection Report - RNIB New College, Worcester. Inspection number 223644, p 37

Gregor P, Newell AF (2000) An empirical investigation of ways in which some of the problems encountered by some dyslexics may be alleviated using computer techniques. In: Proceedings of the 4th International ACM Conference on Assistive Technologies, pp 85-91

Hermsdorf D, Gappa H, Pieper M (1998) Webadapter: A prototype of a WWW-browser with new special needs adaptations. In: Proceedings of the 4th ERCIM Workshop, p15

Jacko JA, Dixon MA, Rosa RH Jr, Scott IU, Pappas CJ (1999) Visual profiles: A critical component of universal access. In: Proceedings of ACM CHI 99 Conference on Human Factors in Computing Systems, pp 330-337

Jacko JA, Sears A (1998) Designing interfaces for an overlooked user group: Considering the visual profiles of partially sighted users. In: Proceedings of Third Annual ACM Conference on Assistive Technologies, pp 75-77

McCann B GOODFEEL Braille Music Translator. Dancing Dots Braille Music Technology, USA. Available at: http://www.dancingdots.com/

Taylor D, Harris C (1999) About nystagmus. Technical report, Nystagmus Network, UK. Available at: http://www.btinternet.com/~lynest/nystag.pdf

Chapter 12

Bridging the Education Divide

M. Pieper, H. Morasch and G. Piéla

12.1 Education Divide as Part of the Digital Divide

A substantial point of research of the FhG-FIT (Fraunhofer Institute for Applied Information Technology) project group TEDIS (Technological Enabling of Disabled and Elderly) is to examine to what extent the potentials of information technology and new media can be used to allow humans with impairments to participate more equally and self-determined in the social and economic life of our future "Knowledge Society." Technology- and society critics in this regard object the progressive informatisation of all areas of life to lead to a new social splitting. Sarcastically they already talk about a new "Internet Apartheid."

Thus, a 1998 inquiry by the US government proves that meanwhile 42% of all US households have a computer. 26% regularly use e-mail or more far-reaching Internet-based services. Gradually the originally extremely remarkable differences in Internet use between men and women, and young and elderly decrease, which is probably primarily due to the increasing user-friendliness and controllability of graphical user interfaces. But at present income-caused, educationally-conditioned differences in Internet use increase dramatically.

In order to reduce educationally caused differences in the use of computer systems by adjusting school instruction, the gap between *what pupils think is fancy* and impressive to know about computers and new media and *what they really have to know* to competently make use of them has to be diminished.

Like all end-users of computer systems, pupils also approach new application software with different technological experiences and different insight ability. Some need only a few minutes, in order to intuitively understand the improved handling possibilities of a new user interface, system version, or application system. Non-intuitive pupils need more time.

In this regard, further research efforts are required in order to be able to offer ability- and talent-adapted help systems and accordingly adapted dialogue interfaces. A major prerequisite, which as a basic architectural principle determines systems design in this respect demands support of target achieving "evolutionary learning" (Shneiderman, 2000). Media competence has stepwise to be enriched based on previously acquired basic knowledge in order to further enrich already enriched knowledge in accordance with individual learning speeds.

12.1.1 Media Competence, Digital Divide and Education Divide in Germany[1]

As in other countries the number of people in Germany who have access to the Internet and make use of it is growing permanently. According to a recent and so far unpublished summary of empirical studies about Internet Access and Utilisation, about 46 percent of the German population, aged 14 to 69, had at least access to the Internet in January 2000 (GfK, 2000; Kubicek and Welling, 2001). Access to the Internet is not automatically followed by utilisation. The same survey, only counted 30 percent of the population (15.9 million) as occasional Internet users (GfK, 2000). However, this share has been increasing rapidly.

Between May 1997 and March 2000, for instance, the number of people, aged 14 and older who were using the Internet at least occasionally tripled from 4.1 million to 13.8 million people (ARD/ZDF, 1999; MGD, 2000). This equals a population share of about 20 percent for the population aged 14 and older.[2]

Basically, all surveys show that Internet utilisation is biased along certain socio-demographic variables like income, age, education, and gender. The average Internet user is still male, well educated, earns a higher income and is aged 20 to 40. Recently, some of the peaks of this uneven distribution declined and the socio-demographic structure of the Internet users is slowly moving towards a more balanced representation of the overall socio-demographic structure of society. But at the same time, there is evidence that particular divides further deepened.

People aged 50 and older are still the most under-represented age group of Internet users, while users, aged 14 to 29 years are still the most over-represented age group. However, even while Internet utilisation declines proportionally for people aged 40 and older, the number of Internet users aged 50 and older increased significantly during the last two years. Between, 1997 and 1999, for instance, the percentage of users aged 50 to 59, increased from 8 to 14 percent (ARD/ZDF, 1999). Thus, special measures to support elderly people to use the Internet seem to show initial positive results.

The gender gap in Internet utilisation did not decrease, despite a growing number of women who went online during the last two years because the number of men who went online still exceeded the number of women. Males are still more likely to be on the Internet than women: approximately 60 percent of the Internet users are men and only 40 percent are female (GfK, 2000; MGD, 2000).

---

[1] This section has in large parts been influenced by previously unpublished studies of the Telecommunications Research Group of the University of Bremen (Kubicek and Welling, 2001)

[2] Kubicek and Welling (2001) point out that "different surveys, which seemingly ask the same questions come to dissenting results. This has several reasons: Surveys apply different samples (size and construction) and use different age ranges for the population represented by the survey. Definitions of utilisation may also vary and cause further deviations. Thus, results should be interpreted with care. Rather than seeing them as exact figures they may point out the basic trends of Internet utilisation."

The probability of Internet utilisation is also influenced by the personal household net income. Generally speaking, Internet utilisation increases almost proportionally with growing household net income. Only people with a household net income, which exceeds a salary of 4,000 DM monthly, account for a share of more than 30 percent of Internet users in their income group (see GfK, 2000).

The sharpest visible divide in Internet utilisation, which also deepened most during the last years, is an educational one. The population share of people with a secondary school qualification who use the Internet, for instance, only increased from 1.5 to around 5 percent between 1997 and 1999. The share of Internet users with a college degree increased from 26 to about 52 percent during the same time.[3]

Kubicek and Welling summarise that "active engagement in form of initiatives and actions is needed to bridge these digital divides" (Kubicek and Welling, 2001). They consider "the creation of equality of opportunity for Internet access and utilisation necessary for avoiding the critical societal polarisation into so-called information-have and have-nots." Especially with regard to the learning disabled the educationally caused digital divide requires the improvement of inclusive didactical measures to educate media competence to face the challenges of the Information Society.

12.2 Educating for the Information Society

In the mid-90's of the last century German society and politicians became aware of the important role of the educational sector for the development towards an Information society. Consequently, a large variety of activities have been started to prepare pupils for this future. Most of these ongoing actions are performed in public / private partnership. The first bundle of actions, to a large extent publicly acknowledged because of many government publications and PR-activities, is focussing on IT-infrastructure in schools, e.g.:

- <u>Schools on the Net:</u> sponsoring Internet access and activities. Very recently, the German Ministry of Education has communicated the successful completion of this program; by the end of the year 2001, 99% of German schools will have access to the Internet (as against only 15% three years before) (see ComputerZeitung, 2.11.2001);
- <u>Market place for schools:</u> sponsoring second-hand PC equipment. There is still a wide gap between the large demand from thousands of schools and the small number of used PCs offered for free by private companies;
- <u>Electronic Classroom initiatives:</u> different actions, often limited to few selected sites or only one school; e.g. equipping a school with mobile units consisting of 4 PCs, or with a notebook for every pupil.

[3] According to Kubicek/Welling (2001) these results are based on the findings of the ARD/ZDF Online-Survey (ARD/ZDF 1999: 405) and own calculations of the authors on the basis of numbers from the *Federal Census Office* about the distribution of educational qualifications throughout the German society (Statistisches Bundesamt, 1999a, p 368).

A second bundle of actions, less known in the public and even among teachers, is orientated towards software equipment and applications, e.g.:

- SchoolWeb: an Internet portal for all types of schools, offering learning materials and communication features;
- NetDays: a competition and exhibition of school projects, organised as a virtual event on the Web, but until now limited to some of the Bundeslaender (German states);
- Learning Software development and distribution: also very recently, the German Federal Ministry of Education has stated that this will become the focal point of future actions; more than 300 Million Euros are provided for this purpose (see ComputerZeitung, 2.11.2001).

Current evaluations of these ongoing actions predominantly show impacts on graduate schools. Special schools like those for the learning disabled are largely neglected. The reasons for this disadvantageous development might be different:

- public awareness of special schools for the learning disabled is smaller and they are not so attractive for education politicians as well as for private companies whose sponsoring activities often depend on image aspects;
- the actors of special schools for the learning disabled (administrators, teachers, parents) have internalised their modest role of a "silent minority" and don't assert their needs in the same way as the actors of graduate schools;
- even if these special schools reach the normal hardware standard, they cannot make use of the offered software because it is not adapted to the special educational needs of the learning disabled.

Thus the well-meant measures for promoting IT at schools contain the risk to intensify the Digital / Educational Divide to the debit of the learning disabled. To avoid this risk it seems necessary to examine their special situation and needs.

12.3 Learning Disability: The Invisible Handicap

In contrast to other disabilities, like blindness, vision, motor or even mental impairments, a learning disability does not become immediately obvious in daily life. Thus normally public awareness of this problem is deficient because a learning disability lacks overt symptoms of physical or mental illness.

Nevertheless, learning disabilities occur more frequently than assumed and affect different cognitive and sensory-motor skills, e.g.:

- perception;
- memory;
- concentration;
- motion;
- reading / orthography;
- math skills, etc.

Often a learning disability becomes a complex problem when several of these handicaps bundle in one person and nearly as often other (social) problems contribute to or result from learning disabilities, e.g.:

- low income household or unemployment;
- lower class neighbourhood;
- broken family;
- foreign cultural origin (language / religion).

Regularly learning disabilities have a negative impact on:

- school career;
- social acceptance;
- chances on the labour market;
- and (last, but not least) self-confidence of the young person.

It is obvious that – under the circumstances and demands of the upcoming "Knowledge Society" – especially the learning disabled are suffering from a key handicap to which the society must pay more attention than ever.

12.4 Special Education for the Learning Disabled

Usually learning disabilities do not reveal themselves before becoming confronted with systematic learning requirements during the (first) school years . Once perceived, pupils with a learning disability (to be confirmed by individual pedagogical and psychological tests and a corresponding expertise) get the chance to move from the regular school to a school specialised to counteract their problems. Here they find individual support, including therapeutic approaches, and lessons in small classes with an average of 15 pupils.

The current situation in Germany can be outlined as follows (Kultusministerkonferenz, 2000; Statistisches Bundesamt, 2000; NRW, 2001):

- Pupils with learning disabilities 230,000 [1.8%] [total 12,700,000];
- Special Schools 1,500 [3.6%] [total 42,000];
- Teachers with additional training 25,000 [3.5%] [total 720,000].

The figures show that compared to the non-disabled pupils, roughly double the educational effort is currently being invested for the learning disabled in terms of schools and teachers.

On the other hand, looking at the total number of pupils, the learning disabled are only a small minority. This might explain why the special needs of the learning disabled to gain media competence have so far been neglected with regard to development and marketing strategies for corresponding educational software by the leading publishers in the school book and educational media market.

Thus, against the background of the upcoming Knowledge Society extended research efforts seem necessary to examine more closely the situation in the domain of the learning disabled to stimulate a better media education for them.

12.5 Research Project - KOMM@SCHU.LE

The Fraunhofer Institute for Applied Information Technology (FhG-FIT) has a strong tradition to focus on IT support for people with disabilities. Its research group on *Technological Enabling of Disabled and Elderly* (TEDIS) started the new research project KOMM@SCHU.LE (Educating Media-Competence at Schools for the Learning Disabled) in the beginning of 2001. The mission of this project is to take up the scientific discussion about Digital Divide and focus it on the Education Divide which actually is especially threatening to the learning disabled.

Project partner in the practice field of the subject is the *Gutenberg School for the learning disabled*, located only a few miles from Fraunhofer-FIT. This partnership is promising because the Gutenberg School:

- is for many years a pioneer in IT school equipment;
- has PCs in every classroom and an additional PC-room;
- is running a school-wide Intranet with Internet access;
- has besides Ecology and the Arts "Technology" as a focal point in its official educational program.

In the current school year 2001/2002, the Gutenberg School has 260 pupils with learning disabilities (age 7-17 years) in 16 classes (12-18 pupils per class) and 24 specialised teachers. KOMM@SCHU.LE aims at:

- creating awareness about Education (Digital) Divide in Information Society, especially concerning the learning disabled;
- yielding empirical background studies on pupils' and teachers' private media competence and the demands of parents and employers;
- initiating, collecting and evaluating Best Practice examples;
- combining Best Practice with a "continuing further educational studies" for teachers about didactical approaches to educate media competence for the learning disabled;
- equipping the school with more and better hardware and software.

12.5.1 The Basics: Media Competence of Teachers

Certainly, educational content competence of teachers is the most important precondition of education. Common preoccupations however frequently call the competence of teachers concerning I T and modern media in question.

To verify this assumption (among others), KOMM@SCHU.LE has carried out an own empirical study, based on oral interviews (30 min.) with 23 of the 24 teachers at the Gutenberg School. The results were surprising; hard facts illustrated a very high level of "private" IT equipment and experience among the teachers:

- 100% have a personal computer at home;
- 75% have Internet access;
- 50% use already the PC at home for preparing lessons.

A deeper evaluation, taking into account four indicators (technical knowledge, Internet use, frequency of PC use, self-confidence concerning IT know-how), shows a high level of modern media competence: 83% are highly competent [44%] or at least medium competent [39%]. The detailed figures reveal that competence of teachers depends on age (Table 12.1). So the relatively young body of teachers gives us reason to look forward with optimism to further developments of the KOMM@SCHU.LE project at the Gutenberg School.

Table 12.1. Media Competence of Teachers

Univ. Graduation	High Competence	Medium	Lower
1960 – 89	1	4	3
1990 – 2001	9	5	1
Total	10	9	4

12.5.2 The Demand: Modern Media Competence

A recent survey in Germany (EMNID 2001) showed that parents are becoming more and more aware of the important role of pupils' media competence:

- 73% of parents think multimedia competence is indispensable at future workplaces of their children;
- 35% are afraid of severe disadvantages to children without appropriate knowledge.

To differentiate these findings with regard to the learning disabled and their parents, KOMM@SCHU.LE has planned in-depth interviews with parents of the Gutenberg School in February 2002.

To prospectively take into account future workplace demands which might affect the learning disabled in a special way, we have carried out an own survey during September/October 2001, with questionnaires to 56 potential employers of graduates from the Gutenberg School. The evaluation of the feedback, resulting from 32 companies (i.e. 57%), is still an ongoing activity.

First findings however already show that 87% of potential employers of the learning disabled expect pupil's computer competence as indispensable or at least desirable.

The four most demanded aspects of such a know-how at future workplaces are:

- handling of a personal computer;
- application of a text processing system;
- use of e-mail application;
- information search via Internet.

Accordingly, most of the new activities at the partner school are addressed to promote these key skills.

12.6 Activities "Bridging" the Education Divide

During the first project year, project initiatives and co-ordinated efforts with the teachers were already successful in many different directions. Preliminary results can be found in a bundle of basic-, Internet related- and didactic measures to support special education at the Gutenberg School and compensate the learning disabilities of its pupils:

Basics:

- every classroom was equipped with 3 – 4 multimedia-PCs with Intranet and Internet access;
- diagnosis software for clarifying different kinds of learning disabilities was made available for regular use;
- procurement, installation and integration of new learning software into subject lessons to support educating basic cultural techniques of reading / writing / math / perception.

Internet activities:

- installation of a new working group (6 pupils with 2 teachers) coping with editing the school's enriched web-pages;
- establishment of regular E-mail correspondence between a Gutenberg School class and another German partner school for the learning disabled;
- set up of an in-house Internet Café which is frequently used by the pupils;
- offering a special educational course to acquire a so called "Internet Surfing Licence";
- installation of a special PC/Internet group with access "for girls only" to additionally avoid the well known co-educative learning obstacle of being urged away by boys tending to dominate technological domains.

Special pedagogic / didactic approach:

- mandatory request for IT recommendations as a standard-support in formally required educational support concept-papers for every learning disabled pupil (in school year 2001/2002);
- development, evaluation and further elaboration of a tutorial system considering the special requirements of pupils with learning disabilities being introduced to IT standard applications (MS-Word).

12.7 Study: Transferring Knowledge on Applying Standard Software for the Learning Disabled

As has been pointed out, applying computers in special schools for the learning disabled is exposed to expectations, which reach beyond pure transfer of school knowledge thereby recovering learning impairments. It considers the value of the computer in our society as a means of communication and work - social domains which are especially problematic for the learning disabled.

Because of its over years further expanding use the Internet offers possibilities of including the computer into almost all learning areas. Thus, the school is no longer an isolated learning place, but may be included by the world open-endedness of this new medium into the surrounding society.

Simultaneously school again becomes interesting and attractive for pupils, who have lost fun and interest in school learning. The highly motivated readiness to learning, which is evoked by computers as a learning tool can hardly be obtained from other learning media. Therefore the computer itself can most easily be used to advance learning disabled pupils' basic IT knowledge.

Of primary importance in this regard is knowledge of how to control keyboards, Windows© GUIs, text processors as well as knowledge about meaningful and responsible use of the Internet.

However, because commercially available instruction programs are too extensive and their dialogue structure is too complicated they are not oriented towards the special needs of learning disabled pupils. Therefore it appeared meaningful to develop a platform independent HTML-based instruction program which could be offered off-line as well as in an Internet-based tele-teaching environment and which is one hand adapted to the learning disabled pupils' special needs and on the other hand as much as possible based on generally acknowledged criteria for learning software (Humboldt Universität, 2001).

12.7.1 A Tutorial System for Standard Software Competence Extension for the Learning Disabled

Because text processing is still the predominant standard application, the Gutenberg School selected "Word for Windows©" (Microsoft) as an example for such a tutorial system to introduce standard applications to the learning disabled.

The necessary tools to design such a tutorial program are either available on PCs with standard office applications (e.g. Internet Browser with an HTML word processor, text processing program) or can be downloaded as Freeware from the Internet (e.g. "Hot Potatoe©" for designing query sequences, "Snap program" to integrate illustrations into sequences of subject learning).

According to the already mentioned criteria of learning software a HTML-based tutorial system, is to a large extent linear organised by hyperlinked instruction sequences for subject learning. Nevertheless there are possibilities of branches within a hyperlinked tree structure which allow e.g. repeating a knowledge query at a self-chosen point in time. The basic structure however remains linear. Thus, pupils have only limited possibilities to deviate from the general learning sequence, which in the case of the learning disabled is intended to avoid confusion caused by getting lost in complicated Human-Computer Interaction structures.

Structurally the tutorial is divided into two parts. First it presents learning orl teaching-subjects, afterwards it checks comprehensibility of these subjects. Thus a typical learning sequence of the tutorial system exists in the presentation of teaching-subjects, which is graphically supported. Graphics however relate only to substantial constituents of subject instructions. They are partly also additionally explained by textual descriptions.

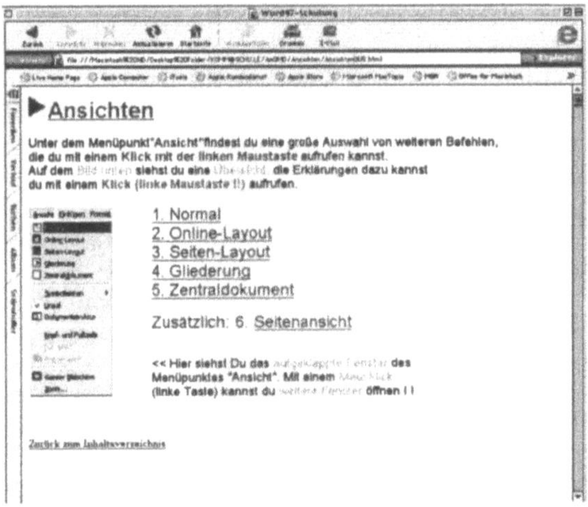
Ansichten
Unter dem Menüpunkt"Ansicht"findest du eine große Auswahl von weiteren Befehlen,
die du mit einem Klick mit der linken Maustaste aufrufen kannst.
Auf dem Bild unten siehst du eine Übersicht, die Erklärungen dazu kannst
du mit einem Klick (linke Maustaste !!) aufrufen.
1. Normal
2. Online-Layout
3. Seiten-Layout
4. Gliederung
5. Zentraldokument
Zusätzlich: 6. Seitenansicht
<< Hier siehst Du das
des
Menüpunktes "Ansicht". Mit einem
(linke Taste) kannst du
öffnen ! !

Figure 12.1. Presentation of learning-subjects concerning "Word for Windows©" main menu "Views"

Subsequently, comprehensibility of taught subjects can be checked. In this context the freeware program "Hot Potatoe©" was used, which offers different possibilities to check knowledge by asking to fill in or allocate gap text, solve corresponding cross word mysteries, answer multiple choice questionnaires etc. Because it follows the same HTML-structure on its application layer "Hot Potatoe©" can easily be integrated with the teaching-subjects module.

Afterwards pupils' responses are analysed. False responses are indicated with possibilities to either return to the subject-presentation module again or repeat the comprehensibility check. Subsequently, the next subject-presentation unit can be accessed

Above all, it is important that single distinctive learning steps have a limited amount of learning subjects and that well defined training objectives are attainable and recognisable for the pupils. This kind of evolutionary target-achieving learning is of high value for learning disabled pupils with many frustrating learning experiences.

However, the advantages of evolutionary target-achieving learning become effective only if the tutorial system complies to appropriate software ergonomic standards, which apply to instructional education of learning disabled-pupils in general (see: Stolze, 2000). First of all these design standards refer to the dialogue structure and HCI modalities, e.g.:

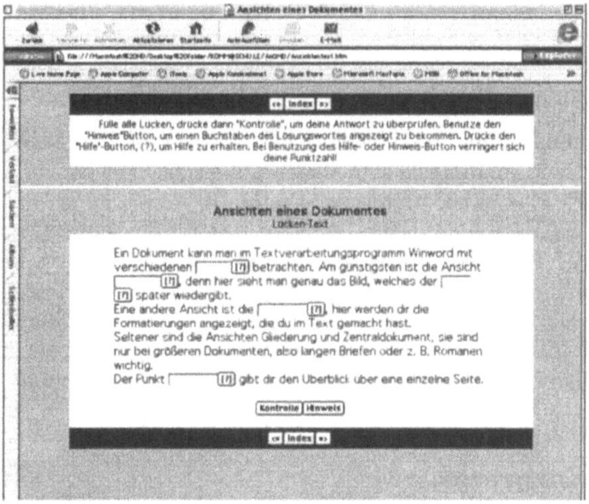

Figure 12.2. "Word for Windows –'Views' " comprehensibility check with "Hot Potatoe©" form filling requests for 'gap text'

- easy operability of the entire program;
- consideration of childlike learning modalities;
- clear task description;
- easy to understand examples for exercises;
- economic use of animation programs for additional assistive instructions only;
- multimodal content representation (image, text , speech);
- clear (multimedia-) instructions;
- context sensitive help;
- UNDO/REDO everywhere and anytime;
- INTERRUPT (pausing) everywhere and anytime;
- adjustable length of the learning sequences;
- adjustable learning speed;
- different degrees of difficulty;
- immediate feedback after (sub-) task accomplishment;
- personalised achievement protocol / achievement related enquiry options;
- conventional instruction handbook to the program.

For the special target group of learning disabled pupils it furthermore turned out to be of relevance that user interface design of tutorial systems is compliant with certain standards for display ergonomics and content adaptation, e.g.:

- clear and unique screen layout;
- cleared up desktop organisation;
- neutral, eye-friendly colours of the background;
- large enough fonts;

- read-friendly, short texts;
- clear paratactical sentences, no hypotactical sentence structure;
- no termini technici or other understanding barriers.

Accordingly, it should be avoided to use most current plug-ins to attract pupils by vivid and fancy multimedia animations as it has become common in large parts of the Internet. It is rather necessary to return to simplicity in software and user interface design. Each additional information disturbs the learning process, which – in the case of the learning disabled is anyway burdened by missing mental flexibility, deficient vocabulary, and deficient evaluation of different syntactic and semantic meanings of letters and words according to their position in a sentence. Much of the multimedia possibilities which fascinate an average user are thus wrongly applied in learning environments of learning disabled pupils.

12.8 References

ARD/ZDF-Arbeitsgruppe Multimedia (1999) ARD/ZDF-Online-Studie 1999. Wird Online Alltagsmedium? Media Perspektiven 8(99): 401-414

EMNID (2001) Internet World. November 2001, p 29

GfK (Gesellschaft für Konsumforschung) (2000) 5. Untersuchungswelle. Präsentation der zentralen Ergebnisse. Available at: http://www.gfk.de

Humboldt Universität (2001) PhilFak IV - Institut für Wirtschafts- und Erwachsenenpädagogik. Available at: http://www.educat.hu-berlin.de/mv/lernsoftware-kriterien.html

Kubicek H, Welling S (2001) Improving InterNet Access and Utilization in Germany as a Precondition for Realizing the Expectations on E-Commerce. Bremen: Telecommunications Research Group, University of Bremen

Kultusministerkonferenz (2000) Schulen im Ländervergleich 1999. Available at: http://www.kultusministerkonferenz.de/statist/ablauf.htm

MGD - Media-Gruppe Digital (2000) @factsBasic. März 2000. Available at: http://www.mgd.de

Shneiderman B (2000) Universal Usability. Communication of the ACM, May, 43(5): 85

NRW Landesamt für Statistik (2001) Sonderschulen NRW. Available at: http://www.lds.nrw.de/stat_nrw/land/daten/d321schul8.htm

Statistisches Bundesamt (1999) Statistisches Jahrbuch für die Bundesrepublik Deutschland. Wiesbaden: Metzler Poeschel

Statistisches Bundesamt (2000) Schulstatistik 1999. Available at: http://www.destatis.de/basis/d/biwiku/schultab1.htm

Stolze J (2000) Lernsoftware-Leitfaden. Available at: http://hbs.hh.schule.de/NeueMedien/prag/pages/Seiten/Softwareleitfaden.html

Chapter 13

Contextual On-line Help: A Contribution to the Implementation of Universal Access

A. Capobianco and N. Carbonell

13.1 Context and Motivations

Universal Design (UD) represents a fruitful concept and a useful body of experiences for promoting universal access (UA) in the forthcoming world-wide 'Information Society.' Guidelines and standards have already been proposed for implementing both concepts, namely: Story (1988) for universal design, and HFES/ANSI (1997), Stephanidis *et al.* (1997) and W3C (1998) concerning universal computer accessibility.

These initiatives address the following major human-computer interaction design issues. That is, how to design interactive software which satisfies the utility and usability requirements:

- of *all* standard user categories (*i.e.*, novices, occasional users, experts);
- in *all* contexts of use, including new contexts and applications (home automation, 'smart artefacts', on-line services for the general public, mobile computing, etc.); and
- which takes into account the specific needs of users with disabilities.

At present, the second and third issues are motivating active research while the first one, which concerns inter-individual cognitive differences, has been overlooked by the scientific community until now. In particular, issues concerning the design of on-line help,[1] most of which stem from the cognitive diversity of users, have not yet been addressed within the framework of the universal design and universal accessibility paradigms.

'Accessibility' here means 'access in the Information Society,' which meaning subsumes the usual acceptation of this term (i.e. 'computer access').

[1] 'on-line help,' here and throughout the chapter, means restrictively 'on-line help to the use of software.' In particular, this acceptation excludes task support.

This chapter aims at motivating research on the design of online help within the framework of the UD and UA paradigms.

First, we point out the strong assets of online help for promoting universal access to 'smart' artefacts and services available in the future Information Society (*cf.* also the emerging concept of 'disappearing computer'). However, in order that these assets may be actually put to use, online help systems must themselves comply with universal accessibility requirements. To meet these requirements, the application of a universal design approach to their design[2] is worth considering.

Next, we list the specific research subjects and issues which need to be address, in order to obtain help systems which satisfy universal accessibility requirements, and therefore could contribute significantly to the promotion and implementation of universal access to software. In particular, the possible contribution of the UD paradigm to the achievement of this goal is examined.

The discussion brings arguments into play, which stem from published empirical evidence and experimental results, ours included. Our results (*cf.* Capobianco and Carbonell, 2001, for their presentation) were obtained from the analysis of a corpus comprising eight oral dialogues[3] between novice users of a standard word processor (Word) and expert users or tutors; experts helped novices to achieve a set of predefined formatting tasks through mixed-initiative dialogues.[4]

Let us note that most arguments put forward here apply both to online help and paper manuals. However, we prefer to focus exclusively on online help, since paper manuals are no longer in current use.

13.2 Online Help Contribution to Universal Access

We first discuss the validity of one current assumption or claim which questions the utility of online help. Then, we illustrate how online help may contribute significantly to the implementation of universal accessibility.

13.2.1 Online Help, a Necessary User Support

After presenting the main argument in support of the uselessness of online help, we describe empirical evidence which invalidates this argument, and demonstrates that novice users need the meta-information provided by online help. To conclude this paragraph, we sum up the various objectives that online help has to achieve as a provider of meta-information on the operation of the associated application software.

---

[2] To our knowledge, the UD approach has not yet been applied to the design of online help.

[3] Dialogues lasted on average half an hour each.

[4] This study (its results, ...) will be subsequently referred to as 'our study' ('our results', ...).

13.2.1.1 The Delusion of Intuitive Interface Designers

One of the main motivations at the origin of direct manipulation was that intuitive, 'transparent,' user interfaces would eliminate the need for specific initial instruction or training to the use of new application software (Shneiderman, 1987).

The argument put forward in support of this assumption can be summarised as follows. The main objective at the origin of direct manipulation was to replace artificial command languages by the intuitive[5] manipulation of meaningful graphical representations of the application objects. The underlying assumption was that users (including the general public) would be able to infer how to manipulate these representations from their *a priori* knowledge of the application domain. Therefore, they would be able to discover and master the operation of any new application software by themselves, simply through interacting with it and exploring its functionalities; they would not need any explicit preliminary instruction.

This assumption is still common among to-day designers, and may explain why on-line help has not yet been considered within the UD and UA paradigms.

13.2.1.2 Empirical Evidence in Support of the Necessity of On-line Help

However, in the eighties already, some empirical studies showed the illusory character of this assumption, and demonstrated that users in the general public are unable to gain, by themselves, a sufficient knowledge of the operation of a new software for achieving the tasks which motivate their use of the software. For instance, according to Mack *et al.* (1983), novice users are confronted with numerous cognitive difficulties which they cannot overcome alone. In particular, they are unable to elaborate by themselves a reliable representation[6] of the capabilities and functioning of a new software. Erroneous or incomplete representations are the source of many errors (semantic errors) which novices can neither detect nor correct for lack of the appropriate knowledge.

Even experts need on-line support. On-line help may spare them the exploration (by trials and errors) of the semantics of a new function, assist them in optimising their interaction with the software, and remind them of syntactic details.

Semantic errors are most difficult to prevent or correct efficiently, since cognitive inter-individual diversity[7] is too high to be fully taken into account by on-line help designers. Therefore, the implementation of the designer's mental representation of the task domain (in the form of software functions) can neither coincide nor be compatible with the mental representation of this domain evolved by each member of a large community of novice users such as the general public. So that beginners have to 'learn' and assimilate the conceptual representation of the task domain implemented by the designer (i.e. the semantics of the available functions), and then, to adapt their behaviours to this representation. Appropriate on-line help can greatly facilitate such assimilation and adaptation processes.

---

[5] *cf.* the underlying metaphor.

[6] or 'system image,' according to Sutcliffe and Old (1987).

[7] This high diversity characterizes users' cognitive capabilities, as well as their knowledge, skills, previous experiences, and current objectives/intentions, all of which influence their representations of the task domain.

Our study confirms Mack's empirical findings, in-as-much as it suggests that the major difficulty encountered by novice users is to establish the necessary relations between their intentions or goals and the software functions or procedures they have to execute for achieving them. One half of the verbal exchanges between subjects and experts were focused on the clarification of these relations (Capobianco and Carbonell, 2001). This result demonstrates the gap between the mental representations of the task domain elaborated by novices, and the software functions implementing the designer's own representation of the task. In other words, this result points to the inadequacy of the semantic representations of the software functions held by novices.

In addition, our results show that the use of so-called intuitive interaction techniques, such as direct manipulation, is a source of difficulties and errors for novice users. Some subjects had difficulty in manipulating the mouse (especially 'drag and drop' actions), and in using menus or dialogue boxes. Almost one third of the subject-expert information exchanges concerned such difficulties which were at the origin of many syntactical and semantic errors.

More generally, the empirical results presented in this paragraph suggest that the design of intuitive human-computer interaction is a difficult aim to achieve. One can even wonder whether it is possible to design user interfaces which require no learning or adaptation effort from the novice user.

In support of this point of view, some intrinsic limitations of the application of Gibson's theory of 'affordance' [8] to user interface design may be put forward. Application software can only reproduce a limited range of human activities accurately by reason of significant differences between human and computer communication or processing capabilities, as well as between the properties of the real physical world where human activities take place and the characteristics of present virtual reality environments. These differences represent major obstacles to the implementation of affordances. To overcome these obstacles, designers of current graphical interfaces resort to metaphors (*cf.* the 'office' metaphor underlying direct manipulation) and natural language (*cf.* menu items and options in dialogue boxes). However, metaphors have limited scopes (similarity is not identity), and natural language is inherently ambiguous (due mainly to lexical polysemy and syntactic ambiguity). In addition, the great diversity of potential users' skills, knowledge and experience is a hindrance to the success of this approach. To conclude this discussion, let us quote Weiser's and Seely's global judgement on affordances, which summarises our point of view accurately:

---

[8] *cf.* Norman's definition of the term 'affordance,' which is easily applicable to interactive software design:

> *"... the term affordance refers to the perceived and actual properties of the thing, primarily those fundamental properties that determine just how the thing could possibly be used."*
>
> (Norman, 1988)

> *"An affordance is a relationship between an object in the world and the intentions, perceptions, and capabilities of a person. ... The idea of affordance, powerful as it is, tends to describe the surface of a design. For us the term 'affordance' does not reach far enough into the periphery where a design must be attuned to but not attended to."*
>
> (Weiser and Seely, 1995)

13.2.1.3 What Kind of Meta-Information Should On-line Help Provide?

To overcome the difficulties described in paragraph 2.1.2, novice users of a given application software need specific on-line support. The main objective of such a support facility should be to provide them with easy access to the meta-information they need to carry out the tasks motivating their use of the application software. In other words, any application software should include a meta-communication facility. Meta-communication refers here to all exchanges of information relating to the conceptual model of the application software functionalities. Although this concept and its implications for human-computer interaction were already presented and discussed in the eighties (*cf.* Tauber, 1986; Waern, 1989), they unfortunately exerted no sensible influence on user interface design. According to Waern (1985), the main objectives of such meta-communication should be:

- to introduce the application software;
- to handle failures caused by the user;
- to provide reminders of the software functions and commands;
- to give information on the current context and the user's previous actions;
- to enable the user to change the current state of the application software.

These objectives are akin to those commonly adopted for on-line help, namely:

- to encourage and implement a 'learning by doing' approach, that is to assist novices in carrying out the tasks they have in mind, and achieving their goals;
- to facilitate the acquisition of the knowledge and skills required to master the use of the application software, without interfering with the novice's task-oriented current interaction;
- to enable novices to acquire easily, rapidly and durably the necessary knowledge and skills, using the potential of interactivity extensively (*cf.* Carroll and Mack, 1992).

To conclude, on-line help appears as a necessity for all users, whatever their cognitive capabilities, knowledge, skills and goals. To be accessible to all potential users, future 'smart' artefacts and services will have to include on-line help facilities capable of adapting to inter-individual cognitive diversity.

13.2.2 On-line Help and Universal Accessibility

On-line help is not only a necessity. It has also the potential to improve software accessibility significantly.

For instance, without appropriate online help, novice and occasional users, especially in the general public, might reject a new software after a few trials, or even shy away from using it. The following observation may explain such behaviours: the authors of Mack *et al.* (1983) observed that novices might experience stress, a major source of errors, during their first interactions with a new software.

By definition, flexible online help could prove very useful for increasing software accessibility. It should indeed have the intrinsic potential to help users with a great diversity of cognitive profiles to overcome the difficulties they are confronted with while discovering a new software or function.

However, these potentialities are still to be exploited. Before initiating research in this direction, it is necessary to solve specific scientific issues, which can be summarised as follows: how to design help systems which are effectively accessible to every potential user in any context of use? Does the UD paradigm represent an appropriate design approach for achieving such a goal? We detail these issues in the following paragraph.

13.3 Towards Designing Accessible Help Systems

13.3.1 Universal Design and Online Help

Universal design being an approach evolved by building designers, it is not surprising that the standard definition of this approach minimises the role of adaptation, and restricts explicitly the scope of UD to:

> *"... the design of products and environments to be usable by all people, to the greatest extent possible, without the need for adaptation or specialised design."*
>
> (Story, 1988; Connell *et al.*, 2001)

Therefore, the seven principles which have been established to guide the implementation of this definition may prove of little usefulness for the design of accessible online help systems, that is systems which have to adapt to the great inter-individual diversity and intra-individual variability of users' cognitive behaviours. Among these principles, only those which are compatible with the implementation of adaptation are applicable to the design of online help systems.

Our claim that adaptivity is an essential feature for ensuring the efficiency and acceptance of online help is supported by the following observations.

Obviously, a restricted set of stereotypes[9] or a few user categories[10] cannot represent accurately the extent of inter-individual cognitive diversity. Adaptive models only have the potential to represent individual cognitive user profiles accurately.

---

[9] *cf.* the taxonomy of user models proposed in Sutcliffe and Old (1987).

[10] *cf.* for instance, the classification of users in terms of their computer knowledge proposed in Shneiderman (1987).

In addition, help systems have also to adapt to the progress of the current user in his/her use of a new software, so as to take account of the intra-individual cognitive variability inherent to learning situations. Such adaptation implies the capability of eliciting, and adapting to, his/her current knowledge and skills dynamically.

Finally, on-line help strategies and messages have to evolve according to the evolution of the current user's intentions and goals during interaction, by reason of the specific attitudes, needs and requirements of users with regard to on-line help – especially those of novices and occasional users in the general public.

Empirical studies dating back to the eighties (Carroll and Rosson, 1987) indicate that most novices concentrate, from the start, on achieving the tasks which motivate their use of the new software, instead of first focusing their efforts on learning how to use the software efficiently. The authors of (Carroll and Rosson, 1987) ascribe the reluctance of novices to consult on-line help to this 'motivational paradox'.

To overcome this reluctance, help systems have to implement user support strategies which promote 'learning by doing' (*cf.* Carroll and Mack, 1992; and the first principle of the minimal manual in Carroll *et al.*, 1987). That is, on-line support should help novices to learn and master the use of a new software through assisting them in achieving the tasks they are bent on carrying out or, in other words, through co-operating with them. Our results suggest that human experts/tutors apply such strategies:

- One half of the experts' speech acts are:
  - attempts at helping the novice to achieve his/her goals and tasks or to plan his/her activity;
  - or assessments of the effects of his/her actions on the interface, in relation to the progress of the current task execution.
- Less than one third of the experts' speech acts are general, non procedural explanations concerning the software functioning or the semantics of its functions.

Therefore, adaptation appears as a key concept and a mandatory requirement for the design of accessible on-line help systems. However, adaptivity, that is the appropriate evolution of the software 'cognitive' behaviour under the influence of the interaction context, is a difficult concept to implement. The main difficulty is to design reliable algorithms for eliciting and interpreting accurately the contextual information (*i.e.*, dynamic knowledge) needed to provide novices with appropriate adaptive support, and more generally, to improve the accessibility of on-line help systems.

In the next paragraph, we outline some major specific issues that researchers should address in the near future, so as to provide designers with efficient guidelines and methods for designing adaptive on-line help systems.

13.3.2 Towards Adaptive Online Help

The trace of the user's actions constitutes the main source of contextual information available to online help systems. How to infer, from such raw data, the dynamic knowledge required for achieving adaptivity is still a crucial research issue.

Sophisticated artificial intelligence techniques (uncertain reasoning, truth maintenance, etc.) have been implemented for modelling, from the analysis of the interaction history, the novice's progress in learning how to use a new software efficiently. However, the resulting prototypes (*cf.* for instance, Paiva and Self, 1994; Brajnik and Tasso, 1994) are too complex and unreliable for meeting the standard ergonomic criteria on utility and usability.

It seems even more difficult to identify accurately the intentions which motivate users' actions, goals and tasks. Approaches based on pattern recognition techniques or statistical learning are basically inadequate, for the following reason mainly.

Co-operation with the user in order to promote 'learning by doing' implies the capability to identify the user's current intention and the task in progress as early as possible, that is after the first elementary action(s) he/she carries out to achieve them. Early identification of the user's current intention is also necessary for the prevention of errors, which requires the capability to anticipate the user's next action or sequence of actions; this information is also necessary for the correction of semantic errors.

However, early accurate identification is often impossible, by reason of the intrinsic ambiguity of the basic software functions, especially in the case of toolkits[11].

The only alternative approach is to induce users to state their intentions before they attempt to achieve them. Our empirical data suggest that human experts often resort to dialogue for eliciting the intentions of novices. The implementation of this approach and the assessment of its ergonomic quality are research subjects worth investigating.

To conclude, appropriate online help strategies are yet to be designed; that is, strategies which help novices to learn how to use a new software efficiently while assisting them in carrying out the tasks they want to perform. The elicitation and implementation of the strategies adopted by human experts/tutors in similar interaction contexts might prove adequate for taking up this longstanding scientific challenge which was first formulated in the eighties (*cf.* Carroll *et al.*, 1987). We are currently focusing the analysis of our empirical data on this elicitation.

[11] For instance, one cannot infer from the selection of a graphical object on the screen, which software function the user wants to apply to this object.

13.4 Conclusion

The aim of the discussion presented in this chapter was to outline the potential contribution of on-line help to the promotion of universal access to the coming Information Society.

We first argued that on-line help, a necessary functional component of any software, may prove useful for overcoming cognitive obstacles to universal access, provided that help systems themselves are accessible to all users, especially the general public, in all contexts of use.

Then, we discussed the claim that some of the seven principles proposed as guidelines for implementing the universal design concept are inapplicable to the design of accessible on-line help systems. Our argument in support of this claim is twofold. While advocates of the UD paradigm strongly recommend to minimise adaptation (*cf.* the overall standard definition of this design paradigm), we demonstrate the necessity of adaptivity for overcoming cognitive inter- and intra-individual variability which constitutes the major obstacle to on-line help universal accessibility.

Finally, we outlined some major research issues pertaining to the design of usable adaptive help systems. In particular, efforts should focus on the definition of strategies capable of inferring accurately, from available contextual information, the dynamic knowledge necessary to achieve flexible adaptation of on-line help to the evolution of the current user's intentions and knowledge (of the software operation) during interaction. Multidisciplinary research, involving mainly cognitive ergonomics, software engineering, and artificial intelligence, is needed on these scientific orientations and issues.

13.5 Acknowledgements

Our study was partly supported by the French Ministry of Defence and the CNRS (DGA/CNRS PhD grant).

13.6 References

Brajnik G, Tasso C (1994) A flexible tool for developing user modelling applications with non monotonic reasoning capabilities. International Journal of Human-Computer Studies 40(1): 31-62

Capobianco A, Carbonell N (2001) Contextual on-line help: elicitation of human experts' strategies. In: Proceedings of UAHCI'01, Lawrence Erlbaum, vol. 3, pp 266-270

Carroll JM, Mack RL (1992) Learning to use a word processor: by doing, by thinking, and by knowing. In: JC Thomas, ML Schneider (eds.), Proceedings of CHI'92, Human Factors in Computer Systems, ACM Press & Addison Wesley, pp 13-51

Carroll J-M, Rosson MB (1987) Paradox of the active user. Interfacing thought, pp 81-111

Carroll JM, Smith-Kerker PL, Ford JR, Mazur-Rimetz SA (1987) The minimal manual. Human Computer Interaction 3(2): 123-153

Connell BR, Jones M, Mace R, Mueller J, Mullick A, Ostroff E, Sanford J, Steinfeld E, Story M, Vanderheim G (2001) What is Universal Design? Available at: http://www.design.ncsu.edu:8120/cud/uni v_design/princ_overview.htm
HEFS/ANSI (1997) Draft HFES/ANSI 200 Standard, Section 5: Accessibility. Proceedings of the Human Factors and Ergonomics Society, Santa Monica (CA)
Mack RL, Lewis C, Carroll JM (1983) Learning to use word processors: Problems and prospects. ACM Transactions in office information systems 1: 254-271
Norman DA (1988) The psychology of everyday things. Basic Books, New York
Paiva A, Self J. (1994) A learner model reason maintenance system. In: Proceedings of ECAI'94, pp 193-196
Shneiderman B (ed.) (1987) Designing the user interface: Strategies for effective human computer interaction. Addison-Wesley, Reading, MA
Stephanidis C, Akoumianakis D, Ziegler J, Faehnrich K-P (1997) User Interface Accessibility: A Retrospective of Current Standardisation Efforts. In: Proceedings of HCI International'97, Elsevier, Amsterdam, pp 469-472
Story MF (1988) Maximizing Usability: The Principles of Universal Design. Assistive Technology 10(1): 4-12
Sutcliffe AG, Old AC (1987) Do users know they have user models? Some experiences in the practice of user modelling. In: Proceedings of INTERACT'87, Elsevier, Amsterdam, pp 36-41
Tauber MJ (1986) An approach to meta-communication in human-computer interaction. In: Klix F, Wandle H (eds.) MACINTER1. Amsterdam: North-Holland, pp 35-49
Waern Y (1985) Learning computerized tasks as related to prior task knowledge. International Journal of Man-Machine Studies 22: 441-455
Waern Y (1989) Cognitive aspects of computer supported tasks. John Wiley & Sons
Weiser M, Seely B (1995) Designing Calm Technology. Xerox Park technical Report (21/12/1995) – Power-Grid Journal (Version 1.01, July 1996)
World Wide Web Consortium. (1998) Web Accessibility Initiative. Available at: http://www.w3.org/WAI/

Chapter 14

3rd Age Interfaces: A Usability Evaluation of the 'Your Guide' Kiosk Prototype from an Older User's Perspective

R.T.P. Young

14.1 Introduction - Consignia and the 'Your Guide' Project

Your Guide is a new service from the Post Office that provides a wide range of useful information and services in a simple way, free of charge and all in one place - the local Post Office branch.

The Government is committed to seeing thriving, profitable Post Offices and to improving accessibility to Government information and services. Your Guide was developed following the Performance and Innovation Unit (PIU) report on the future of the Post Office network which suggested that the Post Office could be an ideal provider of improved access for citizens to Government services. Your Guide is an innovative idea that can achieve these aims, while greatly benefiting customers.

The pilot, currently running in 268 Post Office branches in Leicester City, Leicestershire and Rutland focuses on subjects that Post Office customers said were the most important to them - these include jobs, benefits, retirement, transport and local information.

The Your Guide pilot provides information through a combination of five channels: counter assistance from subpostmasters and staff; leaflets, freephones and touch screens (in 213 branches), along with expert advice sessions at 7 Post Office branches.

The touch screen uses internet technology which allows customers to access information and services held on content providers' web-sites. User enquiries are sent from the 'Your Guide' touch screens to the content provider, and the results are displayed on the touch screen.

More than 30 organisations are providing content and services through the Post Office for the Your Guide pilot, including the Department for Work and Pensions (formerly DSS), National Association of Citizens Advice Bureaux, Leicestershire City and County Councils, Age Concern, Elderly Accommodation Counsel and

Inland Revenue.

The Your Guide pilot will run until 1 March 2002 and the Post Office hopes that if it is successful it will roll out nationally. This study was part of a program of usability tests running through the development lifecycle aimed at achieving accessibility and usability by the target populations. Initial customer feedback results suggests that these exercises have made progress in improving usability with 86% replying that they found the kiosk 'very easy to use' or 'quite easy to use.'

14.2 Description of the Project

The overall aim of this project was to evaluate and improve the Human-Computer Interface of the 'Your Guide' kiosk prototype for the needs of the older population. The kiosk is shown in Figure 14.1 and is supported by a telephone hotline and leaflet rack (on the right of the picture).

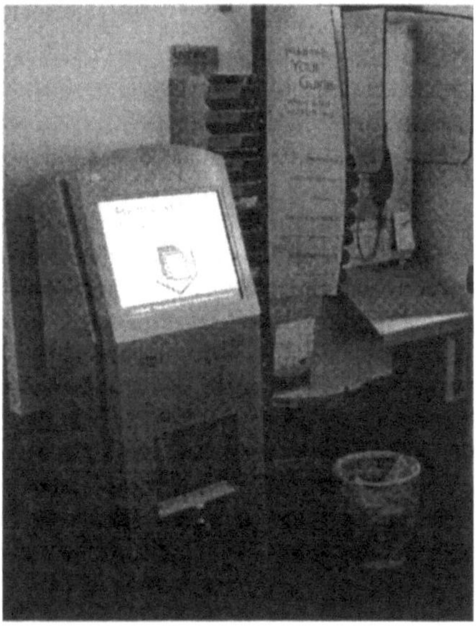

Figure 14.1. Photograph of the 'Your Guide' kiosk situated in the test area.

The older population is only a sub-section of the target user population but was chosen as representing a number of difficult design challenges:

- a prevalence of technophobes - the over 65 age group only account for 4% of the Internet population in the US;
- 69% of adults in UK with some measure of disability are aged 60 or over (Martin *et al.*, 1988);
- of those deemed to be covered by the UK Disability Discrimination Act (DDA) 41% of them are over 65 years of age (Martin *et al.*, 1988).

As well as evaluating the kiosk's usability it also provided the case study to use, compare and assess three usability engineering techniques for their applicability to the areas of public kiosks, touch screens and inclusive design. They were all applied to a prototype kiosk at a fairly late stage in the development lifecycle (working prototype) and therefore acts as a test as to whether these techniques are applicable at this stage of the software engineering lifecycle.

The three techniques used were Guideline Review, Heuristic Evaluation and User Testing (using the 'think aloud' protocol). Four different sets of guidelines were used for the review; Schofield and Flute (1997), World Wide Web consortium (W3C, 1999), Microsoft (1999) and electronic industries association (EIA, 1996). These were chosen because they were all produced with the aim of improving usability/accessibility for physically and mentally impaired users of technology (although each focuses on a different domain). For each set of guidelines, those that were seen as 'not relevant to a kiosk' were discarded from the set and the kiosk was assessed against those that remained. To add a scale for conformance, the kiosk was marked out of five for each individual guideline.

For the Heuristic Evaluations and User Testing the descriptions given in Nieslen (1993) and Mayhew (1999) were taken as the methodology although both protocols used and slightly modified to reflect the user population and the HCI goals of the system. For the Heuristic Evaluation, Nielsen's (1994) revised set of 10 principles were used with the addition of two more, namely:

- ease of use for users with limited hand-motor control;
- ease of use for users with limited visual capability.

These were added to reflect the HCI goals of the kiosk and to include the evaluators experience in designing systems for these groups. They were also given additional information on the intended user profile, kiosk purpose and goals, and the likely task scenarios. These were introduced to try and contextualise the test for the evaluators and hopefully extract more value from the tests. A debrief discussion session and severity ratings were given after the completion of the tests.

In the 'think aloud' approach a mixture of process-based and results-based tasks were used (Wixon and Wilson, 1997). Pre- and post-test questionnaires were also administered to increase the information about the user and their experience using the system. The only major deviation from the methodology was that the tester remained with the user throughout the tests to give support and advice. This was to help over come the initial unease of using the kiosk as all but one user had not even used an Automated Teller Machine (ATM) before. It is however recognised that this may have produced a more artificial situation than if the test had been carried out unaccompanied.

14.3 Profile of the Users and Evaluators

For the Heuristic Evaluation, six evaluators were selected with a range of experience and expertise in the areas of; usability engineering, inclusive design, multi-media design, older or disabled groups, prototype evaluations and Heuristic Evaluations. Each expert had experience in at least two of these areas (most had more).

As for the User Testing, seven users were involved with an age range of 65 to 97, and all but one required some form of sight correction. Each had at least one other impairment and these included; mild and chronic arthritis of one or both hands, congenital and developed hand tremors, cataracts and motion impairments which reduced standing time. In addition, one user had a very low level of English literacy and all bar one had never used a computer or an ATM prior to the tests.

The remainder of this chapter focuses on the types of usability issues found by each technique, a commentary on the usefulness of each technique and then a set of general design principles for designing for older people, extracted from the results of the tests.

14.4 Description of Usability Faults

14.4.1 Guideline Reviews

Table 14.1 shows the kiosk conformed well to the 4 guidelines, achieving between 60% and 73% conformance against those selected as applicable. Out of a total 128 individual guidelines, very few scored a low conformance (0-2). The only areas that did score low were those around personal customisation (of content, control and displays) and it is questionable whether these functions are desirable in a public kiosk. Areas where the guidelines highlighted possible areas for improvement were in button design and screen navigation and layout. However the very one-sided nature of applying guidelines means that they are only good at highlighting areas for future investigation, not definitive evidence of a usability fault.

Table 14.1. Degree of conformance to design guidelines

Guideline name	**J. Schofield**	**W3C**	**Microsoft**	**EIA/EIF**
Degree of conformance to guidelines (actual conformance ÷ max conformance) × 100	73%	60%	64%	73%

14.4.2 Heuristic Evaluation and User Testing

Figure 14.2 shows the percentage of usability faults picked up by each Heuristic (1-10 are Nielsen's (1994) set, 11 and 12 are the additional ones). The second data set shows only those faults that had a mean severity rating of more than 2.5 (4 being a 'usability catastrophe').

The results show that out of Nielsen's original 10 Heuristics the first 4 captured 52% of all the total faults found. These also contain a high proportion of the more serious faults (45%). Alternatively, Heuristics 6-10 detected only 15% of the faults. In the light of this it may prove more efficient in future kiosk applications to concentrate on refining and extending 1-4, 11 and 12 rather than use all 12, which was felt by the evaluator to be a lot to consider during an evaluation.

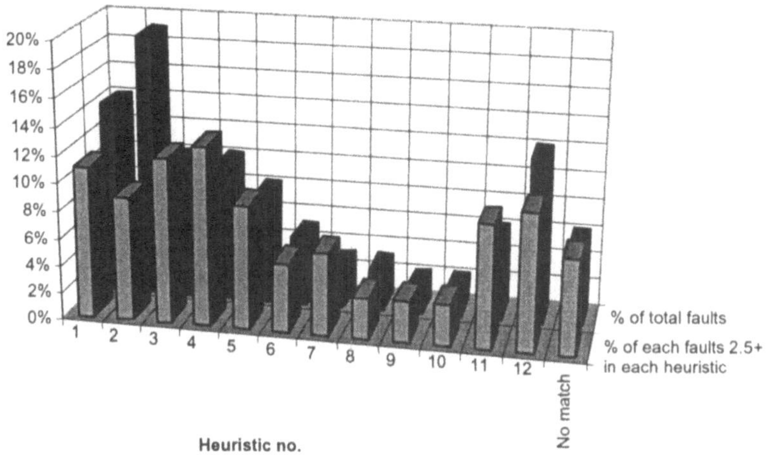

Figure 14.2. Percentage of total usability faults by each Heuristic used

Figure 14.2 shows the percentage of the total number of usability faults found by User Testing and Heuristic Evaluation, grouped together by category. This shows the specific type of faults found. As might be expected the areas where the 2 techniques compared the most closely were in areas of performance, such as understanding text & controls, cognitive load, kiosk design, GUI design and kiosk response. The most common problem using both techniques was the identification of control elements - this represents finding control elements on the screen, distinguishing them from other parts of the screen and then remembering their function from screen to screen.

The most notable difference is that heuristic evaluation provided a wider range of problems with the main area of difference being about elements that are missing from the system, consistency of terminology and button function.

These are generally pulled from the evaluators experience and often closer to design solutions rather than usability faults themselves. For example a user may have problems remembering the directions to a specific page when prompted by the system (e.g. "for ... go to Housing Benefit"). The heuristic evaluator would expect this to be a hot-link directly to the page and record it like that on the observation sheet - but is actually a working memory usability fault and this is a possible solution.

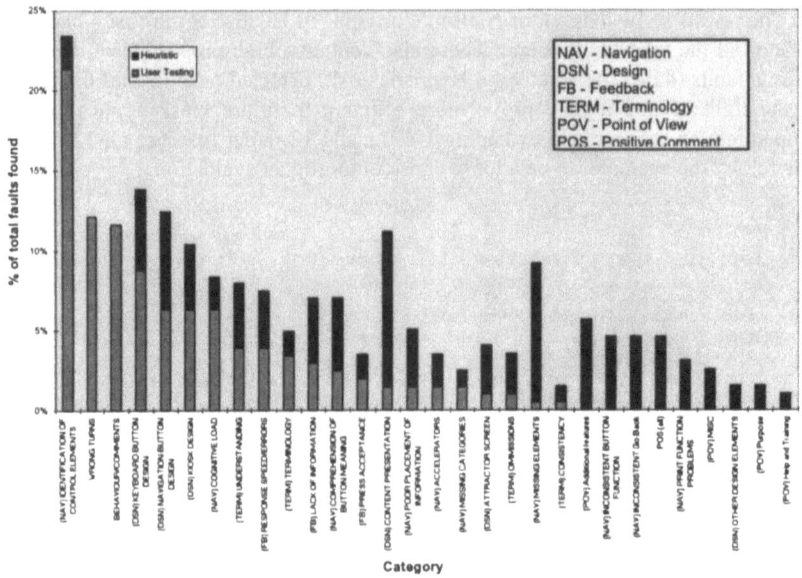

Figure 14.3. Type of usability fault picked up by Heuristic Evaluation and User Testing

The only 2 categories that User Testing picked up that Heuristics did not were the number of wrong turns and comments - these are not usability faults so user testing has only detected a subset of those found through Heuristics. However the advantage that user testing has is in the user performance information that it provides. The frequency, emotional effect and consequences of a particular problem can be seen first hand and a gauge of how severe it is marked against it. Whereas in Heuristics this is only an estimation by the evaluator of how it will effect the users and its likely severity. This fundamental difference is what provides the added value from user testing as opposed to heuristic evaluations and why they can be seen as complimentary, not competing, usability techniques.

14.5 Effectiveness of Tests Used

14.5.1 Guideline Reviews in Evaluations

Guidelines do provide a good, cheap and easily accessible way for designers to appreciate the affect that different impairments may have on the human computer interaction (HCI). Their accessibility also means they are good for briefing less experienced members of the design team and other project staff, allowing them to understand issues that they may have not come across before, especially if designing for media they have not worked with before - such as Touch Screen kiosks.

It was also found that although different guidelines have different depths and focus there is generally very little conflict between them, with a general consensus as to many of the standards. The solutions suggested, however, may be different for each guideline and each application, once use, cost and target population are taken into account. This generally means that if a set of guidelines, well focused to the particular domain, can be found then they are adequate for many purposes.

However, guidelines are generally thought to be more applicable to the start of process as the level of detail is not great enough and the results from this study generally support this. The most important role that they can play is a sense-check during re-design or when adding additional functionality. Reviewing amendments and additions against these guidelines during this processes can help maintain the accessibility that may have been achieved through earlier usability work.

As for the cost/benefit gained from guideline reviews, the time to undertake a thorough guideline review was longer than initially anticipated. Once the guidelines had been read and the relevant ones selected - testing for compliance and defining next steps took between 0.5 and 1.0 days per guideline. This, coupled with the fact that many of the guidelines often lead onto further work to decide on a solution, means that they are more of an educational tool at this stage rather than a evaluation one. As a result it would not be recommended over user testing or heuristic evaluation.

14.5.2 Pros and Cons of Heuristic Evaluations

One difficulty with heuristic evaluation is that the method requires usability specialists, who may not be readily available, and there is evidence that more than one such specialist is needed to gain agreement on the problems present (Budgen and Thomson, 1995). Although Nielsen (1993) argues that these tests can be run by non-HCI specialists, the experience of running these tests leads me to agree more with Budgen, that the experience, knowledge and area of specialism is a critical success factor in heuristic evaluations.

There have also been issues raised as to the quality of the problems found. Although experts often find a large proportion of the inconsistencies quickly and cheaply they often miss some of the most severe problems (Budgen and Thomson, 1995). This carries a risk that expensive development time is wasted on minor issues without providing the evidence to address the more fundamental flaws.

14.5.3 Pros and Cons of User Testing

The main advantage of user testing is that it is not secondary opinion but first hand experience by the people who will actually be using the system. In addition to this the emotions, reactions, fatigue, and thoughts of the user are also captured which can not only assist in determining the severity of particular problems, but also address the underlying problems with the system such as fear, enjoyment, frustration etc.

From the results of these tests it would appear that given the nature of the fault discovery, it is the effect that is recorded, not the cause and therefore it may lead to ambiguity over what exactly has led to the problem (and therefore needs to be improved).

Limitations in the test are mostly around solution development. For minor faults the solutions may be obvious but for more major faults the process does not lead to a immediate solution. In many cases it only succeeds in focusing the attention onto key areas and providing the background for further, more detailed tests which will provide a solution (e.g. correct choice of meaningful icons).

It is generally only a qualitative process and although it can be adapted to be more quantitative, the level of time and effort required generally means that other forms of data collection are usually used (such as interviews/questionnaires). This qualitative nature can have problems when trying to gain buy-in from design teams for the recommended amendments as they may not believe that it is representative of the user population.

This is especially true when looking at users with impairments as it may be difficult to determine the severity of an impairment and therefore can lead to overly optimistic or pessimistic conclusions about a particular groups ability to use a function/element. The results are also rather selective, being somewhat dependant on the tasks chosen - which reinforces the importance of task selection.

User testing can also be very time consuming. Mayhew (1999, p 244). estimates a user test of a moderately complex system takes 144 hours to plan, conduct and analyse. The tests are also criticised for being artificial in that the environment and the 'speak aloud' protocol makes users perform differently than they would do in context. However, on balance the insight that user involvement and direct user testing gives means that it is indispensable in the design and evaluation processes.

14.6 Five Design Principles for Older People

The findings from these tests produced a number of recommendations to improve the usability of the kiosk by the target user group, but it also helps focus thought on what key principles should be borne in mind when designing Information Systems for older people. From the results of the tests, five principles have been distilled that provide worthy goals for all designers of systems for the older population.

Usability Engineering, being a multi-disciplinary subject, deals with many aspects of the user interface, including many of the psychological factors involved. However, the users' motivation for using a system is often ignored by specialists who focus on the components that make up the interface.

Motivation must be seen as a key goal of usability as it adds perseverance and as such is likely to show improvements in many of the measures used in usability engineering (e.g. number of tasks completed, ratio of successes to failures). Motivation, therefore, appears in the key design principles that have been distilled from this work about designing these kinds of systems for older users.

1. There should be a clear function and purpose to the system that is obvious to the user before and during use. This may require reduced and/or more focused functionality (less is more!). Motivation as to why users would want to use the system should be clearly understood by the project team as well as being obvious to the user.
2. Terminology, descriptions and metaphors should not borrow knowledge from the Internet/technology or computer domains (e.g. terms like menu, cursor, delete, enter, kiosk). All text needs to be heavily scrutinised. It must be meaningful and precise, but succinct, with the number of words kept to an absolute minimum. This is to accommodate slow reading speeds and maintain user concentration.
3. User controls and input/output devices that match how older users currently perform these tasks as closely as possible should be chosen. This involves reducing entry to a minimum and probably avoiding some traditional input devices - such as mouse and keyboard.
4. Screen controls should be as large, bold and obvious as possible and grouped within a similar region of the screen as older users tend to concentrate on a particular area of the screen.
5. The level of feedback provided needs to be greater and more obvious than for other user groups as they generally have less of an idea of what to expect from the system. Other users may import knowledge from other systems about response times, what error messages mean, how to correct them and how to interpret cues given by the system. These all help the user make the most of the feedback given by the system. Older users generally do not have this knowledge and therefore require stronger cues. Use of colour change, shape change, tactile & audit cues and textual information are all useful in supplementing the level of feedback.

In summary, designing for older people represents a huge challenge for the designer as they have to overcome a range of not only physical and mental but also psychological barriers. However, designers are becoming more and more aware of the requirements of these groups and the amount of research and advice now available to assist them has grown considerably since the formation of the Disability Discrimination Act (DDA) and Americans with Disabilities Act (ADA). The challenge for the future, however, is to bring this technology into the lives of the older generations through offering products, services and information that can no longer be ignored due to its unrivalled cost, quality and efficiency that are not available through more traditional means.

14.7 References

Budgen D, Thomson M (1995) Experiences with incorporating experimental practice into Software Engineering. Research Index. Available at: http://citeseer.nj.nec.com/219407.html

E-envoy (2001) e-envoy Action Plan. UK Government, Available at: http://www.e-envoy.gov.uk/ukonline/champions/actionplan_menu.htmangible
EIA (1996) Resource Guide for Accessible Design of Consumer Electronics -
Linking Product Design to the Needs of People with Functional Limitations. Available at: http://www.tiaonline.org/access/guide.html#dvisual
Martin J, Howard M, Elliot D (1988) The Prevalence of Disability Among Adults. OPCS Surveys of Disability in Great Britain, pp 1-73
Mayhew DJ (1999) The Usability Engineering Lifecycle. Morgan Kaufmann Publishers, San Francisco
Microsoft Corporation (1999) Microsoft Windows Guidelines for Accessible Software Design. pp 1-157, Available at: www.microsoft.com/enable/
Nielsen J (1994) Enhancing the Explanatory Power of Usability Heuristics. In: Proceedings of CHI '94, pp 152-158
Nielsen J (1993) Usability Engineering. Morgan Kaufmann, Boston, AP Professional
Schofield J, Flute J (1997) Use and Usability - A Guide to Designing Interactive Multimedia for the Public. Multimedia Victoria, Australia
Wixon D, Wilson C (1997) The Usability Engineering Framework for Product design and Evaluation. In: Helender M, Landauer TK, Prabhu P (eds.). Handbook of Human-Computer Interaction. 2nd Edition. Elsevier Science, Englewood Cliffs, NJ
World Wide Web Consortium (1999) Web Content Accessibility. Available at: www.w3.org/TR/WAI-WEBCONTENT

Chapter 15

Virtual Environments for the Training of the Visually Impaired

D. Tzovaras, G. Nikolakis, G. Fergadis, S. Malassiotis and M. Stavrakis

15.1 Introduction

In recent years researchers have started developing force feedback interfaces, which permit blind people not only to access bi-dimensional graphic interfaces (as was the case until now), but in addition to access information present on 3D Virtual Reality interfaces anticipating that the latter will be the natural form of information interchange in the very near future (Burdea, 1994).

The greatest potential benefits from virtual environments (VE) built into current VR systems, are in such applications as education, training, and communication of general ideas and concepts. The technical trade-offs and limitations of the current VR systems are related to the visual complexity of a VE and its degree of interactivity (Burdea, 1994; Colwell *et al,*. 1998).

This chapter presents the applications developed for the feasibility study test developed in the Informatics and Telematics Institute for the EU IST project ENORASI. The main objective of the ENORASI project is to develop a complete training system for the blind and visually impaired based on haptic virtual reality (VR) techniques (Sjostrom, 2001; Yu *et al,*. 2000) the challenging aspect of the proposed VR system is that of addressing realistic virtual representation without any visual information.

In ENORASI our intention is to combine haptic and sound information in such a way as to improve the possibilities for a blind person to obtain overview. By using the computer (and a 3D computer generated world) we may dynamically link the sensation of feeling with sound in ways, which are difficult/impossible with real world models (Scoy *et al,*. 2000; McLaughlin *et al,*. 2000).

The purpose of this chapter is to present measurable results and derive qualitative and quantitative conclusions on the added value of an integrated system aiming to train the blind with the use of virtual reality, based on the CyberGrasp haptic device. The CyberGrasp haptic device (CyberGrasp, 2001) was selected, based on its commercial availability and maturity of technology. In this chapter we have developed a number of custom applications (the Feasibility Study tests) and specific software to support the communication of the applications with the peripheral devices and also integrated a new collision detection algorithm - based on RAPID (1997) and PQP (1999) - in the VHS software library (VHS, 2001) for the CyberGrasp haptic device, in order to improve the performance of the whole system.

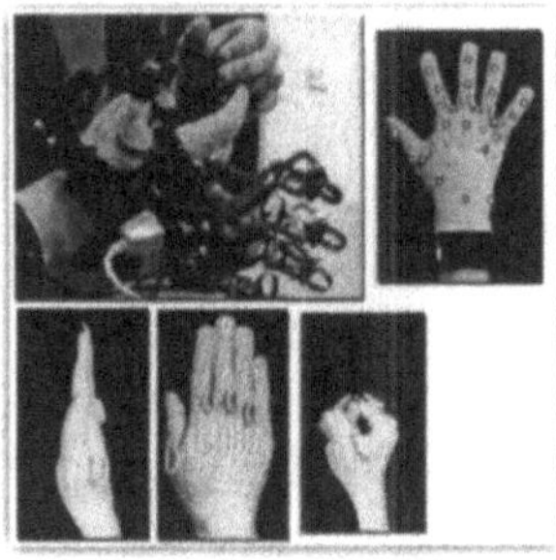

Figure 15.1. CyberGrasp haptic device

The above steps were deemed to be sufficient in order to develop and provide a pilot environment which offers adequate functionality for end users to familiarise themselves with the technology and being able to judge its potential and usefulness. Eight test categories were identified and corresponding tests developed for each category.

15.2 Feasibility Study Tests

The CyberGrasp feasibility study included 26 users from Greece. Each test took approximately 2 hours (including pauses). The test was preceded by a one-hour pre-test that was held the day before the test, in which the users were allowed to get acquainted with the haptic system. The motivation for this pre-test was that the ENORASI system is expected to be a system used more than once by the users. The purpose of the feasibility study was not to test the initial reaction of a user to a haptic system. Rather, the idea was to try to obtain information about the use of such a system by a user who is somewhat familiar with the use of haptics. The pre-test consisted of simple shape recognition tasks, manipulation of simple objects and navigation in the haptic virtual environment using cane simulation.

The tests were implemented by developing custom software applications and their parameters were tuned in two pilot tests performed with users. The majority of the tests in the feasibility study were divided into parts. Those sub-tests were chosen to include tests on similar tasks but with varying expected level of difficulty into the study. The reason for this design approach was that we wanted to use the work put into the feasibility study not only to show that the ENORASI system is feasible, but also to gather information useful in the design of the final system - e.g. a test could consist of an easy task, a middle level task and a complicated task. In the beginning the test sets (below) were designed on this line, but due to time constraints some test tasks were removed after the pilot tests.

15.2.1 Test Set-up

Figure 15.2 shows the layouts of the test equipment used for the CyberGrasp tests. Aside from the material shown in Figure 15.2, tests 1 and 5 used physical models as will be seen in the test descriptions. The backpack for the CyberGrasp haptic device has also been used for tests 7 and 8.

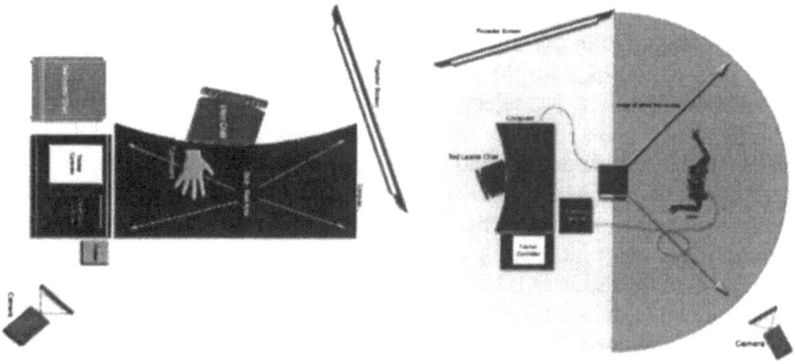

Figure 15.2. Desk and cane simulation setup

15.2.1.1 Test 1 : Simple Objects Test

The user is navigating in a constrained virtual environment (VE) containing geometrical objects. The goal for the user is to recognise the objects and reconstruct the VE using real geometrical objects. FS goals include recognition of shape, knowledge transfer and understanding scale.

Specifically, the VE consists of a table with a number of geometrical objects of different shapes placed in a pattern on a virtual table. On the adjacent desk, there is one box with a number of physical representations of different geometrical objects. The user should feel the VE and try to reconstruct it using the physical models. After completion, the test leader takes a picture of the result, for later analysis (Figure 15.3). Then, the user is informed of the correct placement of the objects.

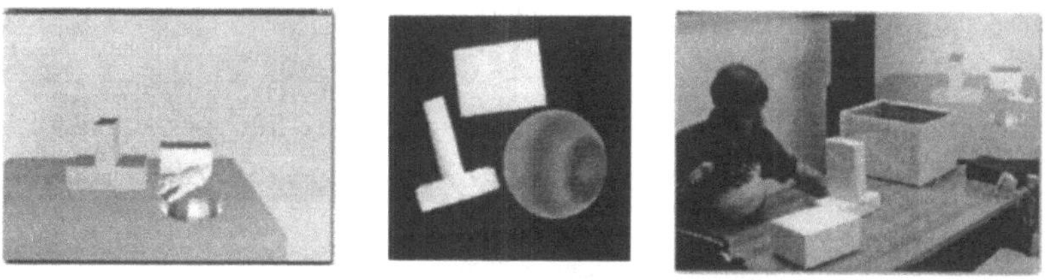

Figure 15.3. Geometrical objects in a pattern test

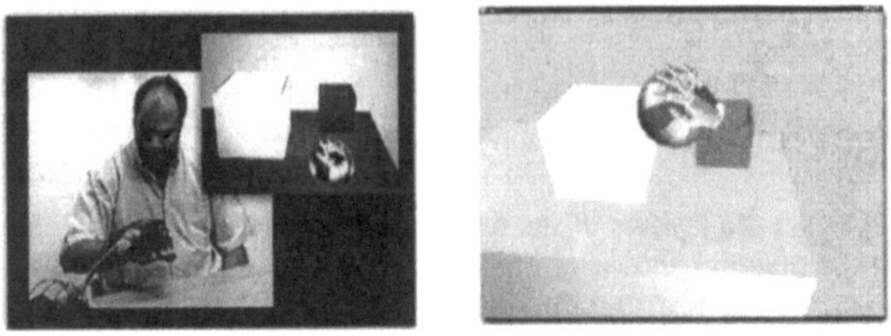

Figure 15.4. A user exploring the VE of Test 2 (Object grasping and manipulation)

15.2.1.2 Test 2 : Object Grasping and Manipulation Test

The user should explore the VE, find the number of objects in it, recognise them and then grasp a pre-selected object and move it to a specific position. Feasibility study goals include recognition of shape, object manipulation into virtual environments, understanding scale and knowledge transfer. The VE consists of a table with three objects (a ball and two empty baskets of different size). One of the baskets is two times bigger than the other. The goal of the user is to find the ball, grasp it and put it into the bigger basket (Figure 15.4).

During the test, the user is asked to feel the virtual models and recognise the ball and the two baskets. He/she should understand the size of the objects and also be able to tell how many times one of the baskets is bigger than the other. This is important, in order to show that scale estimation is possible in virtual environments and also that users can estimate size and scale using only one hand. Finally, he/she should grasp the virtual ball and put it in the bigger of the virtual baskets.

15.2.1.3 Test 3 : Map Test

The maps are representations of house floor plans that the user has to explore and find certain rooms. Sound feedback is provided when the user presses the floor of each room. Feasibility study goals include: navigating in complex environments; knowledge transfer; understanding scale; and interacting with haptic user interface components.

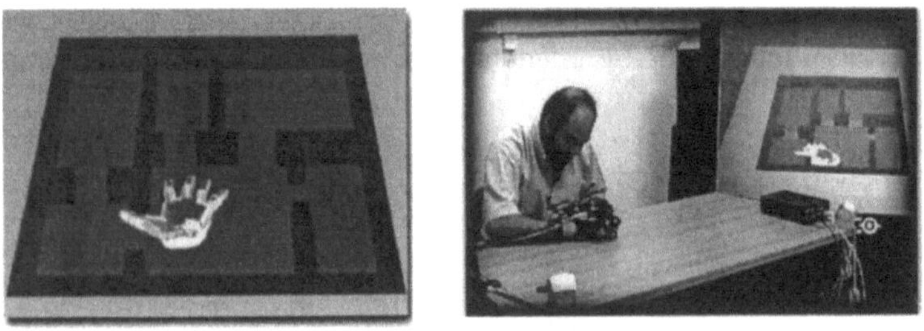

Figure 15.5. A user performing the map test

15.2.1.4 Test 3.1- Flat with 4 Rooms, Kitchen and Hall

The virtual environment consists of a map placed on the floor. The walls are thick and high enough so that the user can identify the difference between the wall and the floor. In the door openings, there is a very thin ridge a lot lower than the walls, to enable the user to feel the difference between walls and doors (Figure 15.5). When the user presses the floor of a room, he/she hears an audible message informing him/her in which room he/she is at the moment. When the user presses the floor again he/she will not hear anything until he/she enters another room.

The user should use a maximum of 7 minutes to explore the map. When the user feels to have an "overview" of the flat, he/she should state the number of rooms that he/she thinks there are in the flat. Following that, the user should use a maximum of 7 minutes to show to the test leaders the relative position of the rooms in the flat and additionally find and accurately follow the walls and the doors.

15.2.1.5 Test 3.2 – Flat with 4 Rooms, Find a Specified Room

If the user needs to walk through the flat again, he/she may explore the flat for less than 2 minutes. When finished, the user should be able to find a specified room, walking from the hall to the room directly. He/she should show this by pressing the floor in the hall, and then go to the specified room and press the floor there. He/she should not press the floors on the way to the room.

15.2.1.6 Test 4 : Mathematics Test

The user works with an illustrative mathematics example designed to teach students mathematical graphs in 2 dimensions. Feasibility study goals include edutainment – use a mathematical educational system and knowledge transfer.

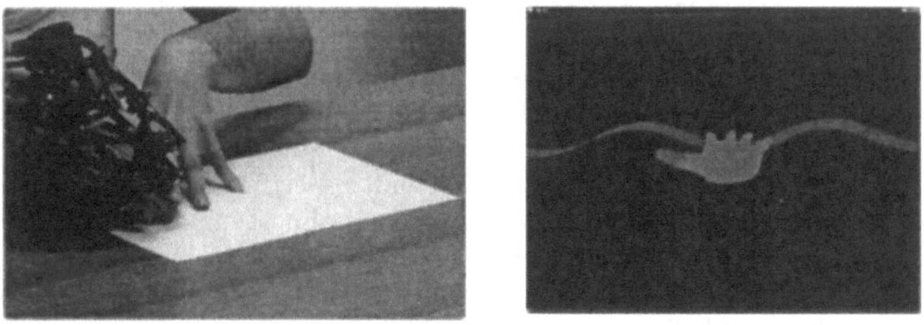

Figure 15.6. A user plotting the curve in the mathematics test

15.2.1.7 Test 4.1- A Sinusoid

The user rests his/her hand on a box located in front of him/her on the test table and the geometrical shape of a specific waveform is passing under his/her fingers (vertical forces are applied to each finger based on the shape of the waveform). A sine of a specific frequency is first simulated by the system (Figure 15.6). The user is asked to leave his/her fingers relaxed and let the device control his/her fingers without applying any resistance to it. Based on the movement of the fingers the user is asked to guess the shape of the waveform.

The user should use a maximum of 3 minutes to feel/recognise the curve that is transferred to his/her fingertips by the system. When the user feels that he/she has understood the shape of the curve, he/she should describe it and try to plot it on a white paper.

15.2.1.8 Test 4.2 – A Sinusoid with Lower Frequency

The frequency by which the sinusoid waveform passes under the user's fingertips decreases and the user is asked if he/she felt any change and what could this change be. The user is again asked to plot the curve.

15.2.1.9 Test 5 : Object Squeezing Test

The user should examine a ball in the virtual space, understand its physical characteristics – specifically, its elasticity and stiffness - and correspond each of the states of the ball with a real object. Feasibility study goals include interacting with virtual objects and understanding their physical properties and knowledge transfer.

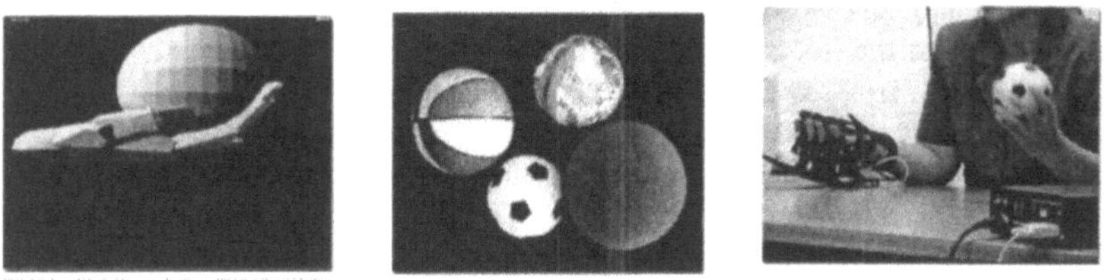

Figure 15.7. A user performing the object squeezing test

The user grasps a virtual ball and squeezes it. The physical characteristics of the virtual ball can be modified, by changing its stiffness and dumping parameters. This is controlled by the test leader, with the press of a button. Initially the ball is very soft (state 3) and the user can squeeze it until a specific point, then it becomes harder to squeeze (state 2) and finally it becomes almost impossible to squeeze (state 1). The four real balls are in a box on the desk (Figure 15.7). Ball 1 is a well-inflated small basket-ball; ball 2 is a less inflated plastic ball; ball 3 is a deflated small soccer ball, and ball 4 is a ball made of sponge.

The user should use a maximum of 4 minutes to examine the virtual ball in all different states. The test leader then changes the characteristics of the ball and the user is asked to describe in detail what does he/she think the ball is made of. Finally, he/she is asked to match each virtual ball with its corresponding real ball lying on the desk.

15.2.1.10 Test 6 : Athletic Event Simulation – Target Shooting

A game-like program has been developed for simulating the participation of a user into an athletic event. Two versions of target shooting for the blind were simulated and evaluated by the users. Feasibility study goals include: edutainment;

participation into a virtual athletic event; interacting with haptic user interface components; and knowledge transfer.

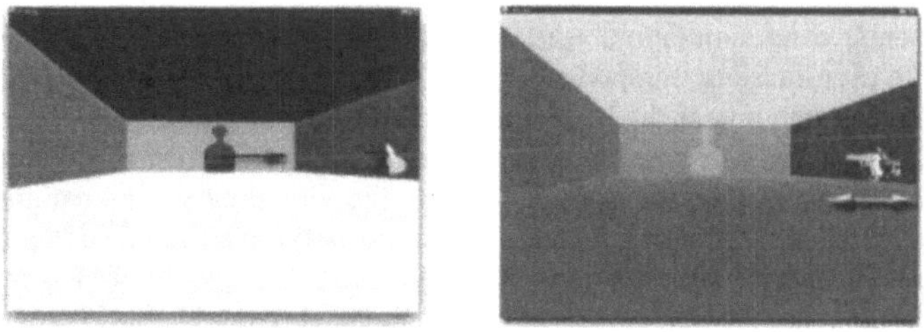

Figure 15.8. Target Shooting-Tests 6.1, 6.2

15.2.1.11 Test 6.1- Target Shooting Using 3D Sound

The user grasps a virtual gun, which fires when you pull its virtual trigger. The virtual gun is supposed to be grounded, i.e. changes in the position and orientation of the hand of the user do not affect the position and orientation of the virtual gun (Figure 15.8). The user can move his/her arm freely, but only grasping and finger movements are affecting the operation of the system. The goal for the user is to shoot the target, which comes from left to right. A 3D sound is attached to the target, which indicates the correct timing for shooting the target (i.e. the sound comes from left to right and the user should fire when the sound approaches the centre).

A shot is considered successful by the system if the user pulls the trigger at an instance differing by less than ±7% from the optimal position. The user is asked to shoot 10 targets and the score is recorded. The objective of this test is to show that 3D sound can be used as an accurate positioning and orientation cue for visually impaired people while force feedback can effectively assist user immersion into the virtual environment. The score of the task is recorded by the system.

15.2.1.12 Test 6.2- Target Shooting for the Blind (Simulation of "Special Olympics" Target Shooting Event)

The user grasps a gun, which fires when he/she pulls its virtual trigger. The user cannot move the virtual gun but he/she can rotate it around an axis perpendicular to the floor, passing from his/her wrist. In this test, changes in the position and orientation of the hand of the user affect only the orientation of the virtual gun (Figure 15.8). The orientation of the virtual gun is converted to a sound frequency, which increases as the gun approaches the direction of the target. Again the sound indicates the correct rotation angle for shooting the target.

A shot is considered successful by the system if the user pulls the trigger at an instance differing by less than ±7% from the optimal position. The user is asked to shoot 10 targets and the score is recorded. The objective of this test is to show that sound frequency can be used as an accurate positioning and orientation cue for visually impaired people, while force feedback can effectively assist user immersion into the virtual environment.

15.2.1.13 Test 7 : Cane simulation test – Outdoor Environment

The user is asked to cross a traffic light crossing using a virtual cane. Sound and haptic feedback are provided by the system upon collision of the cane with the virtual objects. Feasibility study goals include navigating in complex environments, cane simulation, edutainment, knowledge transfer and interacting with haptic user interface components.

The user is standing at the beginning of the test room wearing the CyberGrasp and a waistcoat for carrying the Force Control Unit (FCU) for the CyberGrasp. When the test starts, the user is asked to grasp the virtual cane. The parameters of the virtual cane (size, grasping forces, collision forces) are adjusted so that the user feels that it is similar to the real one. After grasping the cane the user is informed that he is standing in the corner of a pavement (Figure 15.9). There are two perpendicular streets, one on his/her left side and the other in his/her front. Then he/she is asked to cross the street in front of him/her.

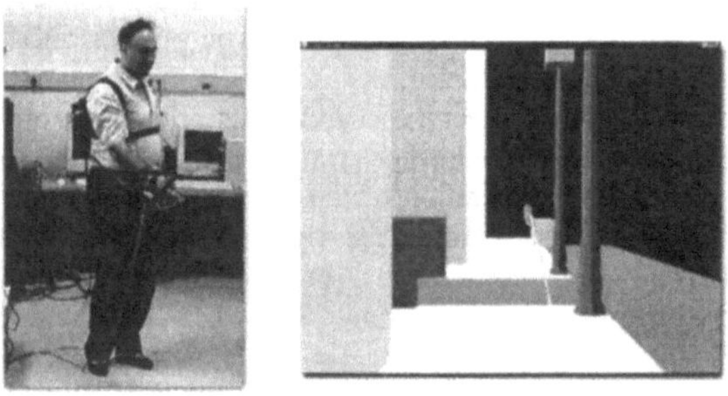

Figure 15.9. Cane simulation - Outdoors (user wearing the CyberGrasp back-pack)

The user should walk ahead and find the traffic light located at about one meter on his left side. A realistic 3D sound is attached to the traffic light informing the user about the condition of the light. The user should then wait close to it until the sound informs him/her to cross the street passage (green traffic light for pedestrians). When the traffic lights turn to green the user must cross the two meters wide passage until he/she finds the pavement at the other side of the street. It is also desirable that the user finds the traffic light at the other side of the street.

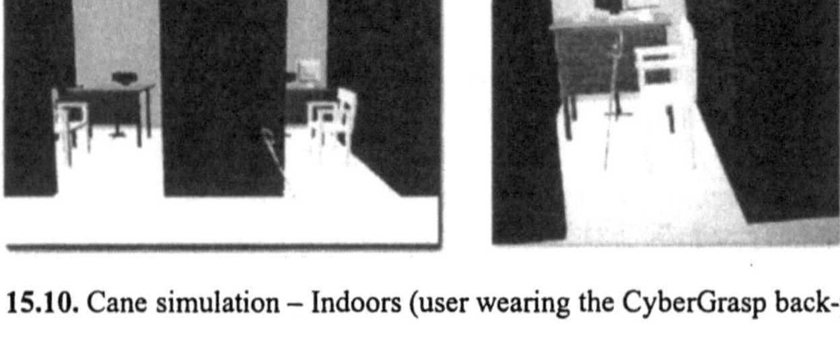

Figure 15.10. Cane simulation – Indoors (user wearing the CyberGrasp back-pack)

15.2.1.14 Test 8 : Cane Simulation Test – Indoors Environment

The user is asked to navigate into an indoor environment using a virtual cane. Sound and haptic feedback are provided by the system upon collision of the cane with the virtual objects. Feasibility study goals include navigating in complex environments, cane simulation, edutainment, knowledge transfer and interacting with haptic user interface components.

The user is standing at the beginning of the test room wearing the CyberGrasp and a waistcoat for carrying the Force Control Unit (FCU) for the CyberGrasp. When the test starts, the user is asked to grasp the virtual cane. The parameters of the virtual cane (size, grasping forces, collision forces) are adjusted according to the characteristics of his/her cane. The goal for the user is to find the second door on his/her left side and enter the room (Figure 15.10). There he/she should find a chair. During his/her walk the user should find successively the wall on his left side, the first door where he/she is not supposed to enter, the wall of the second room and the door where he/she is supposed to enter. After entering the room he/she should find the chair located in his right side. We have also performed the same test without sound feedback.

15.3 Results and Feasibility Study Conclusions

Twenty-six users participated in the tests from the Local Union of the Panhellenic Association for the Blind in Greece. The users were selected so as to represent the following groups: blind from birth, blind at a later age, adults, and children.

Table 15.1. Feasibility study test evaluation results

Test	1.1	1.2	2.1	3.1	3.2	4.1	4.2	5.1	6.1	6.2	7.1	8.1	8.2
Av. Time (min)	4.6	12.8	8.8	10.69	1.26	-	-	5.88	-	-	2	1.96	1.9
Success Ratio (%)	100	92.30	100	96.20	100	100	100	100	100	100	100	96	96.20
Users needing guidance (%)	7.70	26.90	15.38	15.38	3.80	-	-	-	-	-	-	3.80	3.80
Difficulty 1 = v. easy 5 = v. diff.	1.9	2.8	2.1	2.15	2.15	-	1.5	1.38	-	1.7	2.4	2.69	2.88

According to the test evaluation results shown in Table 15.1 the following conclusions were drawn:

- End users participating in the tests faced no general usability difficulty to the pilot system; particularly, when they were introduced with an explanation of the technology and after running some exercises to practice the new software. Little or no guidance at all was needed by the participants, i.e. the users had no difficulties to handle the software and the devices. On the contrary, they enjoyed completing their tasks, showed a lot of commitment and were very enthusiastic.

- The overall result has unanimously been that the prototype introduced was considered very promising and useful, whereas that still leaves a lot of potential for improvement and supplement.
- Provided that further development is carried out, the system has the fundamental characteristics and capabilities to incorporate many requests of the users for a very large pool of applications. The approach chosen for the ENORASI project fully describes the belief of blind people to facilitate and improve training practices, and to offer access to new employment opportunities.
- The most important areas, according to the participants, which can be addressed through the approach of the ENORASI project are: a) mobility and orientation training, b) shape recognition, c) teaching mathematics, d) simulating athletic events and e) map and cane simulation.

15.4 Acknowledgements

This work was supported by the EU IST project ENORASI.

15.5 References

Burdea GC (1994) Force and touch feedback for virtual reality. Wiley-Interscience Publication

Colwell C, Petrie H, Kornbrot D, Hardwick A, Furner S (1998) Haptic Virtual Reality for blind computer users. In: Proceedings of ASSETS '98, ACM Press, New York, pp 92-99.

Sjostrom C (2001) Touch access for people with disabilities." licentiate thesis, CERTEC, Sweden. Available at: http://www.certec.lth.se/doc/touchaccess

Yu W, Ramloll R, Brewster S (2000) Haptic graphs for blind computer users. In: Brewster S, Murray-Smith R (eds.) Haptic Human-Computer Interaction. Springer-Verlag, London, pp 41-51

Van Scoy FL, Kawai T, Darrah M, Rash C (2000) Haptic display of mathematical functions for teaching mathematics to students with vision disabilities: Design and proof of concept. In: Brewster S, Murray-Smith R (eds.) Haptic Human-Computer Interaction, Springer-Verlag, London, pp 31-40

McLaughlin ML, Sukhatme G and Hespanha J (2000) Touch in Immersive Environments. In: Proceedings of the EVA 2000 Scotland Conference on Electronic Imaging and the Visual Arts

CyberGrasp Haptic Device (2001) Immersion Corporation Inc. Available at: http://www.immersion.com/products/3d/interaction/cybergrasp.shtml

RAPID (1997) Available at: http://www.cs.unc.edu/~geom/OBB/OBBT.html

PQP (1999) Available at: http://www.cs.unc.edu/~geom/SSV/

Virtual Hand Suite (VHS) (2001) Immersion Corporation Inc. Available at: http://www.immersion.com/products/3d/interaction/virtualhandstudio.shtml

Chapter 16

User Involvement in the Design of a New Multimedia Communication Service

N. Hine, J.L. Arnott, W. Beattie and P. Sergeant

16.1 Introduction

As human beings, more than two thirds of our conversation is spent in socialising, gossip and story telling (Dunbar, 1996, 1997). Transactional or functional conversation quickly moves on to social interaction, and we constantly recount anecdotes to reinforce a practical point we are making or to reinforce our validity to have an opinion on a subject.

Emler (1994) found that human beings spend more than 80% of waking time in the company of other people. Even when engaged in vocational tasks, people still talk to each other. The vast majority of interpersonal interaction is between people who know each other personally. Only around 7% is either between strangers, or is a business or service transaction. When Emler considered more specifically the content of conversation, he found that around 16% is concerned with exchange of facts and transactional interactions, 10% is concerned with sharing emotions, and the remaining 74% is concerned with discussing, principally as anecdotes and stories, past, present and future activities and opinions about these events, focussing largely on people and places known personally.

Read and Miller (1995) also make the point strongly that humans are social creatures. We learn from others and we share with others what we have learnt. We interact with others in various ways that influence our status and roles in social communities.

Read and Miller's work builds on that of Schank (1990) who explored many aspects of story telling, considering it central to social interactions. Scott (1995), in reviewing the work of Schank and Abelson (1995), makes the point that story telling does not automatically imply the use of words. Other forms of representation are possible, for example using pictures or images, symbols, objects or even mathematical equations.

Csikszentmihalyi and Rochberg-Halton (1981) reported that photographs are the third most treasured possessions in the home of a modern western family after furniture and visual arts. When this is broken down by age, they were ranked sixteenth by children and teenagers, and ranked first by grandparents. The personal value of images was found by Mäkelä *et al.* (2000) to be in socialising and social interactions, and in recording memories. In fact, this study qualified the work of Csikszentmihalyi and Rochberg-Halton (1981), by showing that younger people tended to use images to capture humorous situations or everyday objects that were important to them. This is contrasted with older people who tend to use them to illustrate memories and to recount them in stories.

The life and the communication needs of people with disabilities is changing. Care in the community as a method of delivering care implies that people will not be living in large residential institutions, but will be living in small groups or families, geographically distributed from other people with disabilities. Isolated people with disabilities, therefore, need to be able to interact with care providers, but more importantly, they need to be able to have social interaction with others, using the same set of Internet services that other members of society employ.

A possible means to reconcile the social interaction needs of people, including the desire to share information in different media, and the potential trend towards possible social isolation, is to employ modern telecommunication services, including services such as videoconferencing.

16.2 User Requirements

Given this basic need of human beings to interact socially, and given the changing patterns of community living, there is a need to ensure that new communications services are accessible, in order to promote effective social interaction and to reduce social isolation. One important first step in assessing the user requirements for accessible services, is to determine the nature and scale of the issues involved., ie. to know the users. Sandhu (1997) has investigated the numbers of people within Europe that have impairments that could affect their ability to use telecommunications systems. He concluded that around 10.5 million people within the European Union population of 373 million in 1993 (2.8 % of the population) had a speech/language impairment. This figure was expected to rise to 13.8 million within a population of 379.5 million by the year 2000.

More detailed analysis of the local population of people with speech communication impairments has been undertaken by Brophy-Arnott *et al.* (1992). This study considered a local region and breaks the population down by the nature of the underlying disorder that causes the speech impairment. In this study, 0.65% of the regional population had a significant communication disorder such that professional speech therapy agencies were involved in seeking to deal with the associated implications of that disorder.

Within that set of people, 47% had communication disorders as a result of a condition that was likely to have caused additional physical or sensory impairments. These causes included cerebral palsy (3%), cerebrovascular accident (7%) and other progressive disorders, such as multiple sclerosis, Parkinson's disease and motor neurone disease.

Arnott *et al.* (1990, 1999) state that a cognitive prosthesis is "a system developed to support and augment the cognitive abilities of its user." When the prosthetic function relates to communication, it serves the role of providing Augmentative and Alternative Communication (AAC). The majority of AAC systems are designed to provide the user with the ability to conduct functional or transactional conversations, or for training people towards the use of language. The goal is usually to provide a means by which users can express themselves and their intentions and wishes. Depending on the language ability of the user, the system will provide a more or less comprehensive vocabulary and the means to express ideas according to a more or less complete grammar. This is confirmed by Beukelman and Mirenda (1998), who report:

> *"Most of the research and technical developments in the field of AAC have focussed on strategies for enhancing communication of needs and wants and, to a lesser extent, information transfer. The lack of attention to social closeness reflects both a narrow clinical perspective and the very real difficulties inherent in achieving the goals of social closeness interactions. Nevertheless, from the perspectives of many AAC users and their significant communication partners, this type of interaction may be more important than any other."*

An important parameter in the intervention and provision of an AAC system is the ability of the user to handle the more abstract forms of representation. Millikin (1997) argues that the use of symbols and abstract representations is fundamental to human communication. The more comprehensive the communication, the more we depend on a decreasing number of abstract symbols, but the more powerful and complex are the rules for combining those symbols to represent the concepts and ideas to be communicated.

The more iconic the symbol type, the more restrictive the word class that it conveys. More iconic symbol types tend to be good at representing nouns, but poor at representing verbs and modifiers. The least iconic symbol types can be combined according to recognised patterns to represent nouns, verbs and modifiers.

The situation is still not completely straightforward, however, as those regularly using a symbol type may learn their meanings, but for an unfamiliar user, the symbol may be ambiguous. For example, a photograph may be a very direct concrete representation of a member of a family, but to someone unfamiliar with the family in question, the concrete message of the picture may be completely lost. This property of the iconicity has been characterised by degrees of transparency. Transparent symbols are ones where the symbol is highly suggestive of the concept that it conveys to an untrained observer, whereas an opaque symbol bears no specific resemblance to the concept being conveyed.

So in the field of AAC, pictures or photographs can serve either the purpose of being a representation of a concept or object, or they can convey much more information than simply the noun that they represent. For the user of an AAC device, therefore, a photograph may help the user recognise the information they wish to convey. For the other communication participants, pictures may add a richness to the concept to be conveyed that would require a whole sequence of symbols of another type to represent.

Augmentative and Alternative Communication research and development activities have focussed on the ability to share unique utterances in conversation.

The means to share personal stories that characterise the person's individuality have not received the same amount of attention. Techniques for sharing the multimedia record of these stories have not been provided in any AAC system to date. The research described here, therefore, was to explore a technique for enabling people with impaired speech and language to share personal information, in the form of multimedia items that can be presented as stories. This technique is designed to be part of the solution to the problems faced by these AAC users in successfully interacting socially, both face-to-face and at a distance.

16.3 Initial Concept

In order to investigate the issues of multimedia based social interaction, the research team at Dundee began to design a computer-based multimedia service, Discussions with people with disabilities resulted a the broad design concept where communications services such as telephony, video telephony, text telephony and e-mail were provided in an accessible way for non-speaking people. The overall concept was based on the extension of the conventional telephony service with the extra elements such as text-telephony, video-telephony and picture telephony. Asynchronous interaction is made available using electronic mail, taking advantage of the fact that multimedia elements can be added as attachments or embedded within a message.

This overall concept took into account the different needs of both face-to-face communication, and communication using Internet services. Various functional modules could be located at different places using a distributed technical architecture. In this way, a low-power, low-cost portable device could be used to select and present media items retrieved from a remote server, taking into account the assistance provided by the prediction algorithms running on the server.

16.4 Prototype Evaluation

Following the initial concept definition phase, a prototype assistive communication service was developed that enabled the project team to investigate the possible usability implementation of an assistive communication system that fitted the broad concept explored above. The specific research question that was formulated was:

> *Given that the user interface for a system that allows multimedia items to be retrieved and presented would need to reflect the abilities of the target users, (many of whom have poor manual dexterity as well as speech and language impairments), which aspects of the user interface could or could not be manipulated by non-speaking people, considering that most of the non-speaking people available to evaluate the system also had some physical disabilities?*

16.4.1 Prototype Design

The prototype communication service that was developed consisted of a Java Application optimised to run on a Windows PC platform. Information was stored in a SOLID database, either on a UNIX server, or in the same computer as the JAVA client application. Information was held as blocks of text, JPEG picture files, QuickTime movie clips, or QuickTime audio clips. These media items were organised into topics, and stored in the database with links to five associated items within the same topic. The user interface of the JAVA client application is shown in Figure 16.1 below.

The topics could be selected from a list that appeared when the 'Change Topic' button was pressed on the user interface. When a topic was selected, five media items were loaded into the upper part of the user interface. When the user clicked on a specific media item, that item was presented in the 'Display Panel', and five media items associated with that chosen item were retrieved from the database and placed in the upper portion of the display. A novel feature of this service was that it could be used in a 'conference' mode, with two or more communicating parties exchanging information. Selections made on one interface would be displayed on all the interfaces connected in the 'conference'.

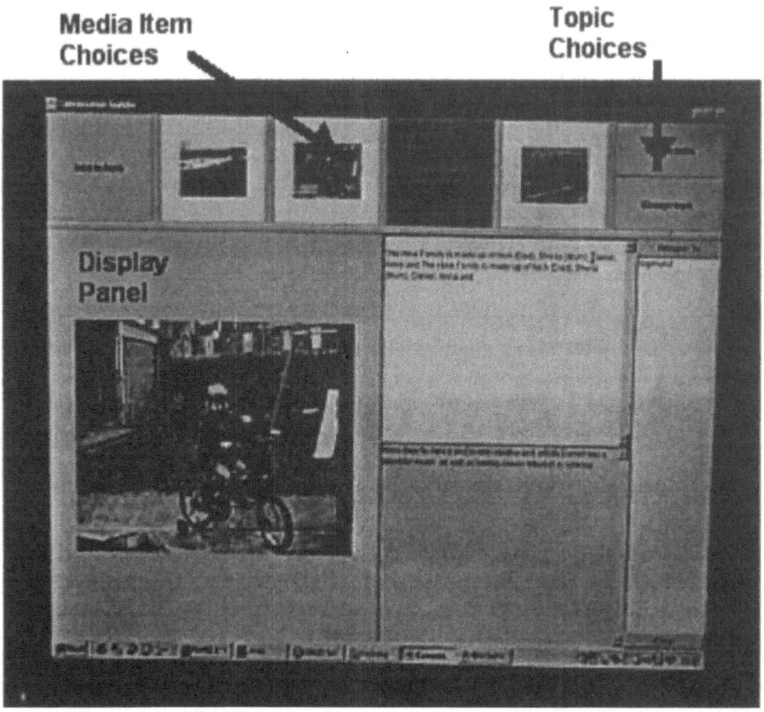

Figure 16.1. User interface of the initial communication service

16.4.2 Evaluation

The purpose of this investigation was to explore with some users with disabilities aspects of the user interface that they found particularly difficult or easy to manipulate.

The user interface of the communication service had been designed and implemented using a broad range of interface elements, including large 'button' areas for selection of media items and text based lists for selection of topics. Another element, however, was a narrow selection field presented in the topic lists that did not persist on the screen once the cursor had been moved off it. One topic of interest was therefore to investigate the usability of all the various interface elements, particularly given that people with disabilities often compensate when encountering difficulties by adopting novel, personal strategies. If the participants could make selections from the topic lists, this might allow more powerful interfaces to be implemented on devices with small screens.

Four clients with impaired speech volunteered to try the service. All four participants also had impaired manual dexterity, three as a consequence of cerebral palsy, and one as a consequence of muscular dystrophy. All four used a wheelchair for mobility.

The trial was conducted on a Stylistic 2300 pen tablet computer. A trial was arranged with each participant. A location was found for the computer that allowed them to interact with it, either on their lap, chair or on a desk close to them. The operation of the software was explained and demonstrated to them, and then they were led through a short sequence involving the selection of media items from the set of items available at the head of the display, and the selection of a new topic. The sequence, based on a predetermined script, resulted in a number of short stories being told whilst the users' interactions with the user interface elements were being observed. Two users selected items for presentation using the stylus on the touch screen, the other two used a rollerball pointing device.

The experience with the participants gave these outcomes.

- All the users considered that the service had the potential to be a useful tool for social interaction, and that the focus of the development activity should focus on that aspect of interpersonal communication, rather than transactional communication, or asynchronous communication. In principle, the users wanted to share their stories in synchronous discussions, and were less interested in asynchronous discussions such as via e-mail.
- In all cases selections of media items from the array of five items at the head of the display could be accomplished. More difficulty was encountered when the selection method involved smaller elements and non-persistent lists.

As far as these users are representative of a significant proportion of non-speaking people, the practical usability issues raised need to be reflected in subsequent versions of the assistive communication service. In particular, non-persistent user interface elements should be avoided. Where the display of the device is small, less user interface elements should be placed on the display, rather than shrinking the size of the user interface elements.

Following the user interface test, the users expressed an interest in collating their own media items for presentation using a revised system. The users supplied pictures, audio and video clips and these were scanned or recorded into the computer. Each media item was given a short label, and was accompanied by a single phrase or sentence to highlight the aspects of interest in the media item. Because the team involved in this activity (users, carers and research staff) were geographically separated, it was decided to host the media items on web pages on a central server, and for the web pages to be updated as media items, labels or accompanying text became available. This provided a very dynamic environment for collating new material, and involved the users in a very proactive way.

These initial user tests were followed by a discussion with carers and research peers that focussed on a review of the user interface presentation and interaction aspects. The general conclusion from this discussion was a requirement to significantly simplify both the interface and the interaction techniques used.

16.5 Communication Service Design

In view of the experience of the users of the prototype communication service, and the experience of collating media items using the web, the service was significantly redesigned. A web-based architecture was adopted based on web pages populated with media items called from a database and presented in a web browser. The client computer and the server may be linked by any Internet Protocol (IP) network, including Wireless LAN. This architecture is shown in Figure 16.2 below.

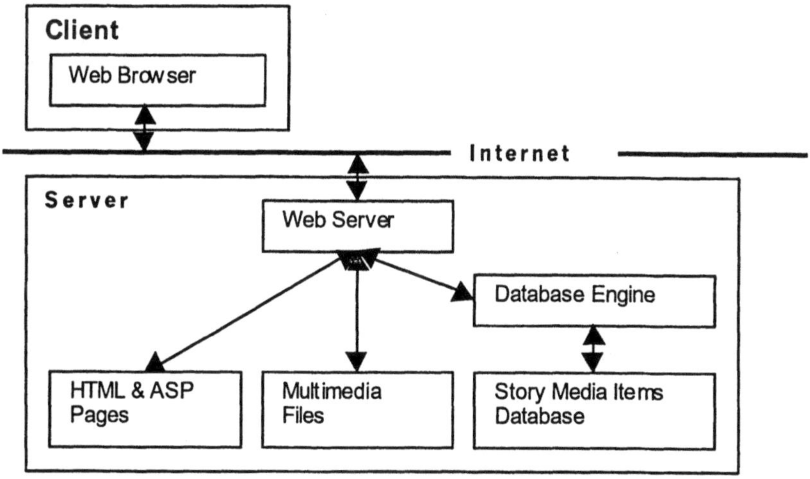

Figure 16.2. Revised architecture of the multimedia communication service

In the revised user interface, the topic and story selection mechanism has be changed from a drop-down list to a set of top level topics always visible on the interface, leading to a dynamic array of sub-topics, stories, and story media items. The media items in the client interface refer to the current story, the other stories in the same topic, and the other topics that the user has stories in, as shown in Figure 16.3 below.

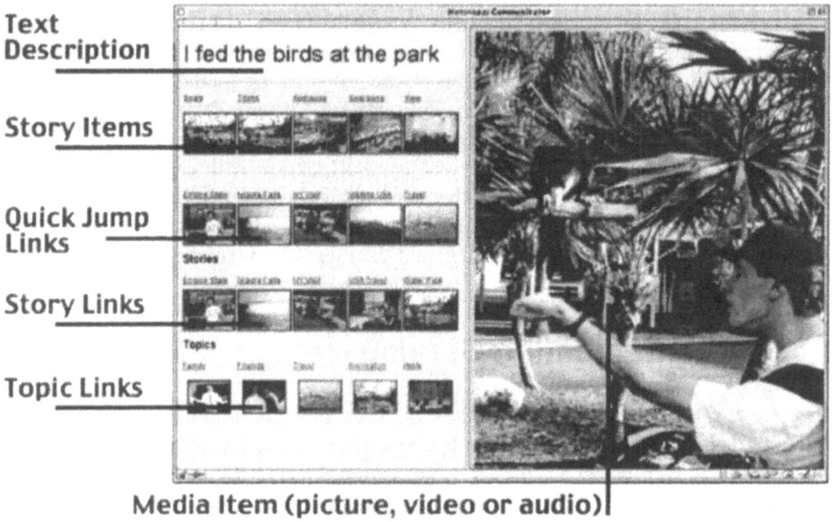

Figure 16.3. Example of the display of the multimedia communication service

The system was populated with media items from two users with impaired speech and with additional motor impairments. The two users were intimately involved in the compilation of the stories within the system, and used the system extensively to verify that the media items reflected the story that they intended to convey. The system was subsequently demonstrated to a group of six non-speaking users and a number of care staff. This demonstration took the form of a workshop where a user presented his stories, and other users who had in interest in the stories commented on the contents and discussed them, using their conventional Augmentative and Alternative Communication (AAC) devices. The workshop was a precursor to an extensive programme of research that has begun to investigate some aspects of the issues that occur when non-speaking people seek to communicate, including the problem of communication breakdown and the aspects of conveying personality attributes during conversations. The validity of the approach as a technique for providing an alternative communication strategy is being explored. Subsequent development of the service will consider the ongoing work in the domains of intelligent and multimedia interfaces (Maybury and Wahlster, 1998) and the domains of cognitive science (Friston and Price, 2001).

16.6 Conclusion

This work has illustrated the key role that users have played in the development of a new multimedia social interaction service. Their requirements have influenced the underlying architecture of the service, resulting in an architecture that enables both users and carers to be involved in a realistic way in the process of adding and managing multimedia items as elements in stories. The users have also contributed to the presentation of the service, the user interface presentation and construction, and the interaction procedures that govern the use of the system. The service therefore reflects the user requirements in terms of fundamental usability, enabling the issues of usage and suitability of the service to meet the social interaction needs of disabled people to be subsequently explored.

16.7 Acknowledgements

Parts of this work was undertaken within the UMPTIDUMPTI Project funded by the European Commission within the ACTS Programme. We would like to thank the staff and clients of Upper Springland, Perth for their assistance during this research and the Fujitsu Company for the loan of a Stylistic pen tablet computer.

16.8 References

Arnott JL (1990) The Communication Prosthesis: A Problem of Human-Computer Integration. In: Proceedings of the European Conference on the Advancement of Rehabilitation Technology, Maastricht, Netherlands, pp 22-26

Arnott JL, Alm N, Waller A (1999) Cognitive Prosthesis: Communication, Rehabilitation and Beyond. In: Proceedings of the IEEE International Conference on Systems Man and Cybernetics, Tokyo, Japan, vol. VI, pp 346-351

Beukelman D, Mirenda P (1998) Augmentative and alternative communication: Management of severe communication disorders in children and adults. 2nd Edition. Paul H Brookes Publishing Company, Baltimore, MD

Brophy-Arnott MB, Newell AF, Arnott JL, Condie D (1992) A survey of the communication impaired population of Tayside. European Journal of Disorders of Communication 27(2): 159-173

Csikszentmihalyi M, Rochberg-Halton E (1981) The meaning of things: domestic symbols and the self. Cambridge University Press, Cambridge, UK

Dunbar RIM (1996) Grooming, Gossip and the Evolution of Language. Mackays of Chatham, Chatham, UK

Dunbar RIM, Marriott A, Duncan NDC (1997) Human Conversational Behaviour. Human Nature 8(3): 231-246

Emler N (1994) Gossip, Reputation, and Social Adaptation. In: Goodman RF, Ben-Ze'ev A (eds.) Good Gossip, University Press of Kansas, pp 117-138

Friston KJ, Price CJ (2001) Generative models, brain function and neuroimaging. Scandinavian Journal of Psychology 42(3): 167-177

Mäkelä A, Giller V, Tscheligi M, Sefelin R (2000) Joking, storytelling, pastsharing, expressing affection: a field trial of how children and their social network communicate with digital images in leisure time. In: Proceedings of the CHI 2000 Conference on Human Factors in Computing Systems, The Hague, Netherlands, pp 548-555

Maybury MT, Wahlster W (1998) Readings in Intelligent User Interfaces. Morgan Kaufman, San Fransisco, CA

Millikin CC (1997) Symbol systems and vocabulary selection strategies. In: Glennen SL, DeCoste DC (eds.) Handbook of Augmentative and Alternative Communication. Singular Publishing Group, San Diego, CA, pp 97-148

Pickering JA, Arnott JL, Wolff JG, Swiffin AL (1984) Prediction and adaption in a computer aid for the disabled. In: Proceedings of INTERACT '84, First IFIP Conference on human computer interaction, London, UK, pp 815-819

Read SJ, Miller LC (1995) Stories are Fundamental to Meaning and Memory: For Social Creatures Could It Be Otherwise. In: Wyer RS (ed.) Knowledge and Memory: The Real Story. Lawrence Erlbaum Associates, Hillsdale, NJ, pp 139-152

Sandhu J (ed.) (1997) A demographic analysis of the number of disabled and elderly people in Europe and related statistics. Deliverable to the CEC from Telematics Applications Programme Project DE3006 MORE, Workpackage WP 1, Deliverable 1.2

Schank RC (1990) Tell me a story: a new look at real and artificial memory. Scribner's, Macmillan Publishing Company, New York

Schank RC, Abelson RP (1995) Knowledge and Memory: The Real Story. In: Wyer RS (ed.) Knowledge and Memory: The Real Story. Lawrence Erlbaum Associates, Hillsdale, NJ, pp 1-85

Scott LM (1995) Representation and Narrative: A Commentry on Schank and Abelson's "Knowledge and Memory." In: Wyer RS (ed.) Knowledge and Memory: The Real Story. Lawrence Erlbaum Associates, Hillsdale, NJ, pp 165-176

Chapter 17

Issues Surrounding the User-centred Development of a New Interactive Memory Aid

E. Inglis, A. Szymkowiak, P. Gregor, A.F. Newell, N. Hine, B.A. Wilson and J. Evans

17.1 Introduction

At the beginning of this research, a participant who lives with memory loss every day of his life attempted to explain what he wanted in a memory aid. "Imagine a memory which is outside you and responsive to you but doesn't control you." This, then was the challenge: to design an effective aid which would be a natural extension to the memory which you and I do not realise just how much we depend upon.

Memory problems are often associated with the ageing process and they are one of the commonest effects of brain injury. Such problems can severely disrupt daily life and put huge strain on family members and carers (Wilson, 1995). Electronic memory aids have been used as a compensatory approach to provide reminders to individuals, and in particular a small pager device has been evaluated with great success. The 'NeuroPage' system was developed in the USA by Hersh and Treadgold (1994). The user carries a telephone pager which alerts them by sound or vibration when a scheduled message is displayed on the alphanumeric screen. The overall operation is performed via collaboration between a local memory clinic and a commercial paging service. In consultation with the user and carers, staff in the clinic decide what messages are appropriate and necessary together with the appropriate time and date for transmitting them, and this information is sent to the commercial service which enters the data into their central paging system.

The aid has been evaluated by Wilson, Emslie, Quirk and Evans (2001) in a study involving 143 clients of ages ranging from 8 to 83 years. It has been found to be very successful, particularly with people exhibiting severe memory, attention and organisational problems.

Based on this success, the current study is to develop an electronic memory aid which will maintain the basic functionality of the pager system, whilst enhancing the service in terms of interactivity and functionality. Enabling two-way communication between a memory aid 'device' and a base station can provide the reassurance to relatives and carers which is required to reduce their workload and worry and increase the independence of the user of the system.

Increasing the functionality of the memory aid presents challenges regarding the usability of the system. These will be addressed by the user-centred design methodology that this chapter describes. This approach to the development also enables investigation of the best way to involve older people in the prototype development. Initial qualitative findings of this process are also detailed.

17.2 Background

17.2.1 Memory Loss

Memory loss can take many forms and affect many people, though it is a decline in prospective memory, the ability to 'remember to remember,' which is particularly relevant to the design of a memory aid. Prospective memory is known to deteriorate in relation to age (McDaniel and Einstein, 1993) and is one of the most common forms of impairment following a brain-injury. Brain-injured users characteristically have difficulty remembering most kinds of new information, including future events, although have normal to near/normal immediate memory (Wilson, 1995). One way to gauge the extent to which these problems can affect the every day life of these people is to look at the messages which users programmed into the NeuroPage memory aid system. Wilson *et al.* (1997) report that the most common messages used on this system were "good morning, it is 'day and date'," "take your medication now," "fill in your diary," and "make your packed lunch." These messages reveal an underlying deficiency in basic memory functioning which has serious implications for day-to-day living.

Older people suffer similar problems. In normal ageing, different degrees of impairment affect different forms of memory. In a population based study of almost 12,000 older participants (65+ years), Huppert *et al.* (2000) found that only 54% of the subjects successfully completed an event-based prospective memory task. Participants were recruited from five centres across the country through their local GPs, with care being taken that the 'very old' (75+ years) were equally represented in the sample. The memory task involved participants being given an envelope and being told that later on they would be asked to write a name and address on the envelope, at which time they should also remember to seal it and write their initials on the back. Ten minutes elapsed between these instructions being given and the task enactment being carried out. Success in this task was strongly and linearly related to age, which is illustrated by highlighting the results in the youngest age group (65-69 years), where 68% succeeded, against the oldest age group (90+ years) where only 19% performed the task successfully. The underlying significance of this research is that just under half the population of adults over the age of 65 in the UK suffer from some form of prospective memory impairment, and that as a consequence the safety and well being of many older people may be at risk. A device to aid memory therefore has huge potential. In view of the reluctance of new-technology uptake which exists amongst many older people, it suggests that a memory aid device may prove even more effective if taken up by the 'young-old' to aid them in later life.

17.2.2 Current Electronic Memory Aids and Usability

Despite the prevalence of prospective memory problems amongst older people, the vast majority of research in this area has focussed on the rehabilitation of individuals from brain injury. A number of ways of improving lost memory functions have been investigated and applied (Harris, 1992). These include strategies such as artificial mnemonics and repetitive practice (a restorative approach to improving memory) and the use of external aids such as calendars and diaries (a compensatory approach). Whilst some restorative methods have been successful (Raskin and Sohlberg, 1996), it is the compensatory approach which shows greater potential, with prospective memory deficits being 'replaced' by prompting the user to carry out tasks and appointments with an external aid.

It is in this area that technology has been used as an aid to memory. Current personal digital assistants (PDA's) and palmtop computers provide time management software which has the potential to be used as a diary/alarm system for people with memory impairment. Kim *et al.* (1999) introduced a Psion Series 3a palmtop computer to a 22 year old man whose memory skills were poor and who was currently undergoing rehabilitation for a closed head injury. Staff at the rehabilitation centre programmed alarms to remind him to attend therapy sessions and ask for medication and the patient was able to carry out all tasks without further cues. In an additional study, Kim *et al.* (2000) reports on a trial involving 12 brain injured patients using a Psion Series 3a computer to assist with memory dependent activities in their day to day lives. In a follow-up interview 9 of the 12 participants judged the device to be useful to them on a daily basis, whilst all patients recommended that the palmtop should be continued to be used in outpatient therapy for brain injured patients.

Further studies by Van de Broek (2000) and Willkomm *et al.* (1997) have evaluated the use of a Voice Organiser device as a memory aid. The Voice Organiser is a handheld dictaphone which can be programmed to replay messages at time periods specified orally by the user. The user is alerted to a message by an alarm, and on pressing a button the message is replayed. Van de Broek asked five subjects with significant acquired prospective memory impairment to perform prospective memory tasks, both with and without the Voice Organiser, over a period of three weeks for each phase. All subjects improved during the introduction of the Voice Organiser, with three subjects establishing a routine which persisted to a certain extent following the removal of the device. Similar results have been obtained by Wilson *et al.* (1999), who reports that a severely memory impaired user of NeuroPage improved on time-based tasks, such as preparing a meal, from 50% success rate pre-pager to 100% during use of the NeuroPage device. For some tasks, the higher success rate was maintained once the pager had been removed due to the establishment of a routine. Other key points to be taken from this study were that the subjects remained in control by choosing the wording of their own messages and that the pager was seen as prestigious rather than an embarrassment.

A common thread within the evidence available is a consideration of who might benefit from such technology. Wilson and Moffat (1984) found that learning to use electronic organisers produces great problems for memory impaired people, and reports from Kim *et al.* (2000) detailing subjects requiring supervised training twice a week suggests that the level of training required is not diminishing as the technology advances. When this is considered in conjunction with recent research (Clare *et al.*, 2000; Wilson and Evans, 1996) which shows that memory impaired people benefit from errorless learning techniques, it is clear that the training required to learn how to use electronic memory aids should be minimal and produce as few errors as possible. In contrast, current time-management software running on PDAs require at least some training for an average user. Although the ease of use of such software applications varies across the range of devices available and the platform on which they run (PalmOS/PocketPC/EPOC), they are not designed for memory impaired people. Wright *et al.* (2001) conducted a study in which an interface specifically designed for brain injured users was employed on two styles of PDAs. It was found that users who had suffered traumatic brain injury could use the PDAs successfully as memory aids, pointing to the need for a custom designed interface for such users.

Usability is therefore a key factor in whether an electronic organiser can be successfully employed as a day-to-day memory aid. A parallel report on WAP usability (the technology used to access the internet from mobile phones) by Ramsey and Nielsen (2000) gives detailed evidence of the problems of creating usable systems for small screen space such as mobile phones and PDAs. Scrolling pages, screen layout and the use of images and text all contribute to a difficult usability problem which can only hamper the use of these technologies as an external memory aid.

Older users provide an additional dimension to the problem. One of the critical points for usable interface design from this perspective is the decline with age in the ability to process items in working memory (Salthouse, 1994). Zajicek (2001) highlights this point by suggesting that memory impairment reduces the ability of users to build conceptual models of the working interface. Further contributory factors to the problems for older people when utilising a small, electronic memory aid are changes to vision, including declining visual acuity, contrast sensitivity and reduced sensitivity to colour, particularly blue-green tones (Hawthorn, 2000), all of which make a small PDA interface difficult or impossible to see. When combined with difficulties in control of fine movement (Vercruyssen, 1996) and the impact this would have on the ability to manage a small touch-screen device, older people present a user group with very specific needs in this design area.

Together these factors point towards an interface with reduced and clearly displayed functionality that minimises the load on working memory. This implies intuitive usability that requires minimal training and visibly maintains the structure of the system at all times.

17.3 Current Study

The approach taken in the current research was to pin-point the deficiencies highlighted in the currently available electronic memory aids and use this as a basis to investigate and formulate the requirements for a new external memory aid. The areas where improvements could be made are perceived to be:

- the lack of two-way communication between user and carer through the aid;
- commercially available software applications being unsuitable/difficult for memory impaired users to learn and interact with;
- devices with small screens displaying small text and making interaction difficult for older users due to poor vision and/or dexterity.

From this platform, the research was undertaken from a user perspective, involving discussions with both older people and brain injured people, together with investigation into suitable technology that is currently available.

17.3.1 User-centred Design Process

17.3.1.1 Methodology: Interviews and Focus Groups

In order to begin designing the prototype under development, 10 older and 7 memory impaired people were interviewed about their current strategies for remembering in their day to day lives. Participants were recruited from sheltered housing and a disability rehabilitation clinic in the local area. Interested volunteers were suggested to the researchers by management or carers, with the interviews being conducted within the homes of the participants or within a day centre that the individuals attended.

Following a structured interview procedure, participants were asked about the memory aids that they currently use, such as a calendar or notebook, together with any other strategies used to help them remember things. They were also questioned on their experience of using technologies such as mobile phones and personal computers, what they considered to be an acceptable size and weight of a memory aid, and what they would ideally like a memory aid to do for them.

In addition to interviewing, 4 focus groups were conducted with older residents of sheltered housing schemes. These proved to be very valuable. The discussion focused on the problems people had with their memory, together with opinions on the PDAs that were passed round to the participants. Interesting findings from these meetings were the responsiveness the participants showed to the technology, despite many of them never having seen devices of this nature before. Interaction with the touch-screens, which are the main input mechanism for the majority of PDAs, proved to be an intuitive concept to which this particular group of older people quickly adapted.

It was also interesting to note that a group of more than 3 individuals within a focus group became hard to manage, as difficulties with hearing, attention and the ability to follow the thread of a conversation proved to be hamper many participants contribution. Future methodology for user-centred design may need to consider this when involving older people in design and prototype development.

17.3.1.2 Qualitative Findings

The findings from these sessions produced several points. Perhaps unsurprisingly, the most commonly used aid/strategy amongst people questioned was a calendar or notebook. The diverse and specific responses to questions regarding the ideal functions of a memory aid made the results hard to categorise. A clear theme, however, was that participants wanted to be reminded not only of what they had to do, but *why* they had to do it.

A further concern voiced by the users was the usability of the system. The need for "big buttons," "clear prompts," "nice and friendly," and "user control" were all statements which revealed the users' awareness of their need for a usable as well as a useful aid. In addition, many of the younger, memory-impaired users were aware of the hardware requirements of a memory aid and asked for "flashing light," "alarm," "voice recognition" and "portability." This technical awareness was not evident in the older group of subjects as one might expect from a generation of people less exposed to developments in technology.

This information produced the general hardware requirements for the prototype memory aid, which gave guidance to investigations of the potential technologies that are currently available to be utilised in the aid. Mobile phone technology is currently being integrated into PDA devices, and new technologies and devices are frequently coming on to the market in this rapidly expanding area. The potential for the use of this technology as a memory aid is enormous as it allows for a truly interactive system which can keep the memory impaired user in contact with a remote, possibly unmanned base, potentially removing the necessity of a call centre for a functional system. Remote access to the device could be provided through a base station that could also be accessed remotely from any PC that was live on the Internet. This would allow reminder messages to be entered into the system from a large number of suitable locations at any time of day, and thus be completely independent of a third-party call centre.

17.3.2 Development Phase: Initial and Future Prototypes

Following the evaluation of these findings, the first prototype was developed as a web-based system that would run independently on a PDA. This provided a measure of what the interface of the memory aid could look like and a basic functionality that allowed users to explore interaction with the system. The prototype aims to reduce the load on working memory by ensuring that all elements of the system are visible at all times. This is in itself a challenge that exaggerates the usability problems presented by the small screen size of the PDA.

The continuation of the development phase will be informed by a series of pilot evaluations with users of this initial prototype. This will involve tracking the users' movements through the system in order to identify potential usability problems or functionality which is redundant or missing, together with videoed observation for interpreting the user feedback. Such interactive evaluation and gathering of feedback will enable design iteration, ensuring that the ideas developed are sound before further prototypes are developed.

The second stage prototype will be implemented for use within an extended informal trial period carried out by the Oliver Zangwill Centre in Ely, who form part of the multi-disciplinary team involved in the current study. Results from this study will be fed back to the design team for a major system revision. The final prototype will be formally reviewed with memory impaired and older users.

17.4 Conclusions

Memory has been shown to decline with age. Although technology has been used and proved to have a positive effect on helping with these kinds of memory problems, usability and technological difficulties have limited the potential in terms of the number of users who can benefit from these aids. These difficulties have also reduced the extent to which the aids can contribute to longer lasting independence and safety of users. The current study is work in progress to develop an interactive memory aid using a user-centred design methodology. Challenges raised include the difficulties in combining usability and functionality on a small device to be used by older people with very specific needs in both of these areas. An additional consideration is how the characteristics of an older user group influence the gathering of design contributions through focus groups and interview techniques. The current study aims to overcome these difficulties and develop a new aid which can be used easily and practicably in everyday situations.

17.5 References

Clare L, Wilson BA, Carter G, Breen K, Gosses A, Hodges JR (2000) Intervening with everyday memory problems in dementia and alzheimer type: an errorless learning approach. Journal of Clinical and Experimental Neuropsychology 22: 132-146

Harris JE (1992) Ways to help memory. In: Wilson BA, Moffat N (eds.) Clinical management of memory problems, 2nd edn. Chapman & Hall, London, pp 59-85

Hawthorn D (2000) Possible implications of aging for interface designers. Interacting with Computers 12: 507-528

Hersh NA, Treadgold LG (1994) NeuroPage: the rehabilitation of memory dysfunction by prosthetic memory and cueing. Neurorehabilitation 4: 187-197

Huppert FA, Johnson T, Nickson J (2000) High prevalence of prospective memory impairment in the elderly and in early-stage dementia: Findings from a population based study. Applied Cognitive Psychology 14: S63-S81

Kim HJ, Burke DT, Dowds MM, George J (1999) Utility of a microcomputer as an external memory aid for a memory-impaired head injury patient during in-patient rehabilitation. Brain Injury 13: 147-150

Kim HJ, Burke DT, Dowds MM, Robinson Boone KA, Park GJ (2000) Electronic memory aids for an outpatient brain injury: follow-up findings. Brain Injury 14: 187-196.

McDaniel MA, Einstein GO (1993) The importance of cue familiarity and cue distinctiveness in prospective memory. Memory 1: 23-41

Ramsey M, Nielsen J (2000) WAP Usability Déjà Vu: 1994 all over again. Nielsen Norman Group

Raskin SA, Sohlberg MM (1996) The efficacy of prospective memory training in two adults with brain injury. Journal of Head Trauma Rehabilitation 11: 32-51

Salthouse TA (1994) The ageing of working memory. Neuropsychology 8: 535-543

Van de Broek MD, Downes J, Johnson Z, Dayus B, Hilton N (2000) Evaluation of an electronic memory aid in the neuropsychological rehabilitation of prospective memory deficits. Brain Injury 14: 455-462

Vercruyssen M (1996) Movement control and the speed of behaviour. In: Fisk AD, Rogers WA (eds.) Handbook of human factors and the older adult. Academic Press, San Diego, CA

Willkomm T, LoPresti E (1997) Evaluation of an electronic memory aid for prospective memory tasks. In: Proceedings of the RESNA 1997 Annual Conference, pp 520-522

Wilson BA (1995) Management and remediation of memory problems in brain-injured adults. In: Baddeley AD, Watts FN (eds.) Handbook of memory disorders. Wiley, Chichester, UK, pp 451-479

Wilson BA, Emslie HC, Quirk K, Evans JJ (1999) George: Learning to live independently with NeuroPage. Rehabilitation Psychology 44: 284-296

Wilson BA, Emslie HC, Quirk K, Evans JJ (2001) Reducing everyday memory and planning problems by means of a paging system: a randomised control and crossover study. Journal of Neurology, Neurosurgery and Psychiatry 70: 477-482

Wilson BA, Evans JJ (1996) Error-free learning in the rehabilitation of people with memory impairments. Journal of Head Trauma Rehabilitation 11: 54-64

Wilson BA, Evans JJ, Emslie H, Malinek V (1997) Evaluation of NeuroPage: a new memory aid. Journal of Neurology, Neurosurgery and Psychiatry 63: 113-115

Wilson BA, Moffat N (1984) Rehabilitation of memory for everyday life. In: Harris JE, Morris PE (eds.) Everyday Memory, Actions and Absent-Mindedness. Academic Press, London, pp 207-233

Wright P, Rogers N, Hall C, Wilson B, Evans J, Emslie H, Bartram C (2001) Comparison of pocket-computer memory aids for people with brain injury. Brain Injury 15: 787-800

Zajicek M, Morrissey W (2001) Speech output for older visually impaired adults. In: Blandford A, Vanderdonckt J, Gray P (eds.) Interaction without Frontiers. Joint Proceedings of HCI 2001 and IHM 2001, pp 503-513

Chapter 18

Games Children with Autism Can Play with Robota, a Humanoid Robotic Doll

K. Dautenhahn and A. Billard

18.1 Background

This chapter discusses the potential use of a small, humanoid robotic doll called Robota in autism therapy. Robota was specifically designed for engaging children in imitative interaction games. This work is associated to the Aurora project where we study the potential therapeutic role of robots in autism therapy. This section provides the necessary background information on autism (18.1.1), and motivates the application of interactive technology in autism therapy (18.1.2). Section 18.1.3 discusses the important role of imitation and interaction games in the development of social skills. Section 18.2 introduces the Aurora project. Sections 18.3 and 18.4 briefly describe the humanoid doll Robota and its potential use in autism therapy. Observations from preliminary trials are discussed in Section 18.5 before section 18.6 concludes this chapter.

18.1.1 Autism

The autistic disorder is defined by specific diagnostic criteria, specified in DSM-IV (Diagnostic and Statistical Manual of Mental Disorders, American Psychiatric Association, 1994). Individuals with autism present a broad spectrum of difficulties and abilities, and vary enormously in their levels of overall intellectual functioning. However, all individuals diagnosed with autism will show impairments in the following areas: Qualitative impairment in social interaction, communication, and restricted repetitive and stereotyped patterns of behaviour, interests, and activities. At the higher functioning end of the autistic spectrum we find people with Asperger Syndrome. Some of them manage to live independently as adults and succeed in their profession, but only by learning and explicitly applying rules to overcome the 'social barrier' (e.g. Grandin, 1995) which demonstrates the benefit of explicitly learnt/taught social knowledge. Instead of picking up and interpreting social cues 'naturally' they can learn and memorise rules about what kind of behaviour is socially appropriate during interaction with non-autistic people.

Many theories exist trying to explain and understand the primary causes of autism at the psychological or cognitive level of explanation. Much attention has recently focussed on the significance of early impairments in imitation (e.g. Rogers and Pennington, 1991) and shared attention (e.g. Baron-Cohen, 1995). Results by Jacqueline Nadel have shown very positive responses when children with autism were imitated by other children (1999). These results are confirming Nadel's view of imitation as a *format of communication* (see Section 18.1.3), a means to express interest by imitation, and a means to engage others in interaction. Based on this paradigm, our working assumption is that an interactive, doll-shaped robot that can imitate will be able to engage children with autism in playful behaviour that can be used to teach basic imitative interaction skills.

18.1.2 Interactive Technology in Autism Therapy

For over thirty years researchers have been investigating the usage of robots in education (Papert 1980; Druin and Hendler, 2000). The potential use of computer and virtual environment technology in autism therapy is increasingly studied (e.g. Colby *et al.*, 1971; Strickland 1996; Powell, 1996; Blocher, 1999). People with autism often interact very 'naturally' with computer technology and use it in an exploratory and creative manner. A few projects have also investigated robotic devices (Weir and Emanuel, 1997; Michaud *et al.*, 2000; Plaisant *et al.*, 2000), and it has been proposed that a humanoid robot might be used as a therapy aid for children with autism (Kozima and Yano, 2001). Teaching methods for children with autism are often based on highly structured teaching sessions (Watson *et al.*, 1989) where the children are explicitly encouraged to make eye-contact, take turns in a social setting, associate facial expressions with emotions etc. (Howlin *et al.*, 1999). Generally, computer technology in education and therapy has the big advantage of *putting the child in control*, under possible guidance of and feedback from the teacher, but with the child learning at his/her own pace.

A humanoid robot, i.e. a robot that can match at least to some extent basic behaviours of human beings (e.g. arm, head and eye movements) is an interesting tool for studying robot-human interaction, and in particular social interaction dynamics. However, research with humanoid robots to date is severely limited by the effort required in terms of required funding, development time, and the necessity to have a large team of highly qualified researchers and technicians maintaining the robot and keeping it operational.

Additionally, humanoid robots are usually not 'mobile', i.e. they can only be studied in the laboratory and cannot be transported easily to different sites, a necessary requirement if such systems are to be used in educational or therapy applications where it is desirable to study people in a familiar environment rather than bringing them to the laboratory. Research into robot-human interaction is often using a commercially available mobile robotic platforms (such as the Pioneer from ActivMedia Robotics, or RWI's indoor robots such as B21r, B14r and Magellan Pro), systems that were historically developed for tasks such as navigation and planning, and therefore have a highly restricted behaviour and interaction repertoire. Robotic toys have become very popular during the past five years (cf. Sony's Aibo, LEGO Mindstorms, Furbys, My Real Baby). As commercial products such toy robots are robust, relatively inexpensive (in comparison to research platforms), and specifically designed for robot-human interaction. Usually, their behaviour and appearance is designed to mimic real biological systems, so as to be 'cute' and popular with people, by appealing to human's tendencies to anthropomorphise. However, such robots are usually limited in terms of their capabilities and provide little freedom for the user to improve those. Either the robot's behaviour is fixed (Aibo, My Real Baby, Furbys) or the complexity of the behaviour that one could program remains very limited because the platform has little computational power (hence affordable by the great public), e.g. LEGO Mindstorms with very few sensors (6) and actuators (3).

In this chapter we discuss possible therapeutic contributions of a humanoid robotic doll to autism therapy. Our approach is based on the assumption that bodily interaction in imitative interaction games is normally an important factor in a child's development of social skills (see next section), and that teaching of such skills (in a playful and exploratory context but nevertheless from an educational point of view focussing explicitly on specific types of interactions) could help children with autism in coping with the normal dynamics of social interactions.

18.1.3 Homo Imitans: Imitation Games People Play

Growing up in a human family means that a lot of time is spent on social interactions. Infants, in particular, receive an important amount of attention. Imitative and rhythmic interaction games (comprising e.g. vocalisations and body movements) between infants and caretakers, such as imitation and turn-taking, play an important part in the development of social cognition and communication in the young human animal (Bullowa, 1979; Piaget 1962; Nadel and Butterworth (eds.), 1999). Infants are born ready to communicate by being able to reciprocate in rhythmic engagements with the motives of sympathetic partners.

Imitation plays an important part in play and social learning in humans, including adults and children. It is necessary for the individual's social acquisition of a variety of skills, ranging from vocal imitation in language games to imitation of body movements (*e.g.* when instructed how to tie shoe laces). Similarly, research in robotics and software agents is trying to employ imitation as a means of social learning, using machine learning approaches such as neural networks. Importantly, the *social function of imitation* in human-human interaction is increasingly recognised as a means to engage others in interaction, to express interest, and to develop co-ordinated interaction that is central to verbal and non-verbal 'dialogues'.

From a neurobiological perspective, given recent discussions on 'mirror' neurons and the neurobiological origin of imitation in primate evolution, one might speculate that *mirror neurons* are nature's solution – at least in some primates – to solving the correspondence problem, namely in creating a common shared context and shared *understanding* of actions and affordances (see below) between two agents (see discussion by Arbib, 2002). Recently a connection between an impairment in the mirror neuron system, imitative skills and autism has been suggested (Williams *et al.*, 2001). However, discussions on deficits of children with autism with respect to imitation are controversial (e.g. Rogers in Nadel and Butterworth, 1999; Charman *et al.*, 1994) and often depend on the particular psychological theories on the nature of autism that particular research groups support. Generally children with autism seem to imitate less frequently, in particular they seem less able to imitate actions and gestures, cf. Jordan (1999).

Although the work that we discuss in this chapter focuses on autism therapy, rather than trying to understand the nature of autism, we would like to point out that robots could also serve as interesting tools for investigating theories and models proposed by autism researchers. Similarly, in biology and cognitive science the usage of robots as research tools in the quest for understanding intelligence has already been widely recognised.

In human culture imitation is an important cultural and social *medium of communication*. Imitation is an important mechanism of social learning in human culture, but also a powerful means of signalling interest in another person, used for purposes of communication. According to Nadel *et al.* (1999) immediate imitation is an important *format of communication* and milestone in the development of intentional communication, linking the imitator and the imitatee in synchronised activity that creates inter-subjective experience, sharing topics and activities. Even unconscious temporal synchronisation and rhythmic co-ordination of movements between people play an important role in communication and interaction in human culture, cf. proxemics (the study of humans' perception and use of space, *cf.* Hall, 1966). Temporal synchronisation of behavioural dynamics has also been implemented in studies with robot-human interaction (Dautenhahn, 1999).

Our work focuses primarily on the *social role of imitation* (Dautenhahn, 1994), i.e. imitation as a format of communication that creates inter-subjectivity in human-human interaction. We propose that the important link between the dynamics of imitation and social interactions can be explored in using a humanoid robot.

18.2 The Aurora Project

The work discussed in this chapter is associated to the Aurora project which has been studying how a non-humanoid mobile robot with very simple interaction skills can be used as a teaching device (a 'toy') in autism therapy. Here, robot-human interactions are unconstrained and unstructured, allowing full-body interactions (see Figure 18.1). Our motivation is that children can explore and 'discover' interaction skills rather than being taught explicitly. For more background on the project's robotic and therapeutic issues see (Dautenhahn, 1999; Werry and Dautenhahn, 1999; Dautenhahn and Werry, 2000, 2001; Werry *et al.*, 2001a,b,c; Dautenhahn *et al.*, to appear). Results are generally encouraging. In a series of trials with 8-12 year old autistic children it was found that: (1) the robot is safe for the children to use; (2) the large majority of children are not afraid of the robot and show great flexibility in coping very well with the new context; (3) the children are very motivated to interact with the robot over a period of five to ten minutes or longer; (4) the children are usually more interested in the robot in 'interactive' mode in comparison to the robot showing rigid, repetitive, non-interactive behaviour; and (5) the children have no problems coping with the robot behaving reactively but not completely predictable. In these trials, the robot showed a few basic behaviours of approach and avoidance. Results also indicate that the children generally showed more interest in the robot (in terms of gaze, touch etc.) and were more engaged in interactions with the robot than with another non-robotic toy. The results showed large individual differences among the children, but it is safe to say that we showed that the robot was able to engage children with autism in interaction dynamics that are important to social interactions in general, and that we can further explore, e.g. in the work described in this chapter. In previous work we studied and adapted different analysis techniques (quantitative and qualitative). The former is based on micro-behaviours (Tardif *et al.*, 1995), the latter uses Conversation Analysis (CA). Such analysis techniques (see Dautenhahn *et al.*, to appear) can also be applied to interactions of children with a humanoid robot.

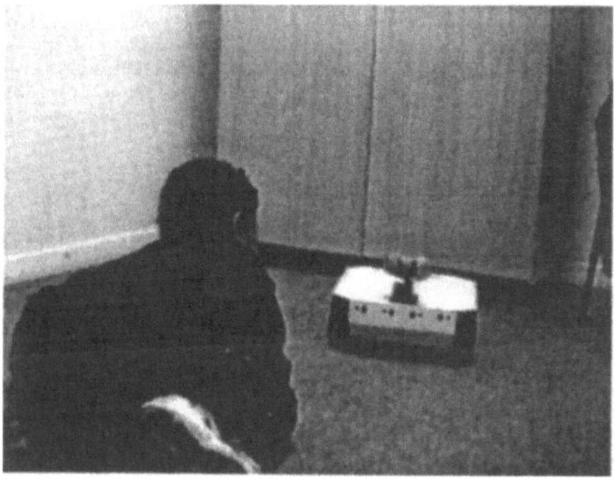

Figure 18.1. A child with autism playing "chasing" games with the mobile robot used in the Aurora project

The main limitation of the (non-humanoid) robot currently used in the Aurora project lies in that it offers only a very small number of interactions with the child, i.e. the type of interactions that can occur are limited to spatial approach/avoidance turn-taking games. The humanoid robot Robota, described in the next section, can complement this work by offering a much larger range of multi-modal imitative interactions, in this way providing new means of interaction such as mimicking movements of body parts (e.g. hands, head), as well as more complex interactions (sequences and combinations of actions). Because of its small size and relatively low price it is also ideal for long-term studies in which the children are regularly exposed to and interact with the robot.

18.3 Who is Robota?

Robota is a doll-shaped robot 50 cm tall, weighing 500 grams, see Figure 18.2. The arms, legs and the head of the robot are plastic components of a commercially available doll. The main body contains the electronics (PIC 16F870, 4MHz and 16F84, 16MHz) and mechanics (5 motors, legs, arms and head, 1 DOF each)[1]. For a complete description of Robota's hardware, see http://www-slab.usc.edu/billard/robota.html. Through a serial link connection to a PC, the robot uses speech synthesising and video processing (based on a QuickCam camera). Using a motion tracking system, Robota can copy upwards movements of the user's arms when the user faces the camera. This game can be used to teach Robota to dance to a specific music, played on the PC. The robot reacts to touch: it detects passive motion of its limbs through its potentiometers and responds with a little jerk of the touched limb. In the present trials, the robot uses speech synthesising to tell its name and describe its behaviour. This is meant to attract the child's attention. In other games, the robot can be taught by the user how to speak (Billard, 1999, 2000, 2002).

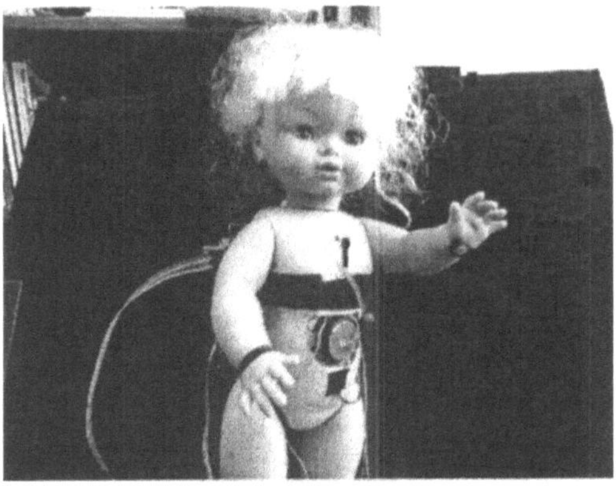

Figure 18.2. Robot, the humanoid robotic doll. The robot's dress is removed in order to show the robotic parts that control its movements.

Robota was designed as an interactive toy for children. The multimedia type of interactions which Robota offers makes it a non-boring toy (not immediately at least). In (Billard, Dautenhahn and Hayes, 1998), we reported initial tests with (typically developing) children of 5 and 6 years old, which showed the potential of the robot as a game for children. The children enjoyed playing with the robot because they could interact with it in different ways. The robot would respond to the children touching specific parts of its body, by making small movements or some sounds. It would mimic the child's head and arm movements. It would speak words that are part of the child's every-day vocabulary (e.g. "food," "hello," and "no"). The level of complexity of the game with Robota can be varied. One can restrict the interactions to built-in behaviours of the robot (a 'baby-like' robot).

[1] Plans to include one motor to drive the eyes in coordinated sideways motion.

18.4 Possible Usage of Robota in Autism Therapy

The previous section discussed Robota's range of behavioural capabilities. In future, the behavioural repertoire will need to be adapted in order to meet the specific needs of children with autism. In particular the 'baby behaviours,' which encourage 'caring' behaviour in typically developing children are not very likely to have the same impact on children with autism. Pretend play, imagination and fantasy which are necessary in order to 'suspend disbelief' and treat the robot doll like a 'baby,' are often impaired in children with autism. Thus, a doll that is too 'humanoid' and 'social' could appear confusing and unpredictable, too similar to human social behaviour. In our work we start with a small behaviour repertoire of the robot. Over time we plan to incrementally change it depending on the children's reactions.

Potentially, a number of different types of robots might be successful in autism therapy. However, the specific nature of autism poses particular requirements and constraints on the robot and its behavioural capabilities. Most importantly:

- **Safety and ethical issues:** It is vital to provide a safe environment where the child can explore as unconstrained as possible the robot's capabilities in an enjoyable and relaxed atmosphere. Since the child should learn through playing, any aspects of the robot that might upset or scare the child need to be avoided by all means. For these reasons we decided to use small, lightweight, toy-size robots.
- **Predictability and control:** Although it is desirable that the child adapts to complex and often unpredictable behaviour, as humans show them, children with autism can easily get overwhelmed by sensory stimuli, e.g. as they occur in human social interactions. Thus, we believe that an important advantage of using robots in autism therapy is not to provide an 'artificial human', but to provide a tool that is *clearly much simpler* than any human being, and that can guide the children through increasingly more varied and complex types of interactions in which they exercise skills (such as turn-taking and imitative skills) that play an important role in human-human interactions. This approach is supported by empirical data which shows the preference of autistic children to 'social' (doll-like) objects with low complexity, in a predictable environment (Ferrara and Hill, 1980).
- **Generalisation:** Any autism therapy method faces the problem that people with autism have great difficulties in generalising learning achievements across contexts, such as applying what was learnt in class to contexts outside the school. For this reason we believe that ultimately a variety of robot designs in autism therapy are useful. The behaviour and appearance of each robot could be tailored toward the particular developmental stage, learning needs, and individual interests of a child. Robots that can 'change shape,' i.e. that can be made more or less machine-like, or anthropo-/zoomorphic could be interesting to study.

By using Robota, a humanoid robot that can engage children in synchronous and imitative interaction games, we hope to develop interaction skills in children with autism, skills that might help them to cope better with daily-life human-human interaction. With Robota we can systematically investigate specific design and behaviour parameters and study how they influence imitative interaction dynamics. Using an enhanced version of Robota with autistic children could address novel research questions that have not been addressed in the above mentioned previous works with robots in autism therapy. Firstly, by varying the shape of the robot from machine-like to doll/human-like one can study the role of human-like features in the social responsiveness of autistic children. In this way, the humanoid robot can be used as a tool to systematically assess the response of autistic children to some basic human features (e.g. directionality of gaze, face expressiveness) and basic social interaction behaviour. Secondly, we could study the effect of repeated and regular interaction between the child and the robot with the robot in the role of a robot 'robotic therapy aid'. Such long-term studies are vital for demonstrating any therapeutic effect or impact the robot might have on the children. Thirdly, with Robota one can study imitation and mirroring behaviour in autistic children. Imitation and mirroring play already an important role in many existing therapies for autistic children. Such behaviours could be studied systematically, intended to guide the child through increasingly complex interaction dynamics. Usually, mirroring/imitation methods are highly time- and labour-consuming and require the teacher to undergo specific training. A robotic therapy aid could provide an economical means that takes some of the strains off teachers and/or parents.

Different from existing projects that use non-humanoid robots for autism therapy, the discussed work investigates a complementary area in the interaction design space, exploring the emergence of imitative interaction dynamics and turn-taking in robot-human interaction, based on research into the social role of imitation. Group scenarios with two children simultaneously playing with the robot, similar to studies we conducted with a mobile robot (Werry *et al.*, 2001c), are also hoped to facilitate social learning and generalisations across contexts.

18.5 Preliminary Trials

The Robota dolls were developed by Aude Billard, originally for different projects (robotics and entertainment applications). In November 2001 a basic version of Robota was available for a few days. Robota was tested with eight autistic children at Radlett Lodge School and six children at Colnbrook School (three of six children played with the robot on two consecutive days). Trials were videotaped. The video data is currently being analysed, detailed results will be published in forthcoming publications. The version of Robota that was used had the following behaviour repertoire: (a) it could 'dance' to one of two pre-recorded songs ('Dancing queen' and 'Rock around the clock'); (b) a camera detected vertical arm movements of the child, Robota responded by lifting the right, left or both arms; and (c) when the child moved the limbs and the head of Robota then the robot could learn and replay the movement sequence. In order to recognise vertical arm movements reliably, the child was required to sit in front of the camera (positioned next to Robota), and s/he had to sit relatively still. Figure 18.3 shows the basic set up. A teacher (background) is sitting next to the child and encourages him to play with Robota. A typical example of such interactions (between a child, his teacher, and Robota) can be described as follows:

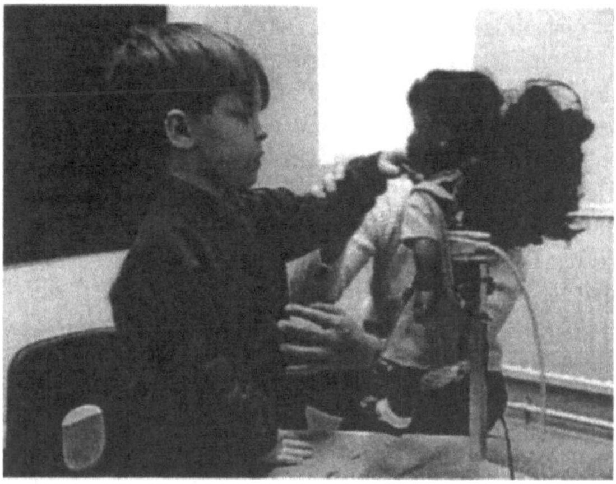

Figure 18.3. A six-year old boy with autism playing with Robota. In this context, he seemed curious about Robota's head movements and so he touches the doll.

- Child and teacher enter the room. Robota is located on a table, an experimenter sitting next to it. Teacher and child sit down on chairs at the table. The teacher 'introduces' the child to the robot, e.g. "Look, this is Robota, you can play with her."
- The teacher demonstrates what the robot can do. For example, the teacher lifts her right arm and tries to encourage the child to do as she did. Robota responds by imitating the arm movements.
- The teacher verbally and with gestures points out the correspondence between Robota's and the child's movements: "Look, Robota imitates you." The teacher then repeats this game using the left arm or raising both arms. The teacher can also initiate a different game where the child moves Robota's arms and head, and where Robota learns this sequence and can replay it (music is used for some children who enjoy music).

Generally, and very different from previous trials in the Aurora project with a mobile robot, the children's behaviour in these trials was very much teacher-directed and teacher initiated. Since the videotapes are currently being analysed, it is at this stage very difficult to draw any general conclusions. We clearly observed many instances in which the children played imitation games with the robot, seemingly enjoying it: we observed clear signs of enjoyment such as smiling, or a boy kissing Robota goodbye before he left the room. Given that children with autism often show less imitative skills than typically developing children, we believe that this is a promising research direction, in addition to using other mobile autonomous robots used in the Aurora project.

18.6 Conclusions

In previous work we studied how a mobile robot can engage children with autism in interaction games. The humanoid robot Robota extends this work by opening up a new and larger range of possible interactions and interaction modalities (involving movements, sounds, remembering and imitating sequences of actions etc.) The games with Robota allow exploring specific therapeutic issues that are relevant to autism therapy. [2] In the long run, this study could contribute to the development of robotic tools in autism therapy, by exploring the space of possibilities offered by different robotic designs (humanoid versus non-humanoid). To this end, the latest development of Artificial Intelligence/Robotics techniques (cf. Billard, 2000; Billard and Dautenhahn, 1998) can be applied for creating games that involve cognitive challenges as well as challenges in motor co-ordination.

In future work with Robota it will be particularly interesting to see how the robot can be used in more 'free-form' play scenarios, without requiring extensive teacher intervention. Note, that sometimes the teacher had to intervene because the child was about to break the robot (e.g. forcefully pulling its arms). We are therefore currently seeking funding in order to develop an enhanced version of Robota that is (a) more robust; (b) more specifically adapted to the needs and abilities of autistic children; and (c) has additional features such as moving eyes. At present only a basic version of robot is available for occasional testing.

The enhanced version of Robota would allow us to study systematically and in-depth the issues that are addressed in this chapter. Most importantly, resources are needed for conducting *long-term studies* where the children are regularly and over an extended timeframe exposed to the robot. Such studies are vital in order to assess the value of the robot in autism therapy. Observing positive interactions of the children with the robot in individual trials is certainly encouraging and informative with respect to the set up of the trials and general issues of robot design and control. However, our long-term goal is to help children with autism and make a contribution to autism therapy, we therefore need to be able to demonstrate therapeutic effects. The second important role of long-term studies is that the robot can be given *adaptive* abilities so that it can change its behaviour depending on the interaction histories with individual children.

[2] We like to thank the teaching staff, parents, and children at Radlett Lodge School and Colnbrook School who participated in the trials. The robot used in the trials reported here was created under the sponsorship of the French National Science Museum, "La cite des Sciences et de l'Industrie," and DIDEL SA (CH). Aude Billard is supported by a personal fellowship from the Swiss National Science Foundation. We would like to thank Stuart Powell, Tim Luckett, Penny Stribling, Paul Dickerson and Tamie Salter for helpful comments on the project.

18.7 References

Aurora (2002) Available at: http://www.aurora-project.com/

Arbib M (2002) The mirror system, imitation, and the evolution of language. In: Dautenhahn K, Nehaniv CL (eds.) Imitation in Animals and Artifacts. MIT Press, in press

Baron-Cohen S (1995) Mindblindness. A Bradford Book, The MIT Press

Billard A (1999) DRAMA, a connectionist architecture for on-line learning and control of autonomous robots: Experiments on learning of a synthetic proto-language with a doll robot. Industrial Robot Journal 26(1): 59-66

Billard A (2000) Play, dreams and imitation in Robota. In: Proceedings Socially Intelligent Agents - the Human in the Loop, Tech. Report FS-00-04, AAAI Press, pp 9-12

Billard A (2002) Imitation: a means to enhance learning of a synthetic proto-language in an autonomous robot. In: Dautenhahn K, Nehaniv CL (eds.) Imitation in Animals and Artifacts. MIT Press, in press

Billard A, Dautenhahn K (1998) Grounding communication in autonomous robots: an experimental study. In: Recce M, Nehmzow U (eds.) Robotics and Autonomous Systems, special Issue on Scientific methods in mobile robotics 24(1-2): 71-81

Billard A, Dautenhahn K, Hayes G (1998) Experiments on human-robot communication with Robota, an imitative learning and communication doll robot. In: Proceedings of Workshop Socially Situated Intelligence, Zurich, Switzerland

Blocher KH (1999) Affective Social Quest (ASQ) Teaching emotion recognition with interactive media and wireless expressive toys. MSc Thesis, MIT

Bullowa M (ed.) (1979) Before Speech. Cambridge University Press

Charman T, Baron-Cohen S (1994) Another look at imitation in autism. Development and Psychopathology 1: 1-4

Colby KM, Smith DC (1971) Computers in the Treatment of Nonspeaking Autistic Children. Current Psychiatric Therapies 11: 1-17

Dautenhahn K, Werry I, Rae J, Dickerson P, Stribling P, Ogden B (to appear) Robotic Playmates - Analysing interactive competencies of children with autism playing with a mobile robot. In: Dautenhahn K, Bond A, Cañamero L, Edmonds B (eds.) Socially Intelligent Agents - Creating relationships with computers and robots. Kluwer Academic Publishers

Dautenhahn K (1994) Trying to Imitate - a step towards releasing robots from social isolation. In: Gaussier P, Nicoud J-D (eds.) In: Proceedings of From Perception to Actions Conference, IEEE Computer Society Press, pp 290-301

Dautenhahn K (1999) Robots as Social Actors: AURORA and The Case of Autism. In: Proceedings of the 3rd International Cognitive Technology Conference, pp 359-374

Dautenhahn K, Werry I (2000) Issues of Robot-Human Interaction Dynamics in the Rehabilitation of Children with Autism. In: Proceedings From Animals To Animats 6, Paris, France, MIT Press, pp 519-528

Dautenhahn K, Werry I (2001) The Aurora Project: Using Mobile Robots in Autism Therapy. Learning Technology online newsletter, publication of IEEE Computer Society Learning Technology Task Force, vol. 3(1)

Druin A, Hendler J (eds.) (2000) Robots for Kids: Exploring New Technologies for Learning. Morgan Kaufmann Publishers

Ferrara C, Hill SD (1980) The responsiveness of autistic children to the predictability of social and non-social toys. Journal of Autism and Developmental Disorders 10(1): 51-57

Grandin T (1995) Thinking in pictures. Doubleday Publisher

Howlin P, Baron-Cohen S, Hadwin J (1999) Teaching Children with autism to mind-read. John Wiley and Sons

Hall ET (1966) The Hidden Dimension: Man's Use of Space in Public and Private. The Bodley Head Ltd, London, UK
Kozima H, Yano H (2001) Designing a robot for contingency-detection game. Working Notes Workshop on Robotic and Virtual Interactive Systems in Autism Therapy. Hatfield, UK, University of Hertfordshire, Technical Report No 364
Nadel J, Butterworth G (eds.) Imitation in Infancy. Cambridge University Press
Jordan R (1999) Autistic Spectrum Disorders - An Introductory Handbook for Practitioners. David Fulton Publishers, London
Michaud F, Clavet A, Lachiver G, Lucas M (2000) Designing toy robots to help autistic children - An open design project for Electrical and Computer Engineering education. In: Proceedings of American Society for Engineering Education
Nadel J, Guerini C, Peze A, Rivet C (1999) The evolving nature of imitation as a format of communication. In: Nadel J, Butterworth G (eds.) Imitation in Infancy, Cambridge University Press, pp 209-234
Papert S (1980) Mindstorms: Children, Computers, and Powerful Ideas. Basic Books.
Piaget J (1962) Play, dreams and imitation in childhood. Norton, NewYork
Plaisant C, Druin A, Lathan C, Dakhane K, Edwards K, Vice JM, Montemayor J (2000) A Storytelling Robot for Pediatric Rehabilitation. In: Proceedings of ASSETS, ACM, New York
Powell S (1996) The use of computers in teaching people with autism. In: Autism on the agenda: papers from a National Autistic Society Conference. London
Rogers SJ, Pennington BF (1991) A theoretical approach to the deficits in infantile autism. Development and Psychopathology 3: 137-162
Strickland D (1996) A virtual reality application with autistic children. Presence: Teleoperators and Virtual Environments 5(3): 319-329
Tardiff C, Plumet M-H, Beaudichon J, Waller D, Bouvard M, Leboyer M (1995) Micro-Analysis of Social Interactions Between Autistic Children and Normal Adults in Semi-Structured Play Situations. International Journal of Behavioural Development 18(4): 727-747
Watson LR, Lord C, Schaffer B, Schopler E (1989). Teaching spontaneous communication to autistic and developmentally handicapped children. Irvington Publishers, New York
Weir S, Emanuel R (1976) Using Logo to catalyse communication in an autistic child. DAI Research Report No. 15, University of Edinburgh
Werry I, Dautenhahn K, Harwin W (2001a) Investigating a Robot as a Therapy Partner for Children with Autism. In: Proceedings of 6th European Conference for the Advancement of Assistive Technology, Ljubljana, Slovenia
Werry I, Dautenhahn K, Harwin W (2001b) Evaluating the response of children with autism to a robot. In: Proceedings of Rehabilitation Engineering and Assistive Technology Society of North America, Reno, Nevada, USA
Werry I, Dautenhahn K, Ogden B, Harwin W (2001c) Can Social Interaction Skills Be Taught by a Social Agent? The Role of a Robotic Mediator in Autism Therapy. In: Beynon M, Nehaniv CL, Dautenhahn K (eds.) Proceedings of Cognitive Technology: Instruments of Mind, Springer Verlag, pp 57-74
Williams JHG, Whiten A, Suddendorf T, Perrett DI (2001) Imitation, mirror neurons and autism. Neuroscience and Biobehavioral Reviews 25(4): 287-295

Part III

Assistive Technology and Rehabilitation Robotics

Chapter 19

Progress of a Modular Prosthetic Arm

A.S. Poulton, P.J. Kyberd and D. Gow

19.1 Upper Limb Prostheses - Design Restraints

Active prosthetic devices to replace missing hands or arms have much in common with robotic dextrous manipulators for industrial tasks (Gruver, 1994). However, the design of an upper limb prosthesis presents a set of restraints which may differ considerably from those in other robotics applications. A mass-produced robot of standardised design may be usable in many different situations, while the needs of prosthetics users are highly individual. The degree of loss can vary from a partial hand up to a complete arm including the shoulder. Variants are needed to cater for different sizes and for the two sides. User surveys (Kyberd *et al.*, 1998a; Kyberd *et al.*, 1999) have confirmed that a prosthesis should be light, reliable, functional, look natural, and be quiet in operation. This contrasts with the requirements of industrial robots where weight, appearance and noise level may be less important than repeatability. If the prosthesis does not make life any easier for the user, it is likely to be rejected. A functional prosthesis must, then, offer real advantages over a purely cosmetic one for it to be accepted. Indeed, the majority of users have one good hand, and become quite adept at performing tasks one-handedly, with little involvement of the prosthetic hand.

In engineering terms, prostheses have developed considerably in recent years. The motors and gearboxes used can be small and unobtrusive, and the batteries can be small, with the energy density increasing with each new development. Modern materials such as carbon fibre are used for strength and lightness. Cosmesis has improved, with realistic looking silicone gloves. However the major problem remains one of control. Powered prostheses are commonly controlled using electromyographic (EMG) signals, which are generated when muscles contract. It is often difficult to find a control strategy that works effectively, as the number of degrees of freedom to be controlled may be greater than the number of independent signals that the user can easily generate.

The introduction of microprocessors to prosthetic applications has greatly increased their potential and simplicity in fitting and maintenance (Poulton *et al.*,

2000). Prosthetic controllers which can be adapted to different needs through field programming have been introduced by a number of manufacturers. They allow the prosthetist to try different control strategies or even invent completely new ones, using graphical software programming tools (Kurtz *et al.*, 1999; Wallace and Williams 1999; Farnsworth and Stevens, 1999; Hanson and Farnsworth, 2001). However the current microprocessor solutions are added to existing prostheses, there are no systems based approaches and so the manufacturers have created a mixture of different technologies with little inter-joint or device compatibility. The ToMPAW solution presented here attempts to address this problem.

19.2 The Control Problem

Good dexterity requires individually movable digits rather than a simple open/close grip; and depending on the degree of loss, there may be wrist and elbow movement as well. Typically, everything has to be controlled through the employment of two muscle sites in the residual limb, which generate EMG signals or possibly actuate some other type of sensor or switch. This normally requires a period of training. It can be difficult to easily control two separable signals, and for these cases the users are limited to very basic control strategies. Additionally the EMG signals may not be very stable, as they can change as the user and prosthesis moves around or they sweat within the confining socket.

There are two main lines of attack to this problem. One is to get more information out of the EMG signals that the user generates. Multiple electrodes can be used, with the user maybe not able to control them individually, but able to generate a pattern of activity that can be detected by techniques such as neural networks. This was the basis of the Swedish SVEN hand (Herberts, 1978; Almstrom, 1981). At that time the computing power needed could not be built into a practical prosthesis, but recently several researchers have revived the idea, now that the technology is becoming possible (Hudgins, 1993; Fermo *et al.*, 2000). Also, the raw EMG signals have been studied to see whether any improvement can be made over the standard technique of amplification, rectification and filtering to give a high level voltage signal that can be used for control purposes. Methods that have been studied include neural networks (e.g. Farry *et al.*, 1996; Asres *et al.*, 1996; Atsma *et al.*, 1996), wavelet-based classification (Englehart *et al.*, 2001), Hilbert transforms and fuzzy logic (Taffler, 1999a, b).

The second, complementary, line of attack has been to approach the control problem from the other end and build some intelligence into the hand itself. It is not easy for the user to judge the amount of force applied to an object purely by visual feedback, and this requires concentration. The amount of grip force applied may be controlled automatically, as in the commercially available Otto Bock SensorHand™. Slip detection can be done by measuring changes in forces (Kyberd 1990; Winkler *et al.*, 1992; Mingrino *et al.*, 1994), or by detecting an acoustic signal with a microphone (Salisbury and Coleman 1965; Chappell *et al.*, 1987).

The type of grip pattern adopted may also be determined automatically, as in the Southampton Hand (Nightingale 1985; Kyberd and Chappell, 1994), which provided two basic forms of grip: precision (pincer) grip and power (fist) grip. The concept was later developed at the Oxford Orthopaedic Engineering Centre in the successful clinical version, the Oxford Intelligent Hand (Kyberd *et al.*, 1998b). The type of grip adopted is determined by the point of first contact. If an object touches the palm first, a power grip is applied; while if the fingertips are touched first, a precision grip is used. The hand closes until the object is held in the lightest possible grip. If slipping occurs, this is detected by acoustic sensors in the fingertips and the grip is automatically tightened.

Current generations of clinical prostheses with microprocessor control have focused on the limited intelligence of detecting slip at a single point and controlling a single degree of freedom device, or in making the selection of simple control philosophies more easily available to the clinical teams (Kurtz *et al.*, 1999). Beyond the Southampton philosophy, the research arena has only recently begun to discuss adding intelligence to multi-degree of freedom prostheses (Shultz *et al.*, 2001).

19.3 The ToMPAW Project

ToMPAW (Totally Modular Prosthetic Arm with high Workability) is a project to design and manufacture a set of modular and flexible standardised hand and arm prostheses, with a very high functionality and cosmesis. The system will be applicable to losses from a complete hand through to the upper arm, and will enable the users and the clinical teams to customise the device to the user with the minimum of effort and time. ToMPAW is a European Union project under the Telematics initiative.

19.3.1 Main Features of the ToMPAW Arm

The ToMPAW hand has four independently controllable digits (the fifth finger follows the movements of the fourth finger). The wrist has two degrees of freedom, flexion/extension and rotation. As well as having low weight and power consumption, a primary design feature of ToMPAW was that it should be as modular as possible, both physically and in terms of the control strategies that are supported. Reliability and ease of maintenance are key issues, and modularity helps to simplify servicing and reduce stock-keeping. For example, the fingers can easily be replaced individually. The modular approach of the mechanical system is reflected in a similarly distributed approach in the controllers. While it would have been possible to use one relatively powerful microprocessor to do everything, this would have meant that conductors from all the sensors and actuators would have to run along the length of the arm. The cables and connectors that would be needed to carry all these signals would need to cross a number of active joints and this would be a significant weakness in a system where conductors are subjected to repeated movement. The preferred option was to use a network of microprocessors, each controlling one or two joints. Each processor is close to the sensors and actuators that interface with it. There are only six conductors in the bus which links the processors, and this makes for a more reliable system. The distributed system also has some in-built robustness, in that it allows a degree of graceful degradation, where if one processor fails the others can continue. The form of control that was adopted is mainly hierarchical. This has the advantage that decisions are taken closest to where they are actually needed, maximising processing speed and avoiding communications bottlenecks. The distributed approach extends the advantages of modularity to the electronics as well as the mechanics. Any degree of loss from a hand to a complete arm can be accommodated using a small standard set of components. Stock-keeping costs are kept to a minimum and modules can be easily replaced.

19.3.2 The LONWORKS® Protocol

Protocols for small scale networks supported by small low-power microprocessors were compared at the beginning of the design process. Echelon's LONWORKS® was adopted as it is a realisation of the full OSI seven-layer communications protocol model rather than a 'cut-down' system. It is supported by Neuron® microprocessor devices from Toshiba and Cypress. Each device has two processors which are microcoded to operate the bus protocol, and these are inaccessible to the applications engineer. A third processor controls the applications, running programs that are written in a Neuron® C, a variant of C that provides multitasking and supports the I/O features of the Neuron® device. Thus the programmer needs to be concerned only with those elements of the system that are important to the application; the details of the communications protocol are invisible. Neuron® devices are capable of driving short network links between themselves on twisted wire pairs with few passive components, simplifying the hardware.

The ToMPAW arm uses a LONWORKS® network to connect a number of Neuron® devices or "nodes". The node that handles top-level control is referred to as the proximal node, as in most cases it will be physically the most proximal (nearest the shoulder) node in the system. The other nodes are referred to as distal nodes. The data on the network is represented by standard network variable types. This data may be categorised as:

- outputs from distal nodes to the proximal node giving current actual positions, forces, and the state of any digital inputs - this data is supplied when requested by the proximal node;
- inputs to the distal nodes from the proximal node for variable data such as demanded positions or forces;
- digital control inputs to the distal nodes from the proximal node - these determine the control strategy to be adopted by the distal node.

The proximal node controller software takes user input, e.g. switch/EMG, and distributes the input over the network, possibly scaling it first to fit it to a standard range. The other nodes control the motors. One node can control one or two motors, so two nodes are needed for the four controllable digits of the hand. This requires positional feedback in each joint. The position of the joint is sensed by a high endurance potentiometer. The nodes in the hand take inputs from force and slip sensors. Force at the fingertips is detected by force sensing resistors, while slip is detected acoustically. Control strategies for each motor include: direct control of motor speed and direction by input variables from the network; proportional control to drive the motor to a desired angle; and control mediated by slip sensors, so that motor drive is incrementally increased in the event of slippage.

These are all tasks that can be scheduled for execution on a distal node without requiring much intervention from the proximal controller, apart from initiating the tasks and monitoring status. Traffic on the network is minimised by designing the system in this way, so that the network normally only needs to handle signals for high-level control. It does not need to transmit fast real-time signals related to EMG, motor control or slip detection.

19.3.3 External Communication

The arm also needs to communicate with external systems. It needs to be able to be driven by the production staff during the initial build and later testing and repair of the system, by the prosthetist during customisation and the control/joint selection process, by the therapist for training, and possibly by the wearer for remote testing and diagnostics. This is done by linking the arm to a clinical support system which runs on a PC. The clinical support system displays the EMG data graphically in real time, and allows parameters such as operating thresholds to be varied. Transceivers for connecting a LONWORKS® bus to a PC are readily available, allowing fast traffic and providing isolation to certified standards. LONWORKS® can also be interfaced to TCP/IP, raising the possibility of remote diagnostics across the Internet. A radio link is another useful option, as the user is not then restricted by cables during set-up and testing. This can be done with standard low-power transmitters and receivers which handle RS-232 serial data (Kyberd *et al.*, 2002). The conversion to this format is done by a Neuron® node. It may be that more advanced technologies such as Bluetooth™ will be used in future.

19.3.4 Practical Implementation

The nodes were designed to make the best use of the functions provided by the Neuron® devices and at the same time meet the wider requirements of the project. The division of functions between three independent processors makes the device ideal for real-time applications of this nature. The I/O subsystem is also designed to be fairly independent of the application processor; it can generate PWM signals for driving motors, and supports an I^2C serial bus for peripherals such as analogue to digital converters (ADCs). From an analysis of the signals used in the system, it was concluded that two basic types of Neuron® node would be needed, one for motor control (with two motor drivers, and analogue and digital inputs), and another with a fast parallel ADC for multiple EMG signals.

In the final design the controller functions were allocated to physical boards to minimise the number of boards and interconnections required. Four-layer printed circuit boards using surface-mount components were produced. A hand board controls a complete hand with four active digits. It contains two motor control nodes, together with the interface electronics for force and slip sensing. A distal board drives two motors in the wrist, and a similar board drives the motor in the elbow joint. Because of the higher current demands of the motors used in these joints compared to those in the fingers, drivers with a higher current rating (3A rather than 1A) are fitted on these boards. A master or proximal board accepts up to eight fast analogue inputs and can be used for overall control of a system. However, the hand board can also accept two EMG inputs, so a hand prosthesis will not normally require a master board in addition. This allocation of nodes to physical functions means that the same node handles the motor and sensors associated with each joint, minimising the network traffic between nodes .

The arm can be powered by lithium polymer batteries, which are light in weight, safe, and have a high energy density. Power is conserved by putting the Neuron® microprocessors into low-power "sleep mode" when the arm is inactive. This is important as studies have shown that users need a prosthesis that runs all day without needing to change or recharge the batteries (Kyberd *et al.*, 1998a).

19.4 Practical Application

The electronic subsystems of the arm were tested prior to integration with the final mechanical hardware, using a development system which consisted of the existing mechanical assemblies of the Oxford Hand and the Edinburgh Arm (Gow, 2001), suitably modified. The modularity of the electronics and control allowed the different systems to be integrated easily. Two users operated the hand alone and two further users employed arm systems composed of hand, wrist and elbow. The control of the arms was very different with one user employing ON-OFF operation with an EMG amplifier and the second employing proportional control. Both used a pull switch to switch between the different axes. Training progressed over several visits, and the adaptability of the system allowed different strategies to be tested in an effort to find the best one for the particular user. The second user could produce myoelectric signals from two muscle sites, but he could not fully separate the two channels and there was some co-contraction. In this case, a "winner-takes-all" strategy was created so that the signal that was smaller in magnitude was ignored, and the larger magnitude signal was used for control. This continued until muscles relaxed and both signals fell below pre-set thresholds.

Assessment of the device is based on a range of criteria. The users informal comments are of use in determining their general satisfaction, also directed questions based on the findings of surveys made prior to the design phase (Kyberd *et al.*, 1999) enable more precise evaluations to be made. Finally, the functional assessment will be made using a hand function assessment protocol that is based on both abstract object handling as well as simulated activities of daily living (Light *et al.*, 1999).

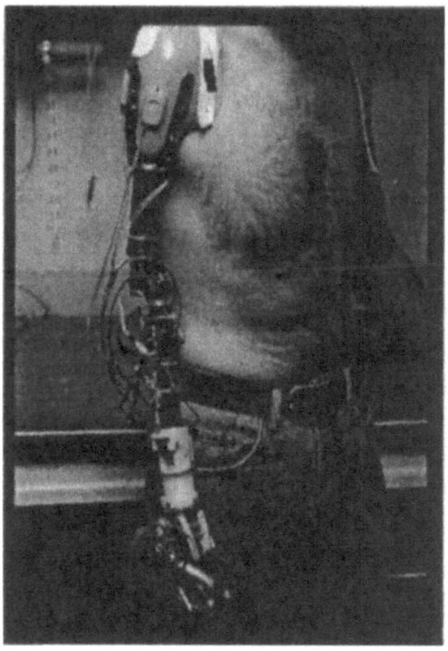

Figure 19.1. Hybrid Edinburgh/Oxford Arm using ToMPAW electronics and control software

19.5 References

Almstrom C, Herberts P, Korner L (1981) Experience with Swedish multifunctional prosthetic hands controlled by pattern recognition of multiple myoelectric signals. International Orthopaedics 5(1): 15-21

Asres A, Dou H, Zhou Z, Zhang Y, Zhu S (1996) A combination of AR and neural network technique for EMG pattern identification. In: Proceedings of 18th Annual International Conference of the IEEE Engineering in Medicine and Biology Society, pp 1464-1465

Atsma W, Hudgins B, Lovely D (1996) Classification of raw myoelectric signals using finite impulse response neural networks. In: Proceedings of 18th Annual International Conference of the IEEE Engineering in Medicine and Biology Society, pp 1474-1475

Chappell PH, Nightingale JM, Kyberd PJ ,Barkhordar M (1987) Control of a single degree of freedom artificial hand. Journal of Biomedical Engineering 9: 273-277

Englehart K, Hudgins B, Parker P (2001) A wavelet-based continuous classification scheme for multifunction myoelectric control. IEEE Transactions on Biomedical Engineering 48(3): 302-311

Farnsworth T, Stevens G (1999) Clinical experience with programmable controllers. In: Proceedings of MEC '99 Myoelectric Controls Symposium, Fredericton, Canada

Farry K, Walker I, Baranuik R (1996) Myoelectric teleoperation of a complex robotic hand. IEEE Transactions on Robotics and Automation 12(5): 775-788

Fermo C, De Vincenzo C, Bastos-Filho T, Dynnikov V (2000) Development of an adaptative framework for the control of upper limb myoelectric prosthesis. In: Proceedings of the 22nd Annual EMBS International Conference, Chicago, pp 2402-2405

Gow D, Douglas W, Geggie C, Monteith E and Stewart D (2001) The development of the Edinburgh modular arm system. In: Proceedings of the Institute of Mechanical Engineers 21(H): 291-298

Gruver W (1994) Intelligent robotics in manufacturing, service and rehabilitation: an overview. IEEE Transactions on Industrial Electronics 41(1): 4-11

Hanson W, Farnsworth T (2001) New digital control technology for powered prosthetic elbows. In: Proceedings of 10th World Congress, International Society for Prosthetics and Orthotics

Herberts P, Almstrom C, Caine K (1978) Clinical application study of multifunctional prosthetic hands. The Journal of Bone and Joint Surgery 60-B(4): 552-560

Hudgins B, Parker P, Scott R (1993) A new strategy for multifunction myo-electric control, IEEE Transactions on Biomedical Engineering 4(1):82-94.

Kyberd PJ, (1990) Algorithmic control of a multifunction hand prosthesis. PhD thesis, University of Southampton

Kyberd PJ, Chappell P (1994) The Southampton hand: an intelligent myoelectric prosthesis. Journal of Rehabilitation Research and Development 31(4): 326-334

Kyberd PJ, Beard DJ, Davey JJ, Morrison DJ (1998a) A survey of upper limb prostheses users in Oxfordshire. Journal of Prosthetics and Orthotics, 10(4): 85-91

Kyberd PJ, Evans M, Winkel S (1998b) An intelligent anthropomorphic hand, with automatic grasp. Robotica 16: 531-536

Kyberd PJ, Gow D, Scott H, Griffiths M, Sperling L, Sandsjo L, Almstrom C, Wartenberg C, Jonsson S (1999) A comparison of upper limb prostheses users in Europe. In: Proceedings of MEC'99 Myoelectric Controls Symposium, Fredericton, Canada

Kyberd PJ, Winkel S, Poulton A (2002) A wireless telemetry system for user training of artificial arms. Prosthetics and Orthotics International

Kurtz I, Heim W, Bauer-Hume H, Hubbard S, Ramdial S (1999) Programmable control: clinical experience at Bloorview Macmillan Centre. MEC'99 Myoelectric Controls Symposium, Fredericton, Canada

Light CM, Chappell PH and Kyberd PJ (1999) Quantifying impaired hand function in the clinical environment. In: Proceedings of MEC'99 Symposium Upper limb prosthetic research and consumer needs, Fredericton, Canada

Mingrino A, Bucci A, Magni R, Dario P (1994) Slippage control in hand prostheses by sensing grasping forces and sliding motion. In: Proceedings of the IEEE/RSJ/GI International Conference on Intelligent Robots and Systems, vol. 3, pp 1803-1809

Nightingale JM (1985) Microprocessor control of an artificial arm. Journal of Microcomputer Applications. 8: 167-173

Poulton A, Boman A, Gow D, Stodne F, Sandsjo, L, Kyberd, P (2000). Use of microprocessor technology in upper limb prostheses. In: Proceedings of 2nd International Conference on Advances in Osseointegration, Surrey

Salisbury LL, Coleman AB (1967) A mechanical hand with automatic proportional control of prehension. Medical Biological and Engineering 5: 505-511

Shultz S, Pylatiuk C, Bretthauer G (2001) A lightweight bionic hand prosthesis. In Proceedings of the 10th World Congress of the International Society of Prosthetics and Orthotics

Taffler S, Kyberd PJ (1999a) The use of the Hilbert transform in EMG analysis. In: Proceedings of MEC'99 Symposium Upper limb prosthetic research and consumer needs, Narrowing the Gap, Fredericton, Canada

Taffler S, Kyberd PJ (1999b) The use of fuzzy logic in the processing of myoelectric signals. In: Proceedings of MEC'99 Symposium Upper limb prosthetic research and consumer needs Fredericton, Canada

Wallace C, Williams TW (1999) New clinically-useful control strategies made possible by the Varigrip II^{TM} multi-device controller. In: Proceedings of MEC '99 Myoelectric Controls Symposium, Fredericton, Canada

Winkler W and Berwirth W (1992) The use of a gliding detector for the control of Prostheses-Hand. In: Proceedings of the 7th World Congress of the International Society of Prosthetics and Orthotics, p 188

Chapter 20

Development of a Novel Type Rehabilitation Robotic System KARES II

Z. Bien, D-J. Kim, D.H. Stefanov, J-S. Han, H-S. Park and P-H. Chang

20.1 Introduction

The future welfare model should meet the needs of the enlarged number of aged and disabled people. Present technology levels increase optimism that the quality of life of the people from these categories can be significantly improved through home-installed mechatronic service devices that provide 24-hour assistance to their everyday movement activities. The design of high effective devices can contribute to the finding of satisfying solutions to this important social and economic problem. The modern research strategies are focused on the development of healthcare systems that fit to real users' needs and preferences.

Research on movement assistance devices is focused on user-friendly interaction and easy adaptation to the home environment. The design concepts follow approaches requiring minimal user participation. To fulfil these requirements, the control algorithms should be based on a small number of commands, relevant to the specifics of the user's motions. The machines should refer not only to the exact user commands but also to user intentions with a high level of "fussiness," treating and executing them correctly. The performance of the assistive device should be harmless for the user and nearby people and devices.

The effectiveness of assistive systems is strongly dependent on the manner of their user interaction. Various input systems, such as a sip-puff switch (Schmeisser *et al.*, 1979), chin controller (Schmeisser *et al.*, 1979), head controller (Coyle *et al.*, 1995), and voice commanders (Rockland *et al.*, 1998) have been developed and applied to different kinds of movement disability. For high-level movement paralysis (e.g. spinal cord injury) only a few pre-defined user's motions can be applied to the command process. Novel interface techniques based on face-feature extraction (Shirai *et al.*, 1994), remote tracking of head motion (Shirai *et al.*, 1998), and user-independent voice recognition in noisy environments (Kasabov *et al.*, 1997) seem to be promising alternatives for people with severe motion restrictions.

When user movements are highly restricted, considerable levels of movement freedom can only be achieved by the use of a set of assistive devices that act in co-operation with each other. Recent concepts for home automation and movement assistance for motion-impaired people are based on home installed rehabilitation robots, intelligent powered wheelchairs, and control devices for the home environment (lights, TV, telephone, doors, home security, etc.). The robotic system is designed to assist disabled individuals in their everyday needs, such as eating, drinking and using simple objects. (Harwin *et al.*, 1995; Van der Loos *et al.*, 1995).

Different robot-user arrangements have been proposed. In simple solutions, the robot is fixed to a desk or to the floor. Using external help, the operator is placed in a suitable position near the worktable and operates the robot, performing pick-and-place ADL tasks unaided (Stefanov, 1995). Independence increases significantly if the user can move freely to different home positions and perform manipulative tasks there with the help of the robot. Wheelchair-mounted robots (Kwee, 1997) can be used both for indoor and outdoor assistance of the user. Drawbacks of such solutions are the inclination of the wheelchair due to the weight of the robot, enlargement of the wheelchair width (which is critical for narrow door passage), and the changes of the dynamic characteristics of the wheelchair. Another solution of indoor robotic system considers desktop-mounted robots and a special wheelchair navigation scheme that can steer the wheelchair automatically to a pre-defined position (Stefanov, 1999). Sitting in the powered wheelchair, the user can access different places within the house and can perform different movement tasks with the robot, controlling it through the same wheelchair interface.

The cognitive load on the user can be decreased significantly if the robot automatically performs repeatable movements (so-called pre-programmed mode of control). Programs can be successfully executed if the robot, the user and the manipulated objects have the same initial position every time when the real task is being performed. For a wheelchair-mounted manipulator the mutual position between the user and the manipulator remains the same, but the position between the manipulator and the object is dependent on the wheelchair position. When the robot is fixed to the desk, the initial position between the manipulator and the object remains the same, but the position of the user is determined by the position of the chair. It can be seen that all variants need accurate wheelchair positioning. Achieving the exact location could be very onerous for the user. It is time consuming, requiring many manoeuvres and considerable mental and physical effort. Such a problem can be solved by the implementation of intelligent automatic controllers with high-level AI that can modify the performed action according to the changes in the home environment and the user's health condition.

20.2 Preliminary Experience: KARES I

KARES I (KAIST Rehabilitation Engineering Service System) project (Bien *et al.*, 1999) developed a wheelchair-mounted manipulator in which a vision-based subsystem determines the mutual position between the gripper and the object, and helps for the navigation of the gripper toward the manipulative object. In case of pre-programmed operation, the vision subsystem is used for compensation of the errors in the wheelchair position and for successful realisation of pre-programmed tasks. The visual subsystem helps in the direct mode for elimination of errors, which are a result of tremor, low-vision, parallax, or non-experience of the user.

KARES can be controlled either the pre-programmed mode or the direct control mode. The vision-based controller is activated every time when the gripper is located in close proximity to the targeted object. A special system, named as "state machine." permanently monitors significant features from the visual scene and passes the control of the robotic arm to the visual-based controller, which performs then fine gripper positioning according to the real position of the object. A small camera (see Figure 20.1, position 1) is mounted on the robotic arm near the gripper. Colour markers are attached on all target objects (position 2), which helps for easy identification of the separate objects.

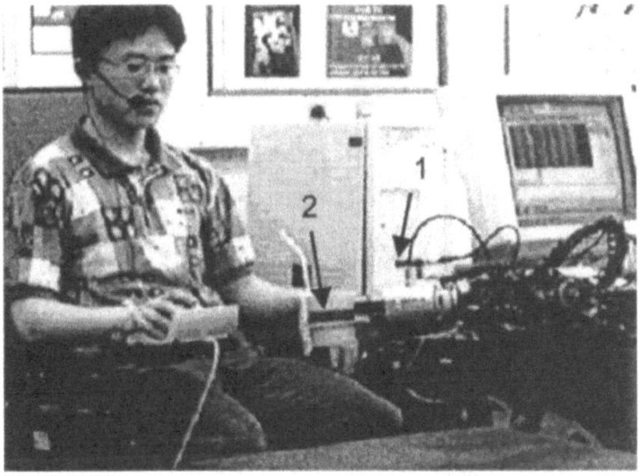

Figure 20.1. KARES I

KARES operates with pre-marked objects. In the TV image, generated by the signal of the TV camera, the sizes of the colour markers change according to the distance between the camera and the marked object. The distance between the camera and the object can be found from the image processing and the depth and orientation information can be obtained on the basis of changes of the size of colour markers. A fuzzy logic algorithm was applied to the image processing.

Based on the preliminary experience with KARES I, in 1999 we started development of the project KARES II. The new system consists of wheelchair, mobile robot and some novel systems for interface and control. Some of the basic ideas and characteristics of the new system will be commented below.

This chapter is organised in the following way: first, the configuration and characteristics of the new system are commented. Then, the control architecture and its I/O relations are described. Next, the wheelchair part and the mobile platform are briefly remarked. The comment on the used human-machine interface includes some basic information about the soft robotic arm, intelligent visual servoing system, eye-mouse, haptic suit and the bio-signal-based control interface.

20.3 KARES II

20.3.1 Configuration and Characteristics

In this chapter, we introduce our new wheelchair-based robotic arm system, KARES II, and its human-robot interaction technologies that assist independent life of the elderly and the disabled that have sensory and motor function impairments.

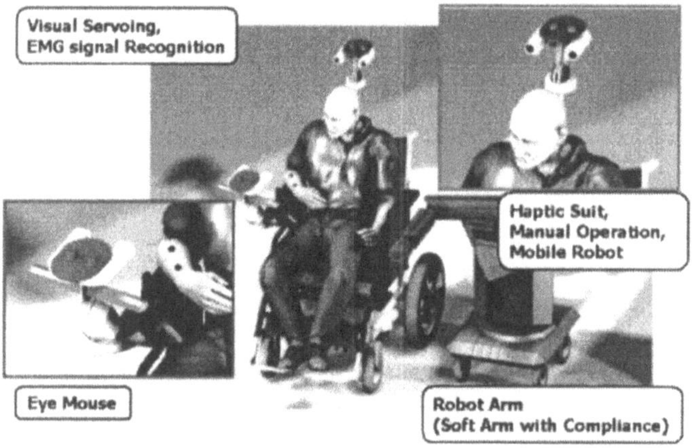

Figure 20.2. KARES II System

The wheelchair robot system consists of a powered wheelchair and a robotic arm (Figure 20.2). It has not only a mobility capability through the motorised wheelchair, but also a manipulatory function with the robotic arm. When a user and robot are in the same environment, safe and comfortable interaction with the robot is important. It is known that many difficulties exist in human-robot interactions with existing rehabilitation robots (e.g. Eftring *et al.*, 1999). For example, manual control of the robotic arm places a high cognitive load on the user, while physically disabled users may have difficulty operating joysticks dextrously or pushing buttons for delicate movements. Therefore, human-robot interaction is an essential technology to be developed for the robot system.

Two factors are essential in intelligent human-robot interaction technology; one is intention reading of the user, and the other is autonomous capability of the robot. Intention reading allows the user to command to the robot system in a human-friendly way possibly by using bio-signal, wearable haptic suit, voice/sound perception, or the "eye-mouse" device that utilises eye movements. Intention that is read can be used as a system state feedback for human-robot interaction. The autonomous capability in controlling the robot system is needed to realise the user's commands when the user has a limited physical ability. A typical example is visual servoing-based or compliance-based control of a robotic arm.

Our rehabilitation system consists of several subsystems such as the eye-mouse, the haptic suit, the EMG- (one of the bio-signals) recognition module, and the compliant robotic arm with visual servoing capability. Figure 20.3 shows the input/output relation of subsystems for human-robot interaction. For example, the task to serve a meal for a user is conducted as follows: the eye-mouse reads the user's intention, and transfers processed information, such as the position of a desired food, to the visual servoing module. Then, the visual servoing module controls the robotic arm to spoon up the food and moves it to the user's mouth. Consequently, the reading of the user's intentions and the autonomous capability of the robotic arm should well be co-ordinated to perform the task successfully.

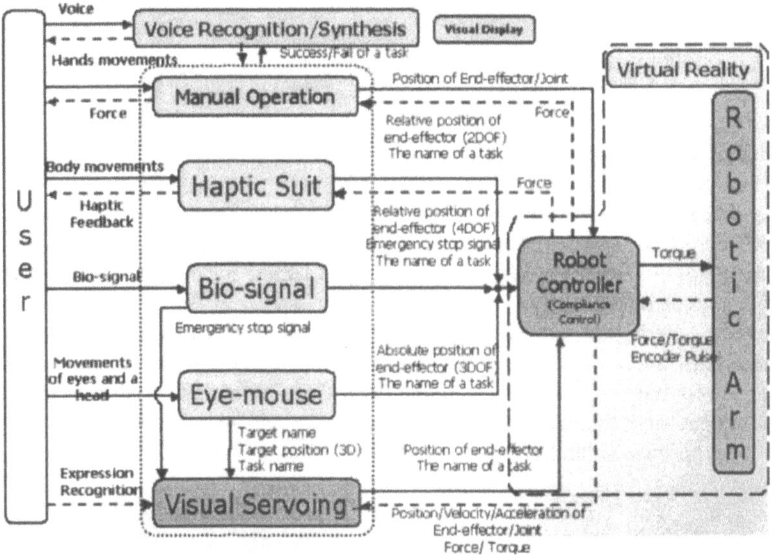

Figure 20.3. Input/output relation of subsystems for human-robot interaction

Figure 20.4 shows a conceptual view of KARES II system. KARES II consists of two subsystems such as a wheelchair part and a mobile platform. Each subsystem is connected by wireless communication device with TCP/IP protocol. Based on these separated structure, KARES II shows better performances than our previous rehabilitation robotic system, KARES I.

For example, using a mobile platform, KARES II is free from various vibration problems. Thus, KARES II can support not only the safety of the users, but also the that of the arm itself. And KARES II can freely locate its robotic base to anywhere. From this advantage, KARES II can serve more broad areas of the daily living activity which is not possible with KARES I. Due to separation of the robotic arm from the wheelchair, the user can move the wheelchair to more narrow area without considering the size and the shape of the robotic arm. Furthermore, the user can control the mobile platform as a remote controlled slave robotic system.

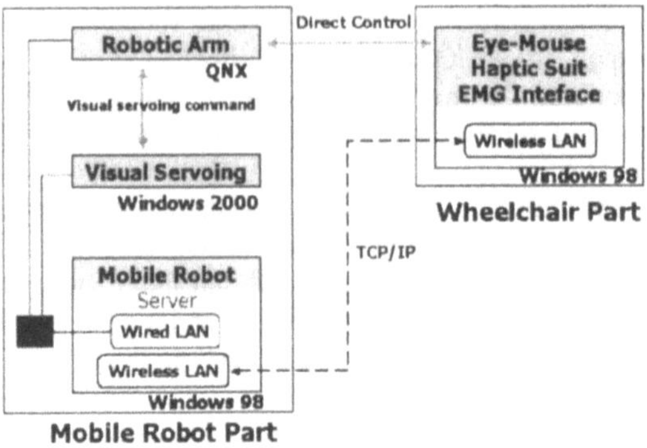

Figure 20.4. A conceptual view of KARES II system

20.3.2 Wheelchair Part

The wheelchair part contains a powered wheelchair with various human-robot interfaces such as eye-mouse, haptic suit, and bio-signal (EMG) based control system (Figure 20.5a). These interfaces are selected by the user with respect to his/her level of disability. For example, if the user can't move the body except above the neck, the eye-mouse system is the only one to control robotic arm, wheelchair, and so on. And in this part, there is a 3D position extraction system with stereo matching techniques. Its purpose are to extract 3D position data around the system and the user, to provide necessary visual information as a visual feedback to the user and the robotic arm during manipulation.

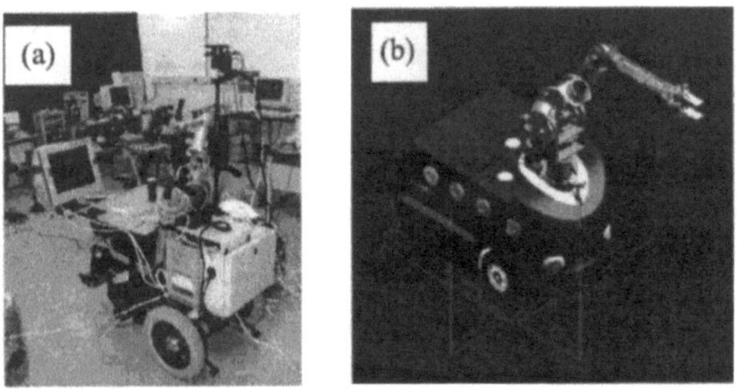

Figure 20.5. KARES II subsystems (a) Wheelchair part (b) Mobile platform.

20.3.3 Mobile Platform

The mobile platform can provide a manipulability with soft robotic arm and a mobility with its own wheel (Figure 20.5b). The user can manoeuvre the mobile platform with his/her own intention through wireless communication.

20.4 Intelligent Assistive Interfaces

20.4.1 Soft Robotic Arm

A robotic arm is developed for giving cares to daily life of the disabled. In our design, we adopt a target-oriented design (TOD) to reduce the cost and effort required for the iterative re-designing process. In TOD, the design targets should be clearly and carefully defined before all the other design activities since all subsequent procedures are aimed to accomplish the targets.

The design targets for the robotic arm are 13 predefined tasks obtained from the careful interview with the users and physicians (Chang *et al.*, 2001). After defining the tasks, they are analysed for clear representation of the target tasks. To make engineering representations of the tasks, each task is translated to task-space and task-trajectory. The task-space gives kinematic targets for a robot arm, and the task-trajectory gives dynamic targets. Each task is observed carefully to obtain realistic representations. Maximum payloads for each task are also determined based on the observations of the predefined tasks. The task-space is a set of via points through which the end-effector or the tool of the robot arm must pass. A via point has six elements, three displacements in directions x-y-z from the fixed base frame, and three angles for orientation of the tool. Of course, the base frames for the displacements and the orientation should be specified to represent such via points. After engineering definitions of the target tasks, we found an optimal kinematic structure for the robotic arm. For given the task-space, the kinematic structure is obtained by using an iterative converging algorithm which is used in finite element methods (Yang, 2000). After finding the optimal kinematics of the robotic arm, the dynamic simulation is performed to determine the maximum torque of each joint. Then, the size of actuators can be selected for detail design.

The robotic arm requires active compliance control, since the target tasks include contact with the users, such as wiping/scratching their faces. These tasks require torque sensing at each joint of the robotic arm resulting in high cost and complex design. To overcome this, we use a cable transmission mechanism that can achieve torque sensing without sensors since it has good back-drivability. The manufactured robotic arm (Figure 20.6) is verified by implementing some of the predefined tasks. Other tasks are going to be implemented and safety will be considered in the near future.

20.4.2 Visual Servoing

Visual servoing is introduced to control the pose of the end effector of a robotic arm relative to a target using visual feedback. A vision sensor allows the robot to obtain non-contact measurement of the environment. A vision system acts as eyes for a robotic arm that interacts with a target on the basis of visual information. Visual servoing in the wheelchair-based robotic arm usually presents many difficulties. For example, it is difficult to process visual information in real-time, to be robust for varying illumination, or to process data under vibration of the robotic arm. Among these difficulties, we primarily concentrate on an efficient image reduction of visual servoing in accordance with the task of the robotic arm.

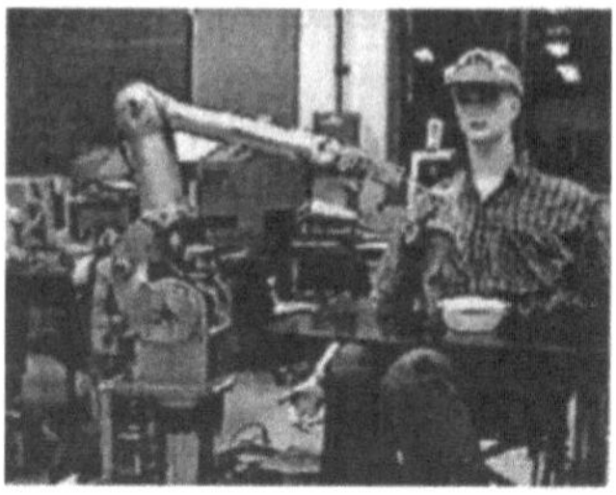

Figure 20.6. Robotic arm serving a meal

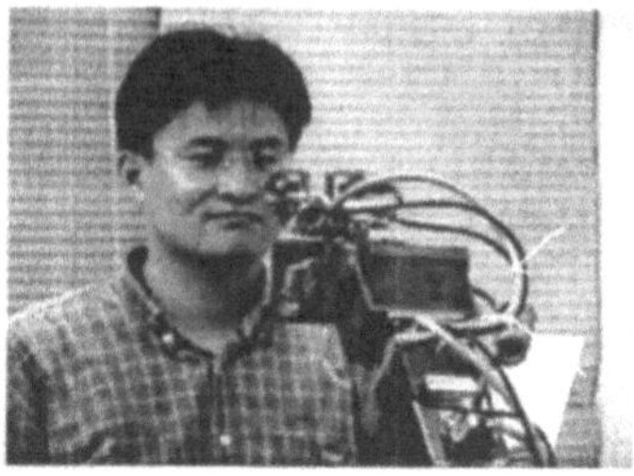

Figure 20.7. User face tracking

An eye-in-hand camera configuration is adopted in the wheelchair-based robotic arm system because it takes images from the standpoint of the robot (Bien *et al.*, 2000). A binocular camera head with vergence movements, which is an action of eye movements that control eye convergence (Capurro *et al.*, 1997), is used to extract the depth of a target. Representative subtasks of visual servoing are "grasping the cup on a table" and "bring the cup to the user's mouth." For this purpose, we have concentrated on three issues: biologically inspired vision techniques for effective visual processing, a small-sized stereo camera head for an eye-in-hand camera configuration, and an intention reading scheme through the shape of the user's mouth for the easiness-to-use and safety. Figure 20.7 shows an example of user's face tracking with our visual servoing system.

20.4.3 Eye-mouse

We have been developing the system that allows the disabled who cannot use their limbs for themselves to control a robot and an electrical wheelchair without using their limbs. It is very difficult or impossible to operate a robot and an electrical wheelchair for the people with the spinal cord injury. Using the Eye-mouse system that we develop, the user can move the mouse pointer that appears on the intersection between the eye-gaze direction and the computer monitor. The user transfer commands to the robot and the electrical wheelchair using this system. Using an iris boundary model, we propose the algorithm that overcomes the problems of the existing limbus tracking methods (Kim, 2000). One problem of the existing methods is that it is difficult to detect the vertical eye movement precisely because eyelids partially cover the limbus. The other is that they use infrared source to be robust to the change of illumination and so, it is expensive (Glenstrup *et al.*, 1995; Arrington *et al.*, 1997). For these reasons, we propose the image-based method that extracts the eye features in real time, tracks the feature points and calculates the eye gaze direction. Using the calculated eye gaze direction, we show that the proposed system is feasible as a new computer input system.

To know the eye-gaze direction including head motion, we must know the head and eye movement data. We designed an eye-gaze tracking system that is head mounted and is composed of two systems: a head and an eye movement tracking system. An eye-gaze tracking system outputs the eye-gaze direction of a user from head and eye movement data that are obtained from head and eye tracking systems respectively. Figure 20.8 shows the designed eye-gaze direction tracking system.

Experimental results showed that application of proposed system to human-computer interface is feasible with mean errors ±3.75mm on the PC monitor. Using this eye gaze-tracking system, the disabled can transfer the commands such as the type of task and the position of target object, to the robot and the wheelchair.

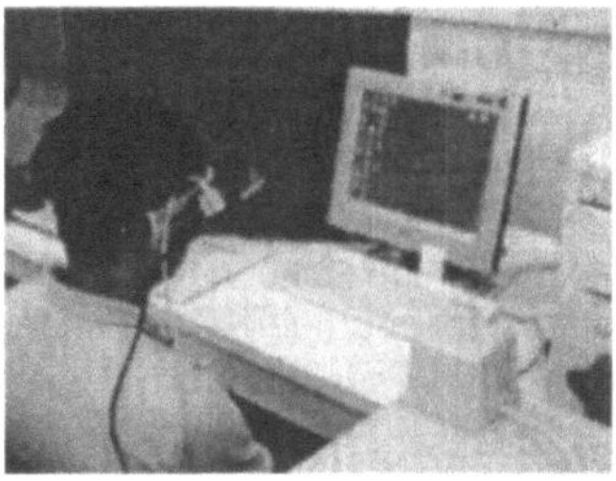

Figure 20.8. Eye-mouse system

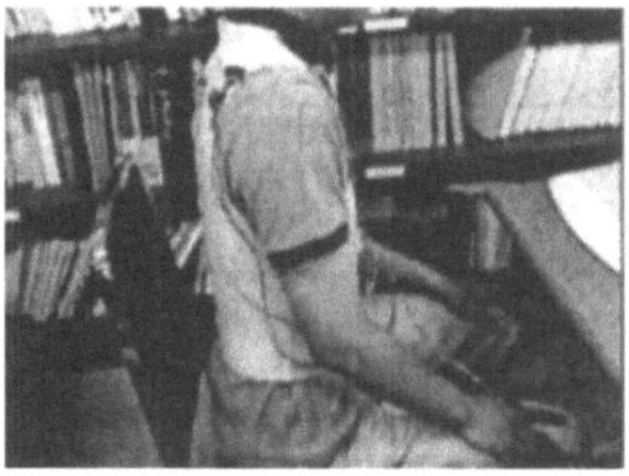

Figure 20.9. Wearable haptic suit

20.4.4 Haptic Suit

Several rehabilitation robot manipulators have been developed (e.g. Song *et al.*, 1998) for handicapped persons. Although the joystick is the most popular of master device for rehabilitation robotic systems, it is not appropriate for those who cannot move their arms. Therefore, it is necessary to develop a convenient and portable master device that can measure human body motion.

Optical fibre curvature sensors are used to measure human body motion and seem to be well-suited to measuring body motion of handicapped persons because of their flexibility, lightness, small size and low cost. Optical fibre curvature sensors are attached to an upper garment. Transmitted light power in the optical fibre decreases exponentially when the fibre is curved (Halley, 1993). Using several optical fibre curvature sensors, it is possible to measure two or more degrees-of-freedom of motion with a mean error ratio of 0.64% during circular movement. The sensors are attached to a tight upper garment, as shown in Figure 20.9. The positions of sensors were experimentally determined where maximum variation of the sensor outputs is met. An experiment to control a mobile robot has been carried out. In the experiment, the first process is calibration. Every time the subject puts on the wearable master, the position of the wearable master with respect to the human body is changed slightly. Since the amount of bending of a human shoulder is quite small, the change of the position of the wearable master causes the change of the co-ordinates of the position command dramatically, so the calibration process is essential. Short calibration time is also important. For instance, the calibration of joysticks is very short and easy.

20.4.5 Bio-signal-based Control Interface

The EMG control is often used to operate prostheses with few DOFs. EMG applications to the user who has severe paralysis are very difficult because the EMG signals of other muscles may interfere with the useful EMG signals.

Soft computing techniques allow us to extract useful information from the EMG signals. Several approaches (Graupe *et al.*, 1975; Saridis *et al.*, 1982; Yang *et al.*, 1996; Fukuda *et al.*, 1998) have been proposed to solve the motion command identification problem when using EMG signals for assistive devices. These studies may be categorised into two groups. The first group (Graupe *et al.*, 1975) tries to find a certain feature, which has high separability between predefined motions. In this method, it is easy to classify predefined motions because there is no overlap in feature values, but the threshold value for successful classification is not universal, i.e. it is often user-dependent. The other researchers (Saridis *et al.*, 1982; Yang *et al.*, 1996; Fukuda *et al.*, 1998) try to find heuristic rules to decrease classification error when the used features have low separability. For example, a probabilistic model (Saridis *et al.*, 1982), an 'if-then' type fuzzy pattern classifier (Yang *et al.*, 1996), and a neural networks pattern classifier (Fukuda *et al.*, 1998) were used as a pattern recogniser. In these methods, however, the threshold value for classification is not user-dependent, but errors in boundaries still are not negligible. Therefore, we propose a method based on soft computing techniques to find a feature set that has high separability and is user-independent.

We developed an EMG signal-based human robot interface and tested it in the controller of the wheelchair-based manipulator. The minimal feature set, which is independent of users, is extracted from the EMG signals of eight predefined motions (Figure 20.10), and users' motion is successfully classified with success ratio 91.04%.

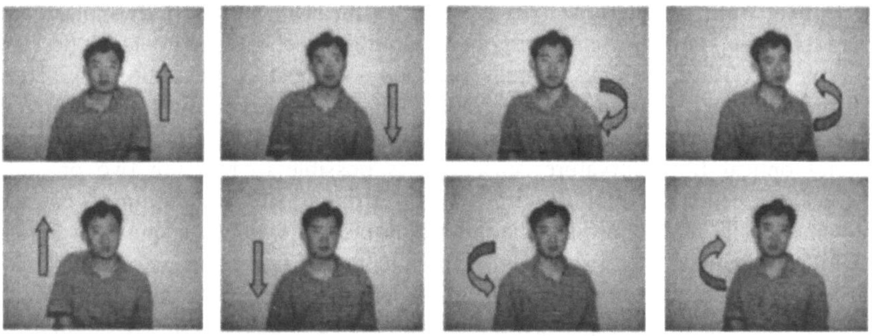

Figure 20.10. The pre-defined motions of user's arm

The classified results are used to execute the pre-programmed motion of the robotic arm. The proposed algorithm can use not only EMG signals, but also other bio-signals, such as EEG and EOG. EMG is a useful input source for an emergency stop switch to prevent the user from injury in a dangerous situation.

20.5 Concluding Remarks

KARES II is a wheelchair robot system to assist the activities of daily life for the disabled. On the basis of the predefined tasks of the wheelchair robot system, the design of the robotic arm and visual servoing techniques to control the robotic arm have been proposed. The experimental results show that the target-oriented design procedure is very effective in designing a robotic arm for the specific tasks.

The new robotic arm, with the cable-driven mechanism, shows good back-drivability to ensure safety. Moreover, the techniques and devices for visual servoing of the robotic arm provide the system with autonomous capability. Then in order to interact with the robotic arm, three types of human-robot interfaces, such as an eye-mouse, an EMG interface, and a haptic suit, well recognise eye movements, electrical signals of muscles, and body motions, respectively.

Spinal cord injured persons can select desirable interfaces in accordance with one's preference. KARES II has a large amount of possibility to assist the disabled. Currently, we are integrating overall systems that are presented in this chapter. And we have been planning to receive the feedback from the intended end-user groups such as the physically disabled and the elderly through the real experiment.

20.6 Acknowledgements

This work is supported by the Ministry of Science and Technology of Korea as a part of Critical Technology 21 Program on "Development of Service Robot Technology." The authors like to thank Prof. Myung-Jin Chung and Prof. Dong-Soo Kwon and other members of our team for their contributions to the program.

20.7 References

Adachi Y, Kuno Y, Shimada N, Shirai Y (1998) Intelligent wheelchair using visual information on human faces. In: Proceedings of IEEE Conference on Intelligent Robots and Systems, pp 354-359

Arrington KF (1997) Viewpoint Eye Tracker. Arrington Research

Bien Z, Song WK (2000) Novel wheelchair-based robotic arm with visual servoing capability for human-robot interaction. In: Proceedings of Workshop on Service Automation and Robotics, Hong Kong, pp 5-17

Capurro C, Panerai F, Sandini G (1997) Dynamic vergence using log-polar images. International Journal of Computer Vision 24(1): 79-94

Chang PH, Park HS, Park J, Jung JH, Jeon BK (2001) Development of a robotic arm for handicapped people: A Target-Oriented Design Approach. In: Proceedings of ICORR, pp 84-92

Coyle ED (1995) Electronic wheelchair controller designed for operation by hand-operated joystick. In: Proceedings of IEE Colloquia on New Developments in Electric Vehicles for Disabled Persons

Eftring H, Boschian K (1999) Technical results from MANUS user trials. In: Proceedings of International Conference on Rehabilitation Robotics (ICORR), pp 136-141

Fukuda O, Tsuji T, Otsuka A (1998) An EMG-based Rehabilitation Aid for Prosthetic Control. In: Proceedings of IEEE Workshop on Robot and Human Communication, pp 214-219

Glenstrup AJ, Engell-Nielsen T (1995) Eye Controlled Media: Present and Future State. B.S. Thesis, Copenhagen University

Graupe D, Cline WK (1975) Functional separation of EMG signals via ARMA identification methods for prosthesis control purposes. IEEE Transactions on Systems, Man, and Cybernetics 5(2): 252-259

Halley P (1993) Optical Fiber Based Sensor for Angular Measurement in Rehabilitation. In: Proceedings of International Conference on Systems, Man and Cybernetics vol. 1, pp 153-157

Harwin W, Rahman T, Foulds R (1995) A review of design Issues in rehabilitation robotics with reference to North American research. IEEE Transactions on Rehabilitation Engineering 3: 3-13

Jung JW, Song WK, Lee H, Kim JS, Bien Z (1999) A study on the enhancement of manipulation performance of wheelchair-mounted rehabilitation service robot. In: Proceedings of ICORR, pp 42-49

Kasabov N (1997) Learning strategies for modular neuro-fuzzy systems: a case study on phoneme-based speech recognition. Journal of Intelligent and Fuzzy Systems 5: 345-354

Kim DH (2000) Development of an Eye-Gaze Tracking System using Video Image Sequence and Magnetic Sensory Information. M.S. Thesis, KAIST, Korea

Kwee H (1997) Integrating control of MANUS and wheelchair. In: Proceedings of ICORR, pp 107-112

Kuno Y, Sakamoto M, Sakata K, Shirai Y (1994) Vision-based human interface with user-centered frame, Proceedings of IEEE/RSJ Conference on Intelligent Robots and Systems, pp 2023-2029

Rockland RH, Reisman S (1998) Voice activated wheelchair controller. In: Proceedings of IEEE Northeast Bioengineering Conference, pp 128-129

Saridis GN, Gootee T (1982) EMG Pattern Analysis and Classification for a Prosthetic Arm. IEEE Transactions on Biomedical Engineering 29: 403-409

Schmeisser G, Seamone W (1979) An assitive equipment controller for quadriplegics. Johns Hopkins Medical Journal 143: 84-88

Song WK, Lee H, Bien Z (1999) KARES: Intelligent wheelchair-mounted robotic arm system using vision and force sensor. Robotics and Autonomous Systems 28(1): 83-94

Song WK, Lee H, Kim JS, Yoon YS, Bien Z (1998) KARES: intelligent rehabilitation robotic system for the disabled and the elderly. In: Proceedings of IEEE EMBS Conference, vol. 5, pp 2682-2685

Stefanov D (1994) Model of a special orthotic manipulator. Journal of Mechatronics 4: 401-415

Stefanov D (1999) Integrated control of desktop mounted manipulator and a wheelchair. In: Proceedings of ICORR, pp 207-215

Van der Loos HFM (1995) VA/Stanford rehabilitation robotics research and development program: lessons learned in the application of robotics technology to the field of rehabilitation. IEEE Transactions on Rehabilitation Engineering 3: 46-55

Yang JY (2000) Development of Unit Workspace Griding Method for the Kinematic Design of Robot. M.S. Thesis, KAIST, Korea

Yang YS, Lam FK, Parker PA (1996) A New Fuzzy Approach for Pattern Recognition with Application to EMG Classification. In: Proceedings of IEEE Conference on Neural Networks, vol. 2, pp 1107-1114

Chapter 21

Improving the Flexibility of an Assistive Robot

M.R. Hillman, N.M. Evans and R.D. Orpwood

21.1 Introduction

21.1.1 Background

At the Bath Institute of Medical Engineering various approaches to assistive robotics have been investigated over several years. Each of these systems has been evaluated by potential users. This experience has been vital in refining the design and guiding the development.

21.1.1.1 Desk-based System – "Wolfson" Robot
This approach (Hillman *et al.*, 1992), while being appropriate for the desk based activities of a person carrying out a vocational task, was found to be restricting for use in a domestic environment. A desk-based system restricts the user to a particular room in the home. Most domestic activities take place in different rooms around the home. It is important that the disabled person can take part in these activities with other members of the family.

21.1.1.2 Trolley-mounted System – "Wessex" Robot
This low cost approach to "mobile robotics" (Hillman *et al.*, 1994) requires a carer to move a trolley-based manipulator around from one room to another. This seems to work well, though users always want greater functionality from their equipment, and often request "could it be mounted on my wheelchair?" or "could the trolley be powered and moved around under remote control?"

21.1.1.3 Wheelchair-mounted System – "Weston" Robot.
This system (Hillman *et al.*, 2001) shares many common components with the trolley-mounted system, but mounted to a wheelchair - this introduces additional design constraints. This approach may be compared with the MANUS wheelchair mounted robot system (Kwee, 1998) where the mechanism was designed from the

start for a wheelchair mounted application. There are many issues involved in integrating the robotic manipulator with the wheelchair. The evaluation of the wheelchair mounted "Weston" robot is described in this chapter.

21.1.2 Requirements for Wheelchair-mounted Manipulator

When considering attaching a robotic manipulator to a wheelchair there are different requirements, compared to either a desktop or trolley mounted system, against which the completed device must be evaluated.

- There must be an adequate range of motion. In the case of a wheelchair mounted system this will include reaching from floor level to head height of a seated user
- The manipulator must not compromise the control of the wheelchair, including such issues as stability, steering, manoeuvrability, user's control and visibility
- The manipulator must not compromise the usability of the wheelchair, including such issues as seat adjustment, pressure relief and transfer into or out of the wheelchair. In addition, the robotic device must be able to be easily removed when not required.
- The manipulator must aesthetically integrate with the wheelchair both in terms of shape, styling and colour.

This chapter briefly describes the system, reports the evaluations that have taken place, and discusses several conclusions that have come out of the evaluations.

21.2 Design Description

21.2.1 General Mechanical Configuration

Users were involved throughout the design of the system. An early consideration was how best to mount the manipulator to a wheelchair. A non-powered mock-up was built to demonstrate one possible approach to users. The mock up could be easily positioned adjacent to the user's wheelchair. As a result of these investigations, the system was fixed near to the rear wheels of the wheelchair such that the vertical actuator was positioned near to the shoulder of the user. Mounting the manipulator in this position on a fixed mounting point is relatively simple to implement, is not too visually obtrusive and does not block the user's line of vision, while still allowing a reasonable forward reach.

The manipulator consists of a single actuator giving motion in a vertical direction and an upper arm, which moves primarily in a horizontal plane. The vertical actuator needs to have a long stroke to enable the manipulator to reach from floor level to head height. A simple actuator would be very tall, and users thought this would be aesthetically unacceptable. The height of the vertical actuator was reduced by the use of a two-stage mechanism.

The upper arm consists of three vertical axes, allowing easy movement in a horizontal plain. The upper arm design is closely based on the trolley mounted "Wessex" robot. At the "wrist" a reverse differential is used, being a very compact arrangement combining roll and pitch. The ability of the wrist to pitch down is an important part of the design as it increases the vertical range. The current gripper is a simple design with two parallel moving jaws.

21.2.2 Mounting

As an initial arrangement the robotic manipulator was mounted to a Scandinavian Mobility (Invacare, US) "Home & Away" powered wheelchair (Figure 21.1). A mounting plate was permanently clamped to the wheelchair. The manipulator was fixed to the mounting plate using three bolts. The manipulator increased the width by 120mm with no increase in overall length.

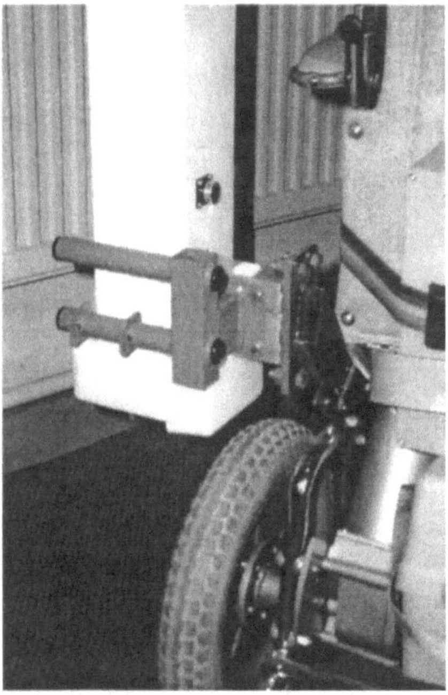

Figure 21.1. Manipulator mounted to "Home and Away" wheelchair

Several volunteers were identified to use the system but it was not feasible at this stage to arrange a custom mounting for their own wheelchairs. Equally it was not appropriate or possible to ask volunteers to transfer into the Home & Away chair. The manipulator was therefore mounted on a trolley, designed so that it could be wheeled close to the wheelchair to simulate the position the manipulator would be in, if mounted to the wheelchair. This allowed evaluation of the general positioning and control of the manipulator, although without either the flexibility or potential compromises of the full wheelchair mounted system.

Of these volunteers one used an Invacare "Storm" wheelchair, and was identified as a suitable person to evaluate the manipulator in a full wheelchair mounted configuration. While the Home and Away chair is of a traditional tubular steel framed design, the Storm is totally different, having an "H" shaped chassis of aluminium box extrusions. This particular wheelchair is also fitted with a large reclining seat, with substantial armrests. The manipulator mounted to the Storm wheelchair is illustrated in Figure 21.2.

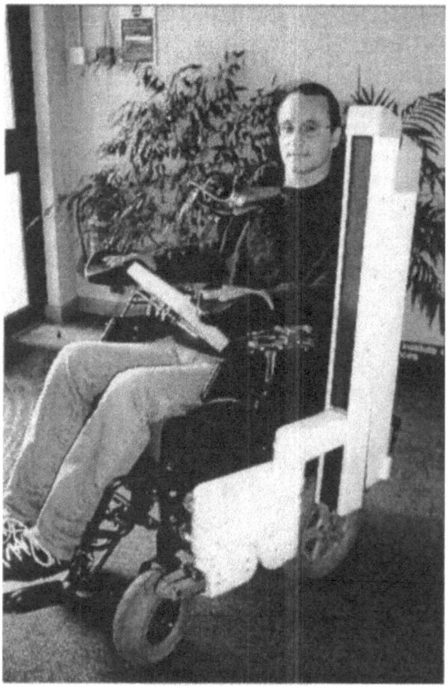

Figure 21.2. Manipulator mounted to "Storm" wheelchair

21.2.3 Electronics & Software Design

The electronics design is very similar to that used in the trolley mounted system. The main processor is a PC card running software for both motor control and the user interface. The processor is housed in a box, which may be hung on the back of the wheelchair. The motor control boards are mounted within the arm. The system is powered from the wheelchair's batteries (24v) or batteries within the trolley.

At the top level the software implements the user interface menu system, calling on lower level software modules for controlling the robotic system.

21.2.4 User Interface

The user interface assumes that the user will be able to use a two dimensional input, such as a joystick, as commonly used for electric wheelchair control. Using the joystick, the user controls a cursor to make selections from a menu screen. Figure 21.3 illustrates the menu layout for controlling the main directions of movement of the manipulator. A similar menu allows control of the wrist and gripper movements. The menu is displayed on a backlit monochrome LCD display.

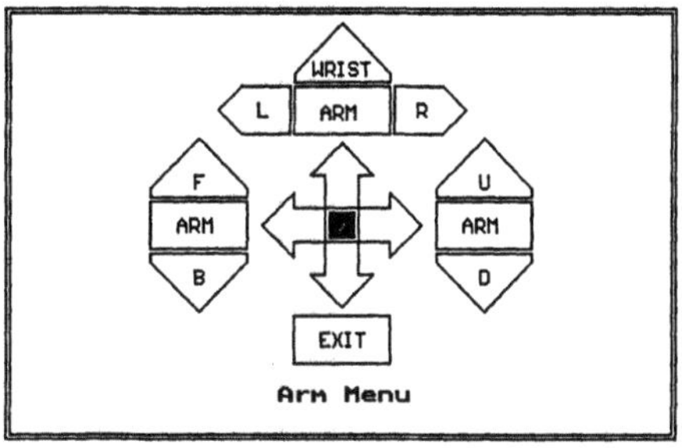

Figure 21.3. User interface menu display

The main emphasis has been on the direct control of the manipulator in real time, by the selection from the menu of different movement directions. There are currently limited facilities for the use of pre-set positions. As reported later in the chapter this has been found to be very valuable by users and so more comprehensive facilities are planned.

Currently the robot interface hardware is independent of the wheelchair. In the longer term it is intended that the robot interface will be fully integrated with the wheelchair control system, and will use the same joystick (or other input device), switching between robot and wheelchair control.

21.3 Evaluation

21.3.1 General Arrangements of Tests

The robotic system was evaluated by four volunteers as detailed in Table 21.1. The priority of these tests was to have been the evaluation of the manipulator mounted to a user's wheelchair. In fact, only one of the four volunteers had the manipulator mounted to his wheelchair, for reasons, which will be described below. In spite of this, the evaluations were very useful and there was particularly useful discussion on the need for flexibility in the mounting of the manipulator.

For each of the volunteers, the operation of the system was demonstrated and explained, both to the user and any carers. The system was then left with each volunteer for a period of a few weeks, in their own home, with an encouragement to investigate different tasks that the manipulator could carry out. We were keen that the volunteers should discover appropriate tasks themselves, rather than have them suggested. When the system was collected there was discussion on the experience of using the manipulator, and wider discussions on possibilities for the future.

Table 21.1. Details of volunteers

	Disability	Age group	Gender	Location
DT	Spinal cord injury	30-40	M	Home
AW	Spinal cord injury	20-30	M	Home
CP	Spinal muscular atrophy	10-20	M	Home
JP	Spinal muscular atrophy	10-20	M	Home

21.3.1.1 Volunteer DT

DT uses an Invacare (US) "Storm" wheelchair, and so it was necessary to make up a custom mounting system for that chair as described and illustrated above. Following discussions with DT it was realised that the manipulator needed to be easily demountable from the wheelchair. This needed to be achieved without risk of back injuries to carers, or the need to undo engineering fasteners. A wheeled trolley is therefore provided which can be wheeled up adjacent to the wheelchair. A simple jack fitted to the trolley lifts the manipulator off the wheelchair onto the trolley. DT uses a chin joystick. For these tests an extra joystick was mounted to the wheelchair, adjacent to the existing chin joystick.

21.3.1.2 Volunteer AW

We were keen to have the involvement of this user even though he uses a manual wheelchair and therefore it was not appropriate to mount the manipulator to his chair. He has been involved in the robot project over several phases and has provided valuable feedback on the Wessex trolley mounted system and also on the development of the interface for the Weston robot.

21.3.1.3 Volunteers CP, JP

These volunteers are brothers, both with spinal muscular atrophy. The younger brother (volunteer CP) uses a powered wheelchair and it had been hoped that the manipulator would be mounted to his chair. The older brother (volunteer JP) is confined to a "bed" mounted on a powered base and it would not be appropriate to mount the manipulator to this. The boys were initially interviewed at home. They were both keen to use it at home, but in that environment they rarely use their wheelchair - instead they are seated in fixed chairs. The manipulator would have been useful at school where the younger brother uses his wheelchair. However the problems of setting up the manipulator on a wheelchair for use by a large number of carers, and the problems of transporting the system to and from school precluded such tests at this stage. Instead it was decided to concentrate on the use of the manipulator in a trolley-mounted configuration in their own home over the school holidays.

21.3.2 Mounting and Integration Issues

DT was the only one of the four volunteers to have the manipulator mounted to his wheelchair. Even though the wheelchair with manipulator attached was able to pass through the doors in his home, he still found it too big. DT often has different carers looking after him at different times and emphasised that transferring the manipulator from wheelchair to support trolley should be totally fool proof. The other area that proved difficult was integrating the robot control input device and LCD screen with the wheelchair and its input device. Since two separate chin joysticks were used, this obstructed the vision of the user.

The other three users used the manipulator mounted to a trolley. All three felt that the manipulator could be useful in this configuration, but wanted more flexibility. CP (who is an electric wheelchair user) could see the benefit of mounting the manipulator to his wheelchair, while JP and AW were more interested in the possible mounting of the manipulator to a remote controlled powered base, or clamping it to a desk top. There was a strong feeling that the system should offer a range of mounting options, and therefore the size and weight are paramount.

21.3.3 User Control of the Manipulator

All four volunteers controlled the manipulator using a switched joystick. DT operated it with his chin, while the other three had sufficient hand function to use their hands. All users found the system easy to use, but sometimes slow to access the required command using a scanning system. Both DT (especially) and also AW thought that this could be overcome with voice activation. DT regularly uses voice activation to input data to a computer and was an enthusiast for using a similar system for the manipulator. AW advised keeping to a restricted number of words in order to improve reliability of recognition.

When designing the system it was assumed that Cartesian control of the gripper would be much more intuitive than joint control. These tests showed that while Cartesian control is often the most appropriate mode of control, it is not always so. Both AW and JP found they used joint control more often than Cartesian control. An alternative to joint mode or Cartesian mode would be to use a polar mode of control. In practice the user should be able to select the most appropriate mode of control for his own preference and the configuration of the manipulator.

The current system allows up to six pre-set positions to be recorded. For example: "parked," "ready to pick up from the floor," and "ready to reach onto a table top." It was felt that this was most appropriate and adequate for a wheelchair mounted system. Both DT and AW strongly argued for the use of pre-programmed tasks (i.e. a sequence of movements of the manipulator). CP and JP were happier to use direct control, although JP found the pre-set positions useful.

21.3.4 Tasks attempted and suggested

DT tested the system on simple pick and place tasks. He did not attempt (or suggest) any more "useful" tasks.

AW had had extensive use of the earlier Wessex trolley mounted system and had shown himself to be a user with a good imagination for ways in which the manipulator might prove useful. During these trials he investigated cleaning his teeth and drinking soups as well as pick and place operations. He also envisaged it being potentially useful for rearranging the sheets on his bed at night-time.

Many of the possible uses discussed with CP and JP were what might be called "play" applications. While not increasing the "independence" of the user they are important for the normal social interaction of children. Among the tasks discussed were reading magazines, painting, various games, opening birthday presents and dropping balls and other objects on your brother or cat!

21.3.5 Overall value of the system

The value of a system combines issues of the cost of the system and the benefit to the user. H.Eftring (1999) in his PhD thesis on the use of the MANUS robot introduces the concept of "useworthiness." He defines this as "the individual user's assessment of the extent to which the technology meets the user's high-priority needs." In the case of DT it was clear that he did not attach any great "useworthiness" to the system. AW however found many more high priority tasks that the robot might achieve. In the case of CP and JP, where the tasks were much more "play" oriented it was more difficult to attach a value to the tasks - however normal play interaction with each other might be seen as "high priority."

The other side of the "value" equation is how much it costs to commercially produce such a system. Our target price is £10000 to £12000. During the evaluations we asked the volunteers and their carers what price they thought would be acceptable. It was generally felt that for many potential users the price needed to be around £5000, although up to £12000 might be justified.

21.4 Discussion

At the start of this project three assumptions were made, each of which has been challenged by the results of our user evaluations. In each case a greater level of flexibility was requested than had been initially assumed.

21.4.1 Mounting of the Manipulator

Assumption: *Mounting the manipulator to a wheelchair is clearly the optimal way forward. It is acknowledged that there will be compromises, but felt that these can be satisfactorily addressed.*

When using the system with volunteers it soon became clear that although a wheelchair mounted configuration was very useful it needed to be combined with other arrangements. The basic manipulator needed to be easily changed from a wheelchair-mounted configuration to other arrangements such as trolley mounted, mounted to a powered base, or mounted to a workstation. This would need to be carried out by carers. The weight and size of the manipulator needs to be optimised. In addition the connections (both mechanical and electrical) need to be as simple as possible.

21.4.2 User Interface

Assumption: *Users of wheelchairs will be able to use a joystick type input device.*

A joystick was found to be a suitable input device, although it needs to be fully integrated with the wheelchair control system. However it should not be the only input device. In particular voice control would be useful, since it offers a much wider bandwidth of information. For this application it would probably be best to use a small vocabulary with carefully chosen words for reliable recognition. Whatever input device is used, varying levels of complexity and degree of control will be required for the user interface depending on the user's experience.

21.4.3 Level of Command

Assumption: *Direct control by the user will be the most appropriate level of control for a wheelchair mounted system, and also that Cartesian (straight-line) control will be the most appropriate mode of control.*

For direct control several of the users preferred to be able to use a polar mode of control. A small number of pre-set positions were provided but most of the users felt that a more comprehensive facility to provide pre-programmed tasks would make the system much easier to use. The currently limited use of pre-set positions, while useful, did not offer the best use of the system. How pre-programmed tasks can best be implemented on a wheelchair-mounted system (with no known environment) will need further consideration.

21.5 Conclusions

Following the evaluation of a wheelchair mounted manipulator by four potential users, the importance of improving the flexibility of such a device has been highlighted. This can be seen in three particular areas.

- Mechanical hardware, in particular mounting arrangements. The device should be able to be mounted not just to a wheelchair, but also other in other configurations, such as mounting to a trolley, mobile base or desk-top.
- User interface. The requirements for the user interface will vary not only with the disability of the user, but also with his or her experience of the robotic device.
- Level of control. Although the primary emphasis of this work was in using the device under the direct control of the user, it became clear that the software functionality should be improved to include pre-set positions and pre-programmed tasks.

21.6 References

Eftring H (1999) The Useworthiness of robots for people with physical disabilities. Doctoral Dissertation, Certec, University of Lund, Sweden, pp 23-28

Hillman M, Jepson J (1992) Evaluation of a robotic workstation for the disabled. Journal of Biomedical Engineering 14:187-192

Hillman M, Gammie A (1994) The Bath Institute of Medical Engineering Assistive Robot. In: Proceedings of ICORR '94, Wilmington, US, pp 211-212

Hillman M, Hagan K, Hagan S, Jepson J, Orpwood R (2001) Integration of a robotic device onto a powered wheelchair. In: Mokhtari M (ed.) Integration of assistive technology in the information age. IOS Press, Amsterdam, pp 192-198

Kwee H (1998) Integrated control of MANUS manipulator and wheelchair enhanced by environmental docking. Robotica 16: 491-498

Chapter 22

Commercialising Assistive and Therapy Robotics

M.S. Colello and R.M. Mahoney

22.0 Summary

This article provides an overview of the commercial efforts of the Rehabilitation Technologies Division (RTD) of Applied Resources Corp., which was formed in March of 1997 with the mission of establishing a product line of assistive and therapy robotic devices. In effect, this mission requires establishing the market for rehabilitation robotics in the United States. In order to be successful in this endeavour, RTD has created a plan consisting of stages for Market Review, Product Development, Market Entry, and Market Growth. A discussion of information gathered during the last five years, and a review of specific product development efforts is also provided.

22.1 Introduction

Two primary areas have been targeted for application of robotics technology to the field of rehabilitation. - personal assistance for people who are elderly and disabled, and devices to assist with stroke therapy. Little of the research and development work, which has been ongoing since the 1960's in both academic research labs and small start-up companies, has achieved commercial success. Over 30 years of R&D have resulted in a collective set of data that demonstrates proof of concept for assistive and therapy robotics, but it remains to be seen if this technology can make a successful transition into mainstream products that are useful in people's day to day lives.

Early development and commercialisation efforts were primarily an outgrowth of research and development (Corker *et al.*, 1979; Mahoney, 1999). A number of commercialisation efforts were made in the 1980's and 1990's, resulting in sales of several hundred units of a handful of different devices (Mahoney, 1997). No significant changes in sales have occurred throughout the last decade.

In most of the world, research and development for assistive and therapy robotics has been sponsored by the government or private foundations. Primary commercial efforts to date have been undertaken by research organisations where the research group or a key individual attempted to perform the transfer. Alternatively, attempts were made by small companies with little financing or business experience. To date, the commercial opportunity for robotics has not been identified by a large established healthcare company with sufficient resources to develop a product and support its entry into the market. The task, therefore, must be accomplished through companies with other expertise and limited resources.

22.2.1 The Market

Although commercial efforts have not reached a satisfactory state, a number of market factors support significant potential for robotics technology in the rehabilitation sector. This position is supported by strong demographic indicators that are largely not known or understood in the context of the implementation of robotics technology. Consider, the demographics of the potential end users of assistive robot products:

In the US, up to 500,000 individuals with severe disabilities, resulting from conditions such as cerebral palsy, spinal cord injury, debilitating muscle disorders, and birth defects, stand to benefit considerably from advances in rehabilitation technology (Stanger and Cawley, 1996). There are between 100,000 and 150,000 students, between the ages of six and 21 with severe disabilities, who require special education services (National Science Foundation, 1996).

The combination of high life expectancy with increased disability ratios (percentage of elderly with a disability) will result in a massive increase in the projected number of moderately or severely disabled elderly persons by 2040. The number would grow from about 5.1 million in 1986 to 22.6 million in 2040, or nearly 350 percent; the elderly population overall would grow by 175 percent during this time (Siegel, 1996).

The market for rehabilitation robots can also be understood in terms of the powered wheelchair market. It is projected that 49,533 powered wheelchairs will be shipped in 2004, with growth continuing at a 7% rate (Frost and Sullivan, 1998). Based on the average powered wheelchair life expectancy of 5 years, it is estimated that in excess of 250,000 users of existing powered wheelchairs also make up the market potential.

The demographic indicators for people with disabilities due to stroke are striking. Stroke is the leading cause of major physical disability in adults in the USA. Stroke survivors represent the most common diagnostic impairment group on many rehabilitation units and almost 40% of these persons have significant disability. 600,000 people a year survive stroke in the USA. The total number of stroke survivors alive in the USA is approaching 4,000,000. Costs for treatment and lost time exceed $7 billion per year. Further, inpatient rehabilitation length of stay following stroke has been drastically reduced due to cost containment. (Stineman and Granger, 1991; Goldstein, 1990; Mayo, 1993; US DHHS, 1995; Wolf *et al.*, 1992).

A recent report on the needs of individuals with chronic care predicts that the ratio of potential caregivers (those aged 50 to 64) to potential elderly requiring personal care (those aged 85 and older) is shrinking dramatically. In 1990 this ratio was 11 to 1. In 2010 it is projected to be 10 to 1, and by 2050 it is projected to be 4 to 1 (Institute for Health and Aging, 1997). All of these market forces represent opportunities that can be addressed by the robot-based products of RT. In most cases, the opportunity triples if the world-wide market is considered.

22.3 RTD-ARC

The Rehabilitation Technologies Division (RTD) represents a combination of market knowledge, engineering design and manufacturing capability, business expertise, and creativity assembled in a unique effort to establish the market for assistive and therapy robotics in the United States.

Formed as a division of Applied Resource Corp. (ARC) on March 17, 1997, RTD has been constructed on its parent company's more than 25 year history as a designer and manufacturer of high reliability, high durability electromechanical components for aerospace, telecommunications, defence and space programs. In 1995, ARC began exploring opportunities to expand and build on its expertise. During this process, it engaged in the manufacturing and technical support for several small companies working to commercialise robotic assistive technology.

This exposure, fuelled by a desire to broaden the business base into more commercial markets, led to the recognition of the opportunity to apply ARC's technical expertise to the field of assistive technology. ARC's research showed that the demographics and the needs of people with disabilities support an outlook of significant market potential. In March of 1997, Richard Mahoney, joined ARC as the Director of Business Development, and became the first academic research scientist in over 30 years of R&D effort to break completely with the research environment to pursue commercialisation of assistive and therapy robotic aids.

Given this backdrop and a broad knowledge of the potential applications, current players, real needs of consumers, and the intricacies of the market, RTD established this mission -- To create a comprehensive line of assistive and therapy products based on robotics technology.

In this effort, RTD identified the following target product areas:

- Wheelchair mounted assistive robots;
- Robotics for upper limb, hand, and lower limb stroke therapy;
- Desktop vocational, educational, and recreational robots;
- Task specific robotic aids, such as for feeding and turning pages;
- Mobile robotic aids for personal assistance and transportation.

In addition to this product focus, RTD has adopted several philosophical guidelines to support its activities. The decision to pursue multiple products was made not only because there was a desire to address the many needs of the target customers, but also so that the success or failure of the company would not verge on the success or failure of one product. Also, the success of any one product would serve to support the introduction of new products that would take advantage of the notoriety and existing organisation.

RTD targeted involving rehabilitation facilities and end users in its product development in order to remain closely connected to real needs, to identify product opportunities, and to establish clinical ties for product testing and introduction.

Although a wide range of products are listed above, RTD's focus is on introducing technology that can have an immediate benefit to the customer, even if that benefit is relatively narrow with respect to the potential for a particular technology. The emphasis is on creating entry level products and then relying on feedback from users to evolve the product.

RTD also targeted creating relationships with existing research programs in order to identify new potential products and to assist with technology transfer.

22.3.1 Plan

Based on the above mission and principles, RTD embarked on a plan consisting of the following stages: Market Review, Product Development, Market Entry, and Market Growth. The various activities of each stage are expanded on further below.

Market Review (Year 1-2):

- assembling the state of the art in commercial and research prototypes and evaluating their suitability for introduction into the US market;
- visiting rehabilitation facilities, primarily along the East Coast, and conducting review sessions with clinicians in order to obtain feedback regarding the utility of the technology and considerations related to marketing and supporting products in this environment;
- visiting research facilities and identifying opportunities for technology transfer;
- performing more detailed market research and investigation;
- identifying and researching regulatory requirements.

Product Development (Year 2, ongoing):

- applying internal resources to develop, design, and manufacture prototypes of key products;
- pursuing government grants and other funds to support development of other product areas.

Market Entry (Year 3, ongoing):

- developing marketing materials;
- carrying out initial marketing and follow up with contacts made during the Market Review stage;
- finalising details for delivery to first customers;
- exploring sales and distribution partnerships;
- finalising pricing and other terms of sale.

Market Growth (Year 5, ongoing):

- escalating sales and marketing efforts;
- expanding sales and distribution resources;
- feeding back first customer experiences into design and service improvements;
- pursuing investment to accelerate sales and marketing and development efforts.

22.3.2 Outcomes

The following information and observations reflects the experiences of RTD as it has performed the activities described above.

RTD recognises that the federal government has always been at the forefront of introducing new technologies, whether this be in defence, telecommunications, or healthcare. In the United States, in particular, the Department of Veterans Affairs (VA), the National Institutes of Health (NIH), the National Science Foundation, and the National Institute on Disability and Rehabilitation Research of the Department fo Education all support research and technology transfer through grants to small companies. Their investment is targeted at improving the lives of their constituents and addressing other issues with respect to the healthcare arena. The VA and NIH are supporting research with respect to technology for stroke therapy. As a company, RTD has pursued these resources in order to meet the objectives of the federal agencies while furthering its own objectives.

Related to this is identification of the need to develop a strong advocacy group for rehabilitation robotics. In short, for this technology to succeed, you need people as a group to say that they want to obtain it and that it has value for them. This also involves educating the entire populace about the availability of robotics technology and the opportunities it brings to people with disabilities. This is a marketing or public relations activity, but it is necessary to move the perception of rehabilitation robotics from forever being on the horizon to being viewed as part of what is available here and now.

To be successful in making this transition, RTD must be run successfully as a business first, and not just as a well-equipped idea. All of the structure and organisational aspects of a business must be embedded in the plan going forward. The speed at which a company can move is then a function of available resources. An existing company with other revenue streams can carry out the early stages without bringing in additional capital. Speed is important because of the desire to bring the benefit of these products to the end user. But as a business, it is important to maximise strategic advantages. The longer it takes, the more likely others will enter the market. In the end, it is unlikely that any small company can achieve this feat bringing in additional resources to support the later stages described above.

A review of rehabilitation facilities shows that the level of knowledge of and experience with technology varies quite a bit. In practice, as the first robotic aids are introduced into real use, it will be necessary to carry out extensive training of therapists and end users in areas related to client assessment, prescription, and protocols to support efficient and safe use of the technology. The first robotic aids will be providing access to a whole new sphere of experiences for the user population that will require early monitoring and support.

Much has been learned about the potential for reimbursement of assistive and therapy robotics. In general, any product that meets the necessary regulatory conditions and is prescribed to a patient by a certified clinical professional will be paid for at some level by a private or government insurance program. It will be necessary early on to follow through on the wide range of reimbursement programs to create the case history that can be used to support later funding. Sales will then become a function of the amount of resources available to support clinical prescription.

It is also unlikely that focusing on cost containment or reduction will provide significant motivation for insurance companies or other third party payers. These organisations are already funding personal attendants and other technologies that meet some of the needs of people with severe disabilities. None of the early products based on robotics technology will be able to completely remove the reliance on these current support mechanisms. Thus, it will take time for the technology to improve and for a greater appreciation to emerge for the value of independence for the end user. For this reason, it is likely that the first adopters of robotic aids will be people who are extremely motivated to obtain the technology.

22.4 Product Development

The Rehabilitation Technologies Division has created a path towards a suite of innovative, creative, and useful products for people who are elderly and disabled. The product development effort may be described in terms of two primary areas, Assistive Robotics and Stroke Therapy Robotics. The products that were selected for development were those identified during the market review stage that had reached a demonstrated level of feasibility and were consistent with RTD's mission of creating entry level value.

The Assistive Robotics area includes devices that support the elderly and those with severe disabilities to live more independently in work, school, personal care, and recreation. Currently, the key product in this area is the Raptor Wheelchair Robot System. Other products or product developments RTD has in this area are discussed further below.

Assistive Robots augment or take the place of attendant care and allow individuals to live more independently. The Stroke Therapy Robotics area includes devices that may be used to replicate, automate, and improve physical therapy for rehabilitation from stroke. Stroke therapy robotics use active and passive constrained motions to retrain lost motor function. Robotics technology allows the therapy device to accommodate improvements in therapy as the person moves through different levels of the rehabilitation process.

RTD has two key products that constitute this area:

ARCMIME: Robotic upper limb stroke therapy assistance; and
Javatherapy: Internet-facilitated therapy alternative for chronic stroke patients.

22.4.1 The Raptor Wheelchair Robot System

The Raptor (shown in Figure 22.1) is RTD's first commercial product offering (Mahoney, 2001). The system permits persons with severe disabilities to manipulate objects in their personal environment and thus to establish a greater measure of functional independence. The target user populations include high-level quadriplegia, neuromuscular disabilities, cerebral palsy, congenital disabilities, and severe rheumatoid arthritis, among others.

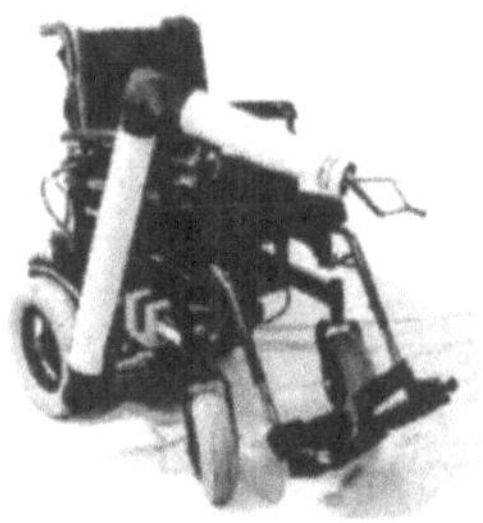

Figure 22.1. The Raptor

The Raptor is controlled through standard switch-based input devices and has been designed for simplicity of operation. After as little as five minutes, users have been able to retrieve an object and utilise it as desired (e.g. pick up a container of water and take a drink). The Raptor is modular in design, can be mounted on either side of most powered wheelchairs and utilises its own controller. The unit is streamlined to permit wheelchair access through standard doorways. The slimness of the arm minimises obstruction of the user's field of vision during operation.

Figure 22.2 shows the Raptor's first user, James Franchino. His purchase in June of 2000 represented the first commercial sale in the United States of an FDA approved robotic aid. The Department of Veterans Affairs has purchased ten units for use in a project to evaluate the efficacy of wheelchair mounted robotics for its population of individuals with spinal cord injuries. More information on the Raptor can be obtained on its web site at www.WheelchairRobot.com.

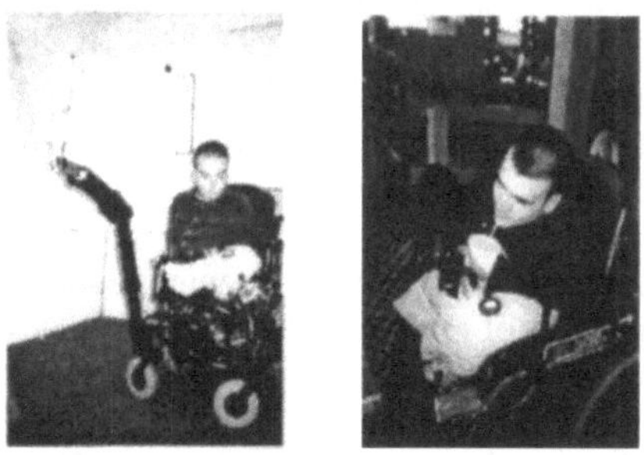

Figure 22.2. The first owner of the Raptor, James Franchino

22.4.2 ARCMIME

ARCMIME is a stroke therapy robotic system that will potentially provide improved rehabilitation outcomes, data on status, cost savings, and extended access to consumers. ARCMIME is the outcome of years of research and development at the VA Rehabilitation RandD Center in Palo Alto, CA. (Lum, Burgar, Kenney and Van der Loos, 1999).

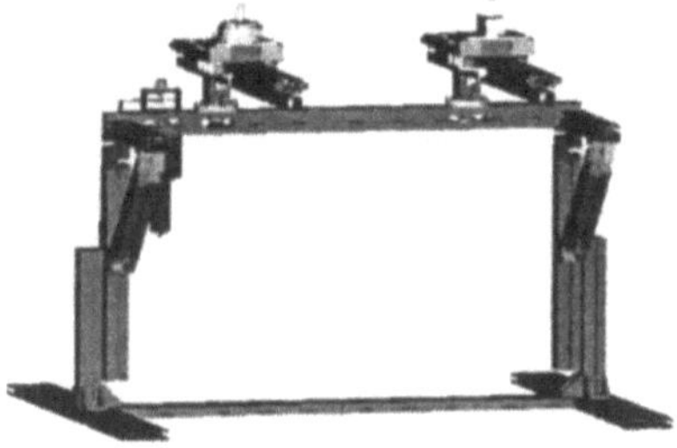

Figure 22.3. A CAD rendering of the ARCMIME system

This research has shown that the robotic stroke therapy replicates to a degree the rehabilitation outcomes for stroke subjects undergoing physical therapy.

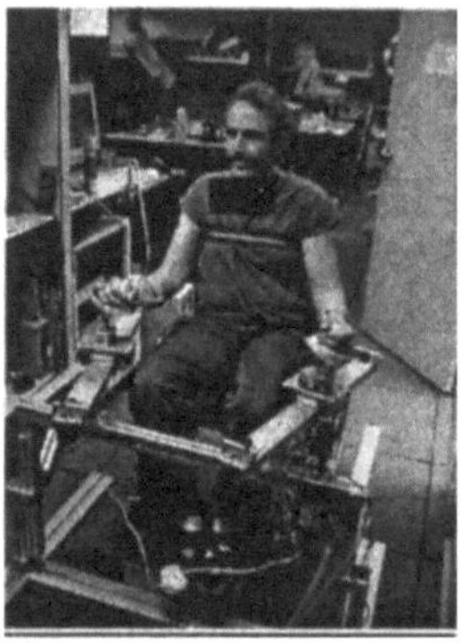

Figure 22.4. User during phase I clinical trials of ARCMIME

ARCMIME provides several modes of operation in co-operation with its sensors, which allows it to adjust with the patient as they progress through their rehabilitation program. In passive mode, it is able to carry the passive limb of the patient through a motion to help retrain the arm. As the arm gains in strength and range of motion, the force sensor and motor provide assisted or resisted motion to extend the strength and range of motion of the patient.

The ARCMIME system was shown to replicate the physical parameters of the experimental system and development of the full commercial system is now underway. (Mahoney, Van der Loos, Lum, and Burgar, 2001)

22.4.3 Javatherapy

Javatherapy is an inexpensive robotic telerehabilitation system for arm and hand therapy following brain injury. (Reinkensmeyer, *et al.*, 2001) Javatherapy will be marketed as a self-paced therapy alternative, providing a low cost therapy option for chronic stroke patients. Users will obtain an account with a monthly subscription. They will then be guided through a number of therapy programs that will be recommended based on their level of disability.

Javatherapy is a web site with a library of evaluation and therapy activities. The web activities can be performed with a commercial force feedback joystick, and the joystick can physically assist or resist in movement as the user performs therapy. The system also provides quantitative feedback of movement performance through the web-site that allows users and their caregivers to assess rehabilitation progress.

RTD has licensed the first prototype system and patent rights. The mechanical components of the system are a low cost force feedback joystick, a custom clip-on splint for individuals without hand grasp, a mobile arm support, and a custom support base. The total cost of these component is less than $200 and they can easily fit on a tabletop.

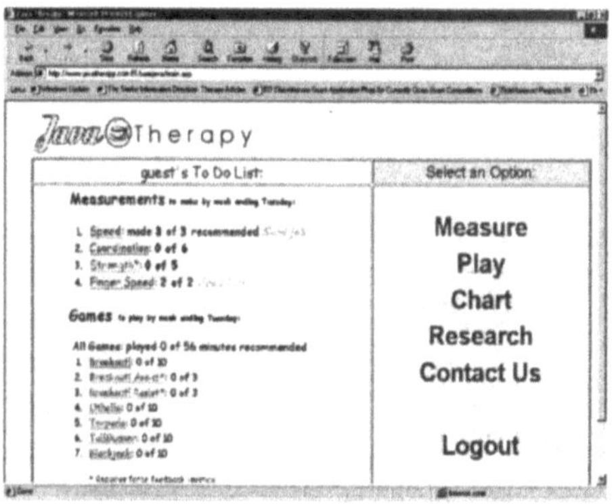

Figure 22.5. Java Therapy main page showing "To Do List" and "Main Menu"

22.4.4 Robox

The Robox is a modular desktop robot that provides access to physical manipulation for children and adults with disabilities for use in education and recreation. The Robox, an original product of RTD, has a simple magnet for a gripper and is controlled through a personal computer.

The software matches the activity board so that the user can interact with objects by requesting locations for them. For example, in a physical science experiment, the user can request, "move the blue block to the ruler." The software would then operate the robot to carry out this task.

Another feature of the Robox is that the activity board is interchangeable and easily designed. The objective is that a wide range of activity boards targeting many different tasks would be developed, such as a sandbox or action figure play area for children, or a hobby module for adults. Development of new activity modules would be carried out by RTD and other vendors, with RTD's primary focus on making the Robox system.

User evaluation of the Robox was accomplished by creating a physical science experiment to be administered to students in a special education class at the Matheny School and Hospital, Peapack, NJ, as part of their normal science curriculum. The lesson plan that was created outlined two levels of proficiency with respect to this system.

Basic proficiency with the Robox. Demonstrate that the student understood how to control the system. In order to accomplish this each student was asked to carry out the following tasks: *Move an object to a location. Repeat. Move objects back to home location. Make independent decisions to move objects where desired.*

Physical science proficiency. Carry out a classroom exercise in a timely fashion. The basic proficiencies to be explored in the physical science experiments relate to simple weighing and measuring. Students were asked to perform tasks such as the following: *Measure the length of objects. Sequencing the size of three objects, longest to shortest. Sequencing the weight of three objects, heaviest to lightest. Find objects that weigh the same.*

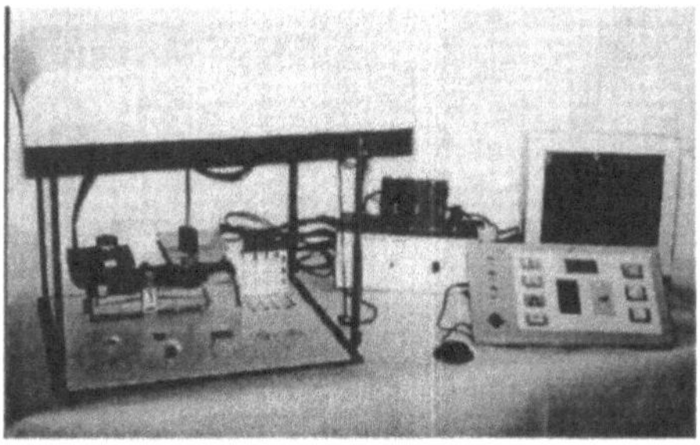

Figure 22.6. The Robox System, including robot work area, a physical science experiment module, the computer interface box, PC monitor, and Intellikeys control interface

The students selected to evaluate the Robox all have severe developmental disabilities and represent a group that on the whole is not physically able to carry out independently the tasks of the physical science experiment. In addition, they all require adaptive interfaces to use a computer

All of the students were able to attain Robox proficiency. All were able to accomplish the basic command of selecting an object and moving it to a desired location. Each student performed to a different degree with respect to proficiency in the physical science experiment. Given robox proficiency, this performance was a true indicator of their knowledge of the experimental activities because there was no other human interaction guiding placement of objects.

22.4.5 Picasso

Picasso, another original product from RTD, is a novel tool designed to provide access to the creation of real visual art by people with disabilities. Picasso is battery powered and remote controlled, so that it is completely portable. It consists of a motorised pallet that can hold a paintbrush (or other medium such as crayons, markers, pencils, etc.) and move it around under direct control of the user. The user is able to dip the paintbrush into a container of paint, bring it to a desired location on the paper, and then apply the brush to the paper while moving it in any direction. Picasso may also hold pens, pencils, markers, and other visual art mediums. Figure 22.7 shows the Picasso prototype system along with ARCSun and ARCFlower, visual art created using Picasso. Current development work is involved with improving and extending the control interface.

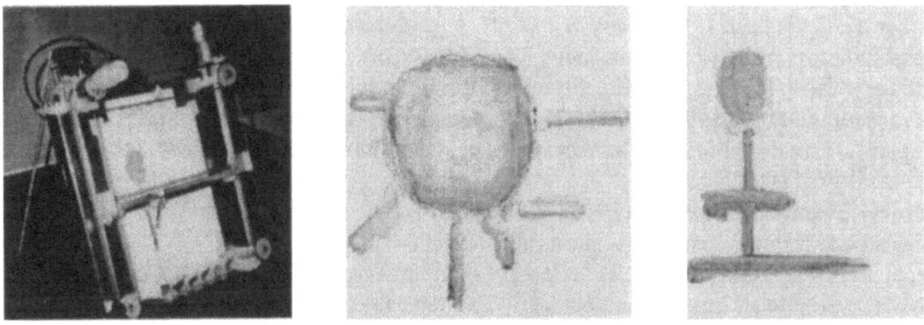

Figure 22.7. The Picasso prototype system, with ARCSun and ARCFlower, visual art created using Picasso

22.5 Conclusions

RTD has successfully emerged from the Market Survey and Product Development stages of its plan with a range of viable products. A great deal of learning has occurred as to the needs of the market and requirements for establishing a successful business model. After more than five years of effort, there is confidence that RTD will be successful in its quest to establish the market for assistive and therapy robotics in the United States. The speed with which this occurs will now be a function of the resources available to support the Product Development, Market Entry, and Market Growth stages.

22.6 Acknowledgements

RTD has reached this level through the efforts and co-operation of a number of individuals and institutions. Special thanks are extended to Machiel Van der Loos, Chuck Burgar, and Pete Lum of the Palo Alto VA Rehabilitation RandD Center; Dave Reinkensmeyer of the Dept. of Mechanical and Aerospace Engineering,

University of California at Irvine; Ken Robey, Gail Darch, and Beverly Bain of the Matheny School and Hospital; Sal Sheredos of the Technology Transfer Division, US Department of Veterans Affairs; Peggy Dellea of the Assistive Technology Center, Spaulding Rehabilitation Hospital. Special acknowledgement is made of the dedication of Craig Wunderly and Aman Siffeti, ARC's mechanical and electrical designers, and all of the members of the engineering and manufacturing staff who are dedicated to high quality in everything they do, and ultimately to the success of this endeavour. RTD acknowledges the support of the U.S. Department of Education, SBIR Grants ED-99-PO-4872 and ED-99-PO-4636, and the National Institutes of Health SBIR Grant 1 R43 HD37301.

22.7 References

Corker K, Lyman JH, Sheredos S (1979) A preliminary evaluation of remote medical manipulators. Bulletin of Prosthetics Research 10(32): 107-134

Mahoney RM (1997) Robotic Products for Rehabilitation: Status and Strategy. In: Proceedings of the 1997 International Conference on Rehabilitation Robotics, Bath, UK

Stanger C, Cawley M (1996) Demographics of rehabilitation robotics users. Technology and Disability 5(2): 125-138.

National Science Foundation (1996) Women, Minorities, and Persons With Disabilities in Science and Engineering. Arlington, VA, NSF 96-311

Siegel J (1996) Aging into the 21st Century. National Aging Information Center, Bethesda, MD, Available at: http://pr.aoa.dhhs.gov/aoa/stats/aging21/

Frost and Sullivan (1998) Wheelchair market/mobility aids industry: Unit and revenue forecasts (US), 1994-2004.

Stineman M, Granger C (1991) Epidemiology of stroke-related disability and rehabilitation outcome. Physical Medicine and Rehabilitation 2:457

Goldstein M (1990) The decade of the brain: challenge and opportunities in stroke research. Stroke 21:373.

Mayo NE (1993) Epidemiology and recovery. Physical Medicine and Rehabilitation: 7(1):1-25.

US Department of Health and Human Services (1995). Post-Stroke Rehabilitation. Clinical Practice Guideline, AHCPR Publcation no. 95-0662

Wolf PA, Belanger AJ, D'Agostion RB. (1992) Management of risk factors. Neurological Clinics 10(1):177-191

Institute for Health and Aging (1997) Chronic Care in America: A 21st Century Challenge. University of California, San Francisco, p 20

Mahoney RM (2001) The Raptor Wheelchair Robot System. In: Mokhtari M (ed.) Integration of Assistive Technology in the Information Age. IOS Press

Lum PS, Burgar CG, Kenney D, Van der Loos HFM (1999) Quantification of force abnormalities during passive and active-assisted upper-limb reaching movements in post-stroke hemiparesis. IEEE Transactions Biomedical Engineering 46(6): 652-662

Mahoney RM, Van der Loos HFM, Lum P, Burgar C (2001) Robotic Stroke Therapy Assistant. To appear in *Robotica*

Reinkensmeyer DJ, Pang CT, Nessler JA, Painter CC (2001) Java Therapy: Web-Based Rehabilitation. In: Mokhtari M (ed.) Integration of Assistive Technology in the Information Age. IOS Press

Chapter 23

Improved Assistive Technology Prescription via Usage Log Analysis

C. Roast, P. O'Neill and M. Hawley

23.1 Introduction

The study of human-computer interaction can be viewed as aiming to ensure that users can efficiently and effectively access the functions that technology enables. The focus of this chapter is to describe the exploration this objective for a specific class of technology designed to support users with severe disabilities. The assistive technology of interest provides key functionalities that are central to the quality of life of its users – such as, providing independent access to: speech synthesis facilities for users with vocal impairment or motorised wheelchair control for mobility. In contrast to a considerable amount of work focused upon supporting users with disabilities, the assistive technology interaction of interest here represents a dedicated system for dedicated usage. Hence, we are working in a context where the solution provided to the user is what they have to live with on a daily basis, and thus effective and efficient interaction are strongly linked to the quality of life of the end user.

The design and configuration of assistive technology is a product of a prescription process involving a variety of clinical experts. The goal of the process is to ensure that the user has efficient and effective access to the required assistive technology. The process as a whole is also an iterative one in which the ongoing assessment of the suitability of a given prescription is valuable in identifying changes in a user's condition, abilities and needs. The process of evaluating the configuration of these products, to ensure they are meeting the user's requirements, mainly relies upon expert assessment with some field observation. Both expert assessment and field observations are not ideal, being: resource intensive, intrusive and often subjective, and the need for additional evaluation methods and frameworks has been widely recognised (Cherry *et al.*, 1996; Churchill, 1998; Keates *et al.*, 2000; O'Neill *et al.*, 2000b).

This work is concerned with enhancing the information available to clinicians by analysing logs of system usage. The goal is to enhance prescription activity through the availability of more objective quantifiable information about assistive technology use (Hawley *et al.*, 1999; Rosen and Goodenough-Trepagnier, 1989; Vanderheiden, 1988). As with assistive technology in general, exploring any proposition such as this has to follow a methodology that is often by definition observational and single subject. Specifically, even limited experimentation with an individual subject's assistive technology provision can be highly intrusive and disruptive (Zghan and Ottenbacher, 2001). The other traditional methods for evaluating interactive systems would be protocol analysis or interviews with users, in the context considered here outcomes from these can be distorted due to the users having to report upon technology that is inherently of a unique value to them.

By means of a case study we describe potential analysis techniques that have been applied to the logs from these systems building upon prior work and experience (Hawley *et al.*, 1999; O'Neill *et al.*, 2000a, 2000b, 2001). The value of these techniques is discussed and illustrated in terms of their potential impact upon expert prescription process.

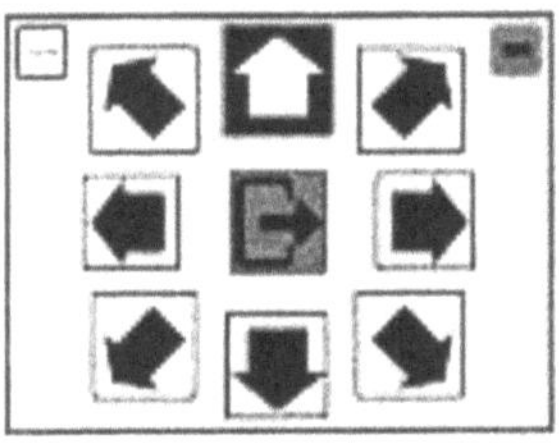

Figure 23.1. Barnsley Wheelchair Interface display

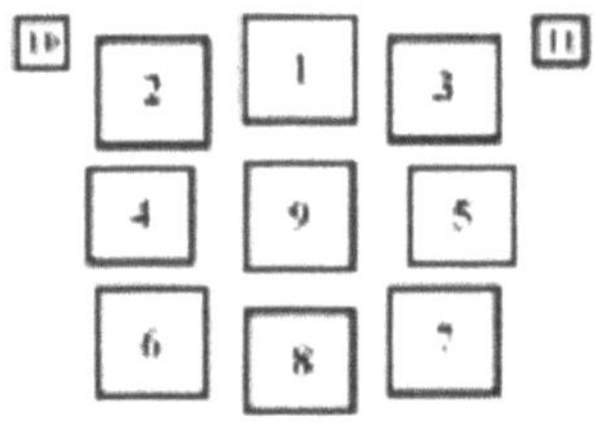

Figure 23.2. The BWI highlight order for configuration: "Forward First, Left-Right Step"

23.2 BWI - An Assistive Technology Case Study

The Barnsley Wheelchair Interface (BWI) is configured by the clinician to meet the individual's perceived needs (see Figure 23.1). When configured in one switch mode each of the items is highlighted sequentially at a set scan rate. When the desired direction is indicated and the user holds the switch closed, and the wheelchair drives in the chosen direction. Releasing the switch de-activates driving. The central icon is an 'exit' icon, allowing the user to exit the application, and a 'setup' icon provides primary user access to configuration options.

23.2.1 BWI Congifuration

The BWI can be configured to highlight the items displayed on the screen in any order chosen by the rehabilitation clinician. While the switch is open the system repeatedly follows the same order. After the switch has been held down to select a direction, the switch release can be configured to continue in order or to re-start the highlight sequence with the forward selection, this is termed forward bias:

- *Forward Bias* means the selection sequence returns immediately to the forward direction after the selection of any of the directions. Non-forward bias means the scan continues with the next item in the sequence following a specific selection.

Although any order can be used in principle, it is common for BWI to start scanning with forward being the first in the order – this choice reflects the most common task that wheelchair usage is likely to initially involve. In addition to the ordering of the sequence, the timing of the paced menu and switch responses can be configured; in particular, there are three key real-time parameters:

- *Pace* – the amount of time each item remains highlighted, while the switch is open;
- *Hold-down-time* – the amount of time the switch has to be closed before the system responds to the switch close;
- *Release-time* – the amount of time the switch has to be open before the system responds to another switch close.

The hold-down-time and release-time are both used to "dampen" switch activity in order to limit the BWI being activated by involuntary actions of the user. It is important to note that the choice of the specific highlighting method is the result of a clinical assessment, as are the specific timings and pace of the selection interface. The highlight sequences that have been most frequently considered in the configuration of BWI have followed a systematic and easily predicted manner. Specifically, the highlight order has been: (i) highly systematic; or (ii) more task oriented, termed 'left right step':

- *Left-right step* – the selection sequence progresses from the forward towards backwards alternating between left and right. Hence, left-right step, would follow the sequence: Forward, Forward-Left, Forward-Right, Left, Right, Backward-Left, Backward-Right, Backward (see Figure 23.2).

The rationale behind the left-right step is that it is sufficiently systematic to be predictable but is not strongly biased towards a particular lateral movement being more easily accessed. The choice of orderings generally reflects a balance between what orderings can be predicted (or discovered) about a user's general movement needs, and what is a suitable order in the absence of such information.

23.2.3 BWI Logging

In the work described here we are interested in using information about specific BWI users in order to configure the BWI most effectively. We explore the information that can be obtained from BWI usage logs and its value for the clinician responsible for assistive technology prescription, configuration and re-configuration. Such feedback has the potential to improve configurations for individuals, further inform clinicians and provide comparative objective methods for determining user needs. Compared with many assessment and evaluation techniques, usage logs have the benefit of easily providing extensive objective data with little intervention.

All selections made by a user of BWI are recorded in a log file recording: selection number, session number, date, time application and action, (Figure 23.3).

```
1,1,Thu,Aug,19,16:29:56,1999,drive,Start
2,1,Thu,Aug,19,16:35:59,1999,drive,Scanning
3,1,Thu,Aug,19,16:36:04,1999,drive,forward
4,1,Thu,Aug,19,16:37:29,1999,drive,Scanning
5,1,Thu,Aug,19,26:37:29,1999,drive,forwardleft
```

Figure 23.3. An example extract of BWI log data.

23.3 Log Analysis Techniques

Although log files provide objective data that is obtained with relative ease, the utility of the resulting information is relatively poor. Given a log some information can be reliably derived, such as selection durations, where as the derivation of other richer information goals, such as the number of user errors, have to be treated speculatively (Hilbert and Redmiles, 2000). In the intended context of use the log analysis is to supplement other, more traditional, assessment methods, hence one of the future goals is to examine the mapping and overlap between traditional outcomes and those of log analysis. However, within the work reported here our primary concern is exploring the information derivable from usage logs.

23.3.1 Analysis Information Levels

The potential value of analysing usage logs, such as that from BWI, is that the information derived can be fed into the prescription process for assistive technology and that the information obtained is additional to that already available to the clinicians involved in prescription. Three levels of information are used to structure the log analysis:

- *Whole system information* is concerned with obtaining an overall view of assistive technology utility and utilisation. Aggregates of technology use are used to ensure uptake, identify periods of familiarisation, learning and other possible trends in usage. For prescription activity this level is significant at a basic level of ensuring the technology is adequate (Hawley *et al.*, 2001). At a more sophisticated level, whole system information is relevant in assessing trends and fluctuations in usage that may be indicative of changes in a user's condition or environment. For instance, a change of physical accommodation may be reflected in a profile of overall usage time.
- *Functional level information* is concerned with the match between a user's assistive technology needs and the assistive applications and functionality

provided. For example, in the case of BWI, we could ask whether the eight distinct directions are those needed – both more directions and fewer directions are valid alternatives. Functional level analysis of logs is reliant upon abstracting over log events in order to map them to domain-orientated activities that are suitable for consideration by clinicians.

- *Interface level information* is focused upon the effectiveness with which required functions can be accessed. Hence, the configuration of a device such as the scanning menu of BWI will be the finest level determinant of whether the required assistive functions are accessed when in fact needed by end users. In this case, analysis is primarily focused upon the reliability of the log characteristics, that is, do log events correspond to actions intended by the user?

Effective analysis at each of these levels is reliant upon some account of expectations about the use of the system. For instance, overall usage may be assessed with respect to upper and lower bounds, or in terms of comparative usage over long time periods. In terms of BWI, a model of likely directions of travel can be employed to analyse and assess logs in terms of the functions provided. The analysis methods examined here are summarised below, and can be related to the three levels considered:

- *Target profiling* focuses upon examining the effectiveness of the scanning menu in terms of whether users actions achieve their intended target (such as a specific option or direction). Determining this is reliant upon an account of what the user is intending to do (functional level) and it generates feedback primarily at the interface level.
- *Selection profiling* focuses upon characterising the individual selections made by the user, such as, their frequency and duration. In considering the selection profile, information from target profiling may be used to possibly eliminate selection errors. In general, selection profiling provides an indication of specific biases and preferences at a functional level, these contribute to comprehending system suitability at all levels.
- *Sequence profiling* concerns the characterisation of the order in which selections are made. In our analysis here, we consider pairs of consecutive selections. Given that simple highlight strategies are normally favoured by practitioners for system configuration, specific sequencing information is less likely to direct the configuration of highlight order and more likely to direct a better understanding of functional needs and environmental factors.
- *Path profiling* refers to using visualisation to develop an understanding of the likely physical paths followed by a BWI user. The aim of analysis methods such as this is relatively ill-defined, it relates to early phases of traditional data analysis activities in which re-viewing the data is intended to give an indication of likely properties worthy of systematic or statistical examination. In the case of BWI, the accurate depiction of physical paths followed is likely to be useful in recognising patterns in both the users utilisation of the functions provided and their environment.

23.3.2 Case Study Data

Usage log data examined was collected from a twelve-year-old boy with athetoid cerebral palsy. The particular highlight method used by this boy is 'Forward First, Left Right Step,' as depicted in Figure 23.2, and the scan rate of the BWI was configured to be one second. Data from BWI usage for a single week generated around 1800 log records. On a continuous daily basis the boy had used the system for just under two months. Therefore, the subject could be considered as an expert user, not only because of the duration spent using this system but also because the individual had been using other scanning based systems for a number of years.

23.3.3 Target Profiles

Target profiles focus upon identifying the integrity of specific records within the log, and hence, whether they can be treated as legitimate representations of users intentions. In order to examine this we have to employ some account of intended activity with which we can compare the data. The approaches taken to assessing intended activity have been to identify simple behavioural patterns that are unlikely to be of any use to a user or to not activate any assistive function. These patterns are then used to estimate likely user errors that alternative configurations may alleviate. For instance, in O'Neill *et al.* (2000b) a combination of observational measures and theoretical user reaction times were used to compare the frequencies with which an assistive technology user entered and exited a mode without using any of its functions.

In the case of the BWI data, a similar analysis was based upon when the user ended a movement and then re-initiated the movement in the minimal time possible. This was interpreted as the result of a possibly mistaken, or involuntary, switch release. Under this interpretation, the data shows that just over 50% of the movements can be viewed as being the result of un-intended switch releases.

A similar approach to the analysis of the data is to identify patterns of use that would reflect the intended efficient and effective use of the system. Cases where such patterns are not evident may be indicative of configuration issues limiting effective use. An example of this in the BWI data is if we consider the role of the paced repeating highlight sequence. The configuration intention is that when a required function/direction is highlighted it will be selected by the user, however the logs show that when changing direction the user rarely took the first available opportunity.

Both these analysis techniques have yielded relatively surprising results about the usage of the BWI. In both cases interface re-configuration may alleviate the apparent problem: a longer release-time setting in the first case, and a slower pace in the second. Although it is difficult to "experiment" with such settings for an individual end-user, these target profiles provide a useful basis for comparison and expert re-assessment. In addition, these findings play an important role in subsequent analyses, since they are indicative of criteria that could be used to abstract over the log.

23.3.4 Selection Profiles

Selection profiles have been based upon: the number of movements made in each direction, the amount of time spent in each direction, and the average duration in each direction (see Figure 23.4 a, b and c). Duration and frequency profiles are similar and are, on the whole, proportional as can be seen when we consider the average time spent in each direction shown in (Figure 23.4c).

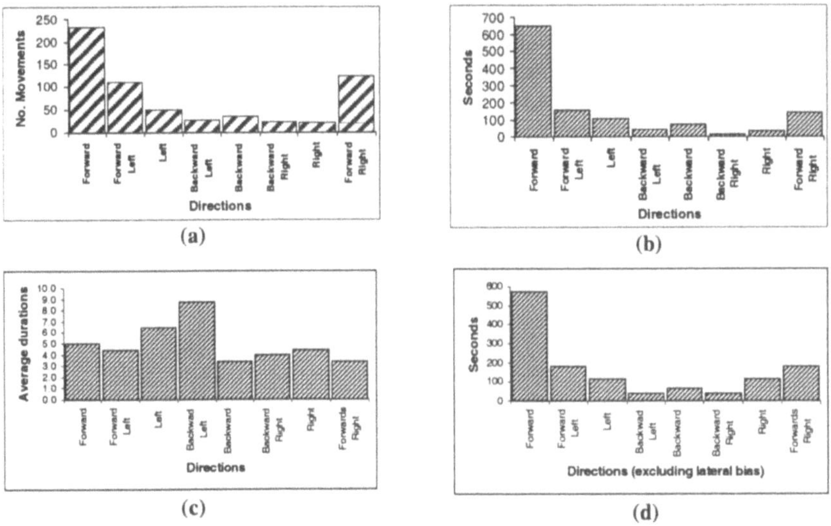

Figure 23.4. Selection profiles for a weeks BWI usage: (a) number of movements; (b) the total movement time; (c) average movement time; and (d) movement time normalised with respect to left and right movement

With the specific BWI data, the profile shows an asymmetry – there is a bias towards the left. Assuming that the users environment is one in which both left and right movement are equality likely to be required, this suggests either a strong bias at the interface level or some feature of the users' condition. The specific highlight order used is largely symmetric and in this particular case the clinician's knowledge of the user has contributed to interpreting the profile. The user activates the switch by the leftward movement of their head, hence, while directing the BWI their right-hand field of vision is limited. This appears to explain the specific asymmetry.

To explore other features of the profile, the data can be normalised with respect to lateral movements (see Figure 23.4d). It can be see that, but for backward movement, direction usages correspond to left-right step ordering of the paced menu. This raises the question as to whether the log is showing the user's direction preferences or the user is conforming to the "preferences" embodied in the specific configuration. The preference for the back direction over those that can provide a similar function, i.e. backward left and backward right, serves as a demonstration that the user is selecting the required direction, as a opposed to an easier compromise offered by the system.

23.3.5 Sequence Profiles

The sequence profiles from the log data have been limited to the consecutive pairing of directions selected. In this case it gives a profile relative to each of the directions. The directional biases of the selection profile are evident, however in addition, it can be seen that there are some behaviours linked with prior directions. Table 23.1 shows the proportion of consecutive directions selected - those entries that are statistically significant (within a column) are highlighted. From our knowledge of the target profile and the re-selection, the fact that like-to-like entries are significant is not surprising.

Table 23.1. Proportion of consecutive directions. The greyed figures are those that are statistically significant within their column.

		First selection							
		FL	L	BL	B	BR	R	FR	F
Total		107	46	23	32	17	19	112	214
Second selection	FL	0.48	0.11	0.17	0.09	0.06	0.11	0.09	0.13
	L	0.04	0.39	0.09	0.09	0.12	0.16	0.05	0.04
	BL	0.01	0.02	0.43	0.0	0.0	0.11	0.04	0.01
	B	0.04	0.07	0.04	0.63	0.0	0.05	0.02	0.01
	BR	0.02	0.04	0.09	0.06	0.47	0.0	0.01	0.01
	R	0.04	0.02	0.0	0.03	0.18	0.26	0.03	0.01
	FR	0.07	0.13	0.04	0.03	0.18	0.32	0.55	0.14
	F	0.32	0.22	0.13	0.06	0.0	0.0	0.21	0.65

With the like-to-like consecutive selections eliminated from the analysis there are only a few significant relationships remaining:

- following Forward, Forward-Left and Forward-Right are the most likely alternative directions to be chosen; and
- symmetrically, following Forward-Left and Forward-Right, Forward is the most likely alternative direction to be chosen.

These consecutive patterns are well supported by the forward bias and left-right step configuration of the BWI in this case study.

The fact there are few strong patterns of successive direction choice by the user is relatively re-assuring. If the data were to demonstrate strong pairings that were poorly supported by the BWI, then they may serve as a basis for further exploration. For example, if backwards was found to often precede forwards, then an examination of the effective control of reversing may be provoked.

23.3.6 Path Profiles

Path profiles were explored as a way of obtaining an overview of the data. Since usage log is recording movement within a wheelchair, depicting the movements taken can contribute to understanding its usage in an holistic manner. Ideally viewing the profile may provoke specific questions regarding the nature of use that can be treated in a more systematic manner. Mapping logs back to a graphical depiction of the path taken is particularly difficult since there are various factors that influence the direction taken by the wheelchair that are not recorded. For example, uneven surfaces and differences in tyre pressure can influence the direction, rate of rotation and speed of the wheelchair.

To develop an estimated path profile from a log, it is divided into sub-paths, where there is a pause in movement of more than a minute. To aid comparison between sub-paths each is plotted independently starting in the same direction (northwards), and juxtaposed along an east-west axis. Finally, pauses in movement shorter than a minute are depicted by a cross on a path, with the size of the cross being proportional to length of the pause. The path profile of a selection of BWI activity is show in Figure 23.5.

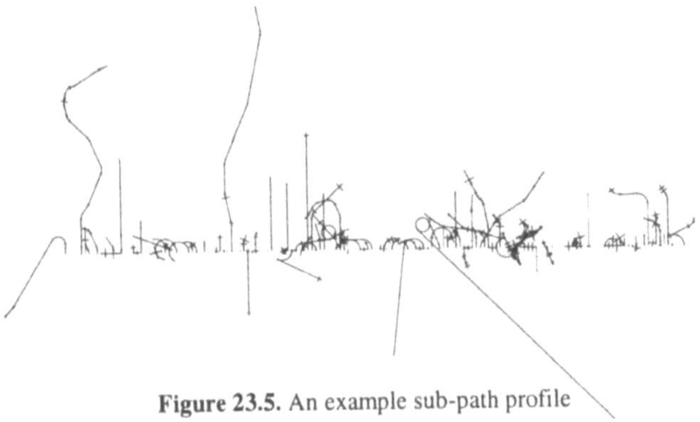

Figure 23.5. An example sub-path profile

The path profile can aid the inspection of diversity and commonality in the paths followed by the user. Taking Figure 23.5 as an example, the manner in which the user orientates and travels is easily observed. It is of interest to see where local orientation takes place; it appears that most dramatic orientation activity occurs at the beginning of sub-paths. This may serve as an indication of the accuracy with which the system is being used; if the BWI configuration was a poor match for in terms of orientation accuracy, then one would expect to see more dramatic turns throughout a sub-path.

The use of path profiles, such as this, is highly exploratory and speculative. Observations drawn from the visualisation require careful consideration and experimentation with the visualisation. For instance, the claim about orientated accuracy is qualified by the sub-path definition employed (i.e. over a minute without movement). In fact, for the case study data examined the same characteristics appear to remain when longer sub-paths were examined.

23.4 Conclusions

This chapter has reviewed various applied log analysis techniques that have the potential to help enhance the prescription of assistive technology. The techniques provide a systematic and consistently re-usable information source that is rarely available to clinicians. Future work will expand these techniques and will focus upon the needs of practitioners engaged in assistive technology prescription. In particular, the analysis outcomes provide interesting data for discussion, and for the motivation of alternative analysis methods. However, within the context of prescription, the benefit of stable and comparable analyses outweighs the availability of sophisticated highly flexible tools. A more complex task of external validation of specific methods in terms of their utility and value will involve extensive consultation with rehabilitation professionals. The analysis methods described, and others, will serve as illustrations for consideration during this process.

23.5 References

Cherry AD, Cudd PA, Hawley MS (1996) Providing Rehabilitation Integrated Systems Using Existing Rehabilitation Technology. Medical Engineering and Physics 18(3)

Churchill S (1998) Greatly Increased Scanning Speed for Switch Users with Slow Reactions In: Procedings of ISAAC'98, Ashfield Publications Dublin, pp 451-452

Hawley MS, O'Neill P, Webb L (1999) A provisional framework and software tools to aid the prescription of electronic assistive technology: results of a case study. In: Assistive Technology on the Threshold of the New Millennium, ISO Press, pp 728-732

Hilbert DM, Redmiles DF (2000) Extracting Usability Information from User Interface Events. ACM Computing Surveys 32(4): 381-421

Keates S, Clarkson J, Robinson P (2000) Investigating the Applicability of User Models for Motion-Impaired Users. In: Proceedings of the 4th International ACM Conference on Assistive Technologies, ACM Press, pp 129-137

O'Neill P, Roast CR, Hawley MS (2000a) Evaluation of Scanning User Interfaces Using Real-Time Data Usage Logs. In: Proceedings of ASSETS 2000, ACM Press, pp 137-141

O'Neill P, Roast CR, Hawley MS (2000b) Evaluating and informing assistive technology from usage logs. In: Turner S, Turner P (eds.) Proceedings of the British HCI Group Conference, vol. II, pp 41-42

O'Neill P, Roast CR, Hawley MS (2001) Scanning User Interfaces: Evaluation Using Real-Time-Data Usage Logs. In: Avouris N, Fakotakis N (eds.) Proceedings of PC-HCI2001, pp 287-292

Rosen MJ, Goodenough-Trepagnier C (1989) The Tufts MIT Prescription Guide: Assessment of Users to predict the Suitability of Augmentative Communication Devices. Assistive Technology 1(3)

Vanderheiden GC (1988) A unified quantitative modeling approach for selection-based augmentative communication systems. The vocally impaired: clinical practice and research, pp 40-83

Zghan S, Ottenbacher KJ (2001) Single subject research designs for disability research. Disability and Rehabiliation 23(1): 1-8

Chapter 24

Virtual Interface Development and Sensor-based Door Navigation for Nonholonomic Vehicles

R.S. Rao, K. Conn, S.H. Jung, J. Katupitiya,
T. Kientz, V. Kumar, J. Ostrowski, S. Patel and
C.J. Taylor

24.1 Introduction

There are numerous examples of partially autonomous systems that are controlled at some level by a human operator or user. Generally control at the lowest levels is autonomous while the human user is primarily responsible for decision making at the highest levels. Examples of such systems include passenger automobiles, HVAC systems in buildings, CNC machines in job shops, and security systems. An important class of systems are mobile agents with embedded computers that are directly controlled by a human pilot or navigator in the loop. This chapter addresses (i) the design of interfaces between the human user and the computer-controlled system and (ii) the design of control algorithms that enable autonomous motion of the vehicle when desired. The performance of such human-in-the-loop systems is very sensitive to the persons ability to interact with the embedded computer and sensors (Rahman *et al.*, 1994).

Our main focus is on smart wheelchairs (Figure 24.1), devices that can potentially benefit over 15 million individuals in the U.S. alone. Current systems have very little computer control, except at the lowest levels of motor control. Interfaces are similar to those found in passenger cars. The rider has to continuously specify the direction, and in some cases, the velocity of the chair using a joystick like device. In cases where the level of neuro-muscular control is poor, joysticks are used to specify directions while the choice of speed is limited to either zero or a safe constant value.

There is extensive research on computer-controlled chairs where sensors and intelligent control algorithms have been used to minimize the level of human intervention (Levine *et al.*, 1990; Orpwood, 1990; Simpson *et al.*, 1999; Wagner *et al.*, 1999). Many efforts have used sensors and low-level controllers to guarantee safety by monitoring human commands that may cause chairs to approach risky states. Attempts to build autonomous chairs have faced many challenges, most of which stem from the lack of robustness of motion planning, perception, and control algorithms (Kumar *et al.*, 1997).

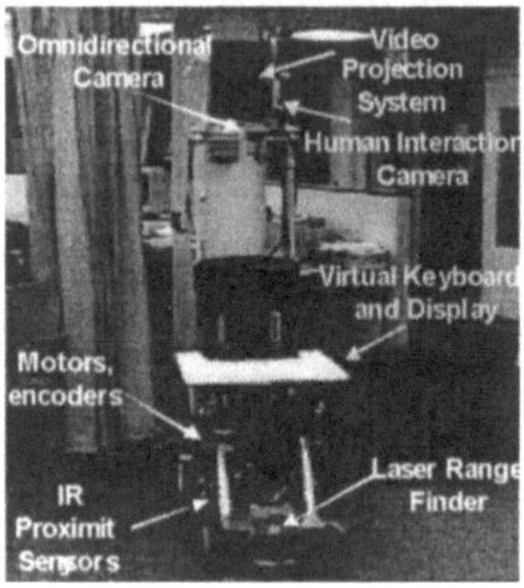

Figure 24.1. A view of the system showing the different components- the projector, the cameras, the motors and the laser

Our research goal is to design and develop a system that allows the user to robustly interact with the robot at different levels of the control and sensing hierarchy. At the lowest level, the user can drive the chair through conventional joystick-like interfaces. At a higher level, the user can select from a range of behaviors such as hallway navigation, or moving forward while avoiding obstacles. At an even higher level, the user should be able to specify goal positions while the system automatically selects behaviors and plans paths to guide the chair to the goal. In intelligent buildings, where maps are available through wireless networks, the user should be able to specify destinations on the map and the chair should be able to navigate to that location. Our smart wheelchair consists of a vision-based human robot interface, a suite of sensors, and a set of intelligent control algorithms that allow for computer-mediated motion control.

24.2 The *SmartChair* System

Figure 24.1 is a view of the system showing some of the components, including a video projector, cameras, laptop tray and laser rangefinder. The main components of the augmentative software and hardware system are shown in Figure 24.2. A standard PC mounted on the chair handles all the required processing. The motion control system consists of a 2 axis controller driving two 150W servomotors. These are coupled to the rear wheels via a 15:1 planetary gear head and a 7:1 belt drive. A digital encoder on each motor provides the feedback in the control loop. The power for the motors is currently obtained from two PWM brush type servo amplifiers.

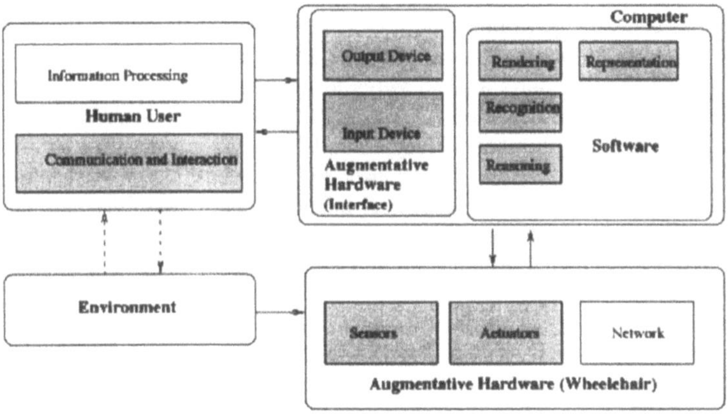

Figure 24.2. The main components and the architecture for the proposed interfaces. Shaded boxes show hardware and software components of interest, while solid arrows show information flow of interest.

24.3 Interfaces for Human-Robot Interaction

User input on the *SmartChair* is accomplished by projecting an image of the interface onto the lap tray, which is monitored by an overhead video camera. Figure 24.3a shows a view of this interface as seen by the user. By analyzing the images acquired from the video camera, the system is able to determine what the user is pointing to on the interface and to respond appropriately. Effectively, the projector and camera systems acting in concert form a feedback system where user interaction is effected by occluding various parts of the projected image.

The scheme hinges on the observation that the relationship between the three surfaces of interest, the work surface, the virtual interface and the image obtained by the camera can be characterized by projective transformations of $\mathbb{RP}^2$(Figure 24.3b). By definition the coordinates of a point in the frame buffer, (x_f, y_f), and the coordinates of its image on the screen, (x_s,y_s), are related by a projective transformation. This relationship can be expressed as $(x_s \; y_s \; 1)^T \; \alpha \; H_{sf}(x_f \; y_f \; 1)^T$ where $H_{sf} \in GL(3)$. Similarly, another projective transformation relates the positions of points on the screen to the coordinates of their projections on the video image, (x_i,y_i).

It is well known that a projective transformation is completely specified if its operation on a set of points which constitute a projective basis for the relevant projective space (in this case the real projective plane $\mathbb{RP}^2$) is known. This suggests a straightforward calibration scheme for determining the mapping between the frame and image buffers. Simply choose four distinguished points in the frame buffer such that no three are colinear, and then locate their correspondents in the image buffer. The projective transformation H_{if} can then be computed from these four point correspondences in a straightforward manner using standard techniques (Faugeras, 1993; Taylor, 1999).

The basic advantage of this vision based interaction technique is that it does not involve mechanical input devices such as keyboards, mice and touch screens. There are no moving parts and no wires to connect to the interface surface. By avoiding a physical instantiation of the interface we gain a level of abstraction that can be exploited in a number of ways. Firstly, the system designer is allowed to specify the layout and action of the user interface entirely in software without being constrained by a fixed mechanical interface. This flexibility can be used to customize interfaces to the needs and capabilities of individual users. Secondly, the interface can be switched off when not in use, freeing the laptray for other uses.

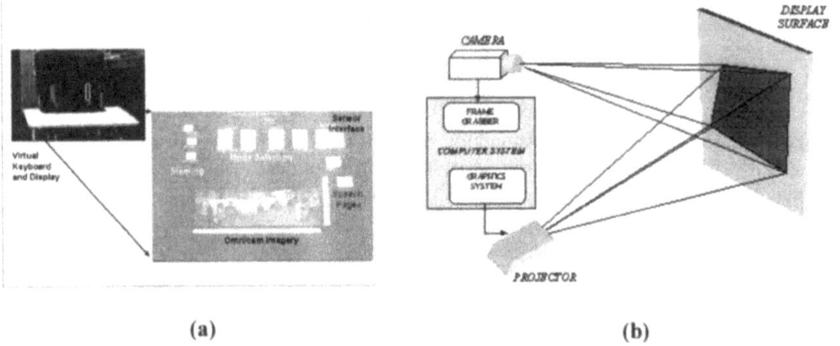

Figure 24.3. The interface as seen by the user, and the transformation of points from the world frame to the camera frame

24.4 Computer-Mediated Motion Control Interface

Figure 24.4 shows the architecture of the computer mediated motion control system. The system is organized into a three level hierarchy and the user interface allows the occupant to interact with the sensors and actuators at various levels. The lowest level of interaction corresponds to direct control of the servo motors and direct access to the sensor data. The second level corresponds to a set of control behaviors that the user can invoke selectively while the highest level of the hierarchy, the navigation level, corresponds to sequences of operations that ultimately guide the chair to a desired location.

The user can interact with the system at the lowest level via the interface shown in Figure 24.3a. The user can steer the chair around by occluding different icons to control the chair's motion.

At a higher level, the user can choose one of many control modes or behaviors (Figure 24.4). Modes are closely coupled perception-action loops with associated controllers and estimators. The control modes or behaviors that we have implemented on our *Smart Chair* include:

- go to relative position and orientation;
- go forward while avoiding obstacles;

- three-point turn (backing up and turning to avoid an obstacle in the front);
- go down the hallway following wall(s);
- navigate through a doorway; and
- make turns while avoiding obstacles.

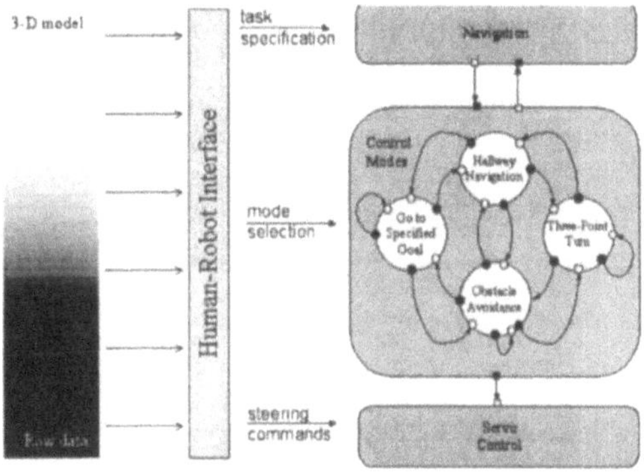

Figure 24.4. The Computer- Mediated control architecture for the system

The interface allows the user to select the desired mode of operation by pointing to buttons on the interface. These modes can also be combined in natural ways, for example the system can be made to avoid obstacles in its path while following hallways or corridors by invoking the obstacle avoidance and hallway following modes simultaneously.

One convenient feature of the interface is that it allows the user to select target locations in the scene by pointing to regions in the unwarped omnidirectional image. For instance, the user can specify a target for the doorway navigation algorithm by selecting two vertical lines in the image. The user can also select arbitrary destinations in the scene for the Go To mode by pointing to locations in the image. This image based human robot interaction provides a powerful, intuitive and convenient mechanism for registering the users intention with the systems sensory devices (cameras and range finders).

There is also a natural "undo" action that is reminiscent of the undo operation in human computer interfaces (Eberst *et al.*, 2000). Sometimes a user might find himself in a corner, without enough room for the system to execute a turn. With this situation in mind, a *Retrace* mode has been added. In this mode the wheelchair returns to its starting point along the same path that it took to get to the current position. Of course, the user has the option to take over control of the system in any emergency or at any point during the retrace maneuver.

The *SmartChair* also allows the occupant to communicate with others through a speech board interface. The interface is divided into a set of pages each of which contains a collection of interactive icons that have been mapped to common phrases used in daily conversation. The occupant communicates by pointing to appropriate icons on the interface that causes the computer to generate the phrase through a speech synthesizer. It is envisioned that such an interface would be useful to persons who have impaired speech but reasonable motor control abilities.

24.5 System Model

In order to analyze the system and develop controllers, we place an inertial coordinate frame at the center of the doorway, with its y-axis aligned with the doorway and x-axis pointing through the door (see Figure 24.5). The heading of the robot, θ, is chosen to be measured with respect to the x-axis. This coordinate frame is slightly unintuitive, but has the advantage that the goal position is the origin, $(x, y, \theta) = (0,0,0)$. Notice, though, that in this coordinate frame the robot's position will generally have $x < 0$.

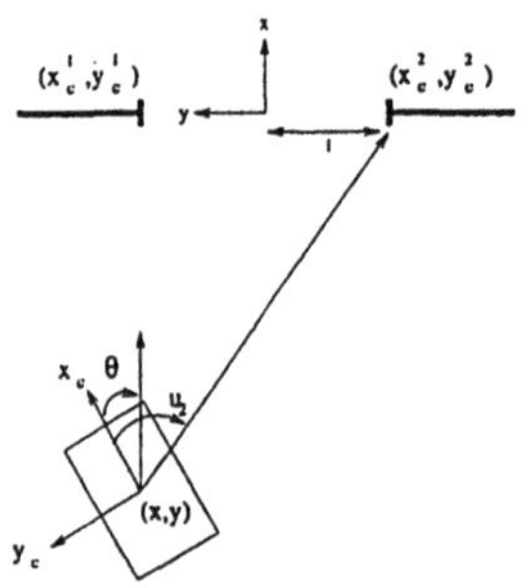

Figure 24. 5. Coordinate Frames of the System

We use as a model for our system a two-wheeled, nonholonomic cart-like robot, with position referenced by the center of the two wheels. A nonholonomic system is one in which the kinematics are expressible with differential relationships only. By contrast, the kinematics of a holonomic system, like a robot arm, can be expressed by algebraic relationships. For this model, which represents the wheelchair's motion quite well, the governing equations are well known:

$$\dot{x} = v\cos\theta \ ; \ \dot{y} = v\sin\theta \ ; \ \dot{\theta} = \omega \qquad (24.1; 2; 3)$$

where the inputs are the forward velocity, v, and angular velocity, ω; (x,y) are the Cartesian coordinates of the center of mass; and θ is the orientation angle with respect to an inertial frame.

The imaging model is based on Cyclovision's omnidirectional camera. In servoing to doors, we make special use of the fact that two strong vertical lines in the image plane characterize doorways. For this reason, we only utilize the projection to the image plane of vertical lines. For a camera mounted on a planar robot, this implies that each feature (vertical line) can be thought of as having a projection to a single point in the image space (this will of course work for other projective models as well). With this assumption, a vertical line can be described by its coordinates in the inertial frame, say (x_f, y_f). If we denote by u the azimuth angle to which the vertical line is projected in the image plane, and write the location of the line in terms of a camera coordinate frame (coinciding with the body reference frame of the robot), (x_c, y_c), $u = atan2(y_c, x_c)$, where

$$\begin{pmatrix} x_c \\ y_c \end{pmatrix} = \begin{pmatrix} \cos\theta & \sin\theta \\ -\sin\theta & \cos\theta \end{pmatrix} \begin{pmatrix} x_f - x \\ y_f - y \end{pmatrix} \tag{24.4}$$

and (x, y, θ) describes the robot's current pose in the inertial frame.

If we denote the locations of the door edges to be at $(0, \pm l)$, then the two edges will project to

$$u_1 = \tan^{-1}\left(\frac{x\sin\theta + (l-y)\cos\theta}{-x\cos\theta + (l-y)\sin\theta}\right); \quad u_2 = \tan^{-1}\left(\frac{x\sin\theta - (l+y)\cos\theta}{-x\cos\theta - (l+y)\sin\theta}\right) \tag{24.5; 6}$$

where u_1 denotes the left-hand door edge, and u_2 the edge on the right. We note that using this information alone, we cannot determine the inertial position of the robot. However, merging this data with the laser range data, we will be able to extract a pose from the data that can be used for pose-based servoing. We will return to the issue of image-based servoing in Section 24.7.1.

24.6 Pose Estimation and Prediction

Three sensors are used to estimate relative position of the robot with respect to the target. Sensor measurements from the different modalities are then fused to produce a unique representation of the target. The omnidirectional camera is aligned with the laser scanner so that each measurement taken can be combined with the azimuth angle of the target. The physical offset, $(x_{off}, y_{off}, \delta_{off})$, between the two sensors is used to form a transformation function which maps depth and azimuth angle estimates from the laser scanner to the corresponding azimuth angle on the image. Given (r_i, ϕ_i) from the laser scanner, the corresponding azimuth angle on the image is calculated by:

$$\begin{pmatrix} x_{im} \\ y_{im} \\ 1 \end{pmatrix} = \begin{pmatrix} \cos\delta_{off} & -\sin\delta_{off} & x_{off} \\ \sin\delta_{off} & \cos\delta_{off} & y_{off} \\ 0 & 0 & 1 \end{pmatrix} \begin{pmatrix} x_{laser} \\ y_{laser} \\ 1 \end{pmatrix}; \quad \begin{pmatrix} x_{laser} \\ y_{laser} \\ 1 \end{pmatrix} = \begin{pmatrix} r_i\cos\phi_i \\ r_i\sin\phi_i \\ 1 \end{pmatrix} \tag{24.7; 8}$$

The offset is obtained by direct measurements. In our case, the offset is (12 cm, 45 cm, 2.6°).

The odometry is used to predict the target position with respect to the inertial coordinate system during navigation. The vision system collects 360 degree view images and unwarps them into panoramic images where the vertical lines are preserved. The target vertical lines marked by the user on the initial state (drawn as two boxes on the unwarped image in Figure 24.6) are tracked to give the target's relative azimuth position. The tracked azimuth angles are combined with depth measurements from the laser scanner to produce relative pose estimates.

The laser sensor can generate depth information at 0.5° increments through horizontal scanning. The vertical line extraction from vision, along with odometric predictions, is used to guide the initial search of the depth map to find discontinuities characteristic of a doorway. This is shown in Figure 24.6, where the dashed vertical lines show the matching of the image and laser data. The azimuth value of the discontinuities is coupled with depth to update the estimate of target position and is correlated with the estimates from the vision to reject bad data. Each estimate calculated from the image and the laser sensor is updated with odometry and the relative position estimate used to predict and update the target position:

$$\begin{pmatrix}\hat{x}(k)\\ \hat{y}(k)\end{pmatrix}=-\begin{pmatrix}\Delta X(k)\\ \Delta Y(k)\end{pmatrix}+\begin{pmatrix}\cos(\Delta\theta(k)) & \sin(\Delta\theta(k))\\ -\sin(\Delta\theta(k)) & \cos(\Delta\theta(k))\end{pmatrix}\begin{pmatrix}x(k-1)\\ y(k-1)\end{pmatrix};\ \Delta\theta(k)=\theta(k)-\theta(k-1) \quad (24.9;\ 10)$$

where $(\hat{x}(k),\hat{y}(k))$ are the predicted target position and $(\Delta X(k),\Delta Y(k),\Delta\theta(k))$are the odometry values at time k.

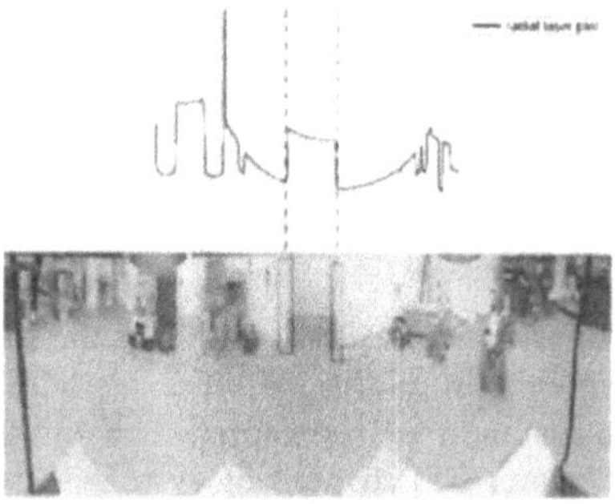

Figure 24.6. Laser (top) and unwarped image (bottom) matching

24.7 Controllers

A wide variety of possible methods for controlling such a system exist, e.g. work by Canudas de Wit and Sordalen (1992). Topological restrictions (often referred to as Brockett's necessary condition) place certain limits on the achievable tasks using smooth, static state feedback. For this reason, we generally pursued controllers that did not seek to stabilize to the origin, but rather whose goal was to drive the robot through the center of the doorway by converging to the x-axis defined by the doorway (see Figure 24.5). Additionally, we explored the use of image-based switched controllers, since these have the potential to provide better overall performance. We describe in brief here a switched, image-based controller.

24.7.1 An Image-based, Switching Controller

Instead of relying on a simple pose-based controller to do the servoing, we explored the potential of an image-based controller that did not rely so severely on depth. This controller uses two basic types of feedback modes: one attempts to maintain one of the features in a fixed location, usually at or near the boundary of the sensor, and the other relies on centering the robot between the two features. Thus, the first controller is used to steer the robot towards (and through) the middle of the doorway, while the second is used to drive the robot through the doorway.

In order to explore these two controllers in more detail, let us look at the effect of the controls on the motion of the features in the image plane. Using the projective model given in Equations 24.5 and 24.6, combined with the equations of motion for the robot (Equations 24.1, 24.2 and 24.3), we find (after some interesting algebraic simplifications) that the equations governing the motion of the features, (u_1, u_2) are:

$$\dot{u}_1 = -\omega + \frac{v}{z_1}\sin u_1 \;;\; \dot{u}_2 = -\omega + \frac{v}{z_2}\sin u_2 \qquad (24.11;\ 12)$$

where z_1 is the distance from the camera to the vertical line being tracked, given by

$$z_1^2 = x^2 + (l - y)^2 \qquad (24.13)$$

(and respectively, $z_2^2 = x^2 + (l + y)^2$). The two proposed controllers can be derived in a straightforward fashion from Equations 24.11 and 24.12 and are discussed individually in detail in the literature (Patel *et al.*, 2002).

The switching controller works quite well in simulation and in practice. In Figure 24.7, we plot the simulation results from a variety of initial conditions. We have not included detailed simulation data for any single run, only because the differences from the experimental data presented below are unremarkable.

In the case that the field of view constraint is not very strict, we see that the first controller is able to steer easily into the center region, at which point the centering control law takes over. The exception to this is when the robot starts out very close to the doorway, as is seen in the simulation results with initial conditions (x,y) = (-500,2000)mm. In this case, the robot cannot fully approach the center line while simultaneously satisfying the sensor constraints. We will return to this case in Section 24.7.2. However, we note that this occurs only for very narrow field-of-view constraints or in situations where the robot is placed at a very shallow angle to the door, which is not generally realistic for doorway navigation scenarios.

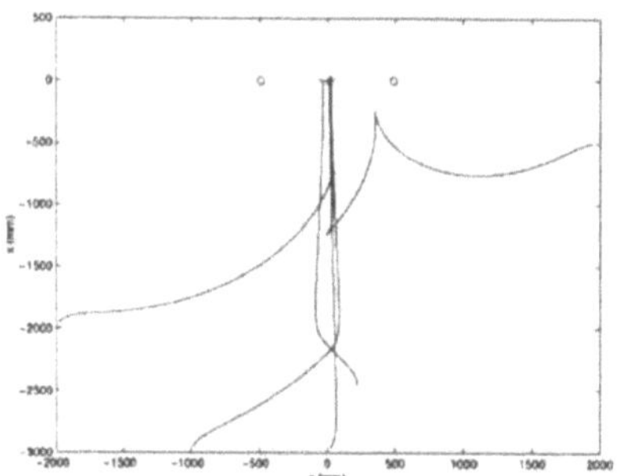

Figure 24.7. Simulation results from a variety of initial conditions

Figure 24.8 shows similar results for the experiment. The left plot shows the (*x*, *y*) position, both given through odometry estimates (dashed curve) and for estimates based on the combined image and laser data (jagged curve). It also shows the curve produced when the data from the different sensors is combined. Note that the pose estimates from the laser and vision data alone, even if outliers were to be removed, are clearly very noisy and were found to be unsuitable for controlling the robot. Likewise, the odometry estimates also cannot be relied on directly since the drift due to the heading error, although small, is unacceptable. Thus, the gradient method proves to be succesful in incorporating the raw information into information that will allow the wheelchair to proceed through the doorway. The key here is to properly mix the relative pose information from odometry with the noisy absolute pose data from the laser range finder. The right plot shows the image features (u_1, u_2) and their center value.

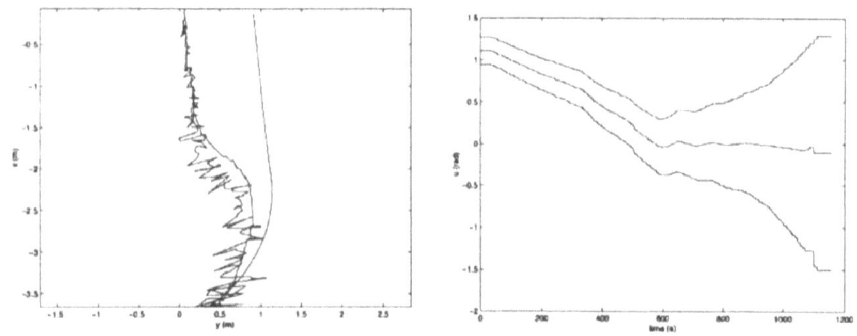

Figure 24.8. Experiment using a switched controller

24.7.2 Obstacle Avoidance

We have implemented a simple obstacle avoidance algorithm on our platform. Although we have yet to prove completeness conclusively, we believe that this will be case under certain basic assumptions about the initial configuration and the free path leading to the doorway. Thus, when the laser senses an object in front of the wheelchair, it sends signals to the controller so that the obstacle avoidance algorithm is activated. The chair smoothly avoids the obstacle by going around it while also continuing towards the doorway destination. During obstacle avoidance, the robot is guided by the new direction, which is the sum of the original heading direction from the controller and the repulsive direction from the obstacle. As long as one of the doorway edges is sensed, the chair is able to move forward towards it. Of course if both edges are obstructed or there isn't enough space for the wheelchair to get through, it will not be able to continue. However, in cases where an edge is visible and there is enough space, the wheelchair is able to navigate through the doorway. See Figure 24.9.

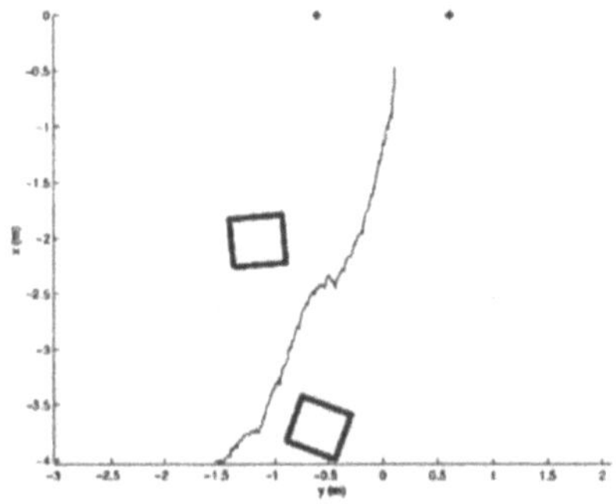

Figure 24.9. Experimental trial of obstacle avoidance

24.8 Discussion and Future Work

We have designed a user interface to allow the wheelchair operator to either control the vehicle or take higher level decisions such as selecting doorway features. A possible enhancement will be to have the computer pre-process the image to highlight possible doorways to make the selection by the user even easier.

We also note that the issues arising in doing visual servoing with nonholonomic robots and image-plane constraints lead to some very interesting challenges. We have chosen a switched controller feedback approach that shows a good deal of promise in tackling these general issues. In many ways we feel this parallels the work of Cowan and Koditschek (1999), where a navigation function approach is used for an omnidirectional robot. The present switched controller provides one potential mechanism for solving this same problem in the presence of nonholonomic constraints. The interface and the software can be adapted to the user and to the level of disability. We believe that the vision-based control interface and the paradigm of computer-mediated motion control are applicable to a large class of smart embedded systems and have the potential to increase the level of access to such systems.

Our future work is directed in two different directions. First we will integrate our system with databases that can be made available through a wireless network and access to the internet. The user can download maps describing buildings and streets, and the onboard sensors (cameras, laser range finders, GPS) must allow the user to designate destinations at the highest navigation level. Second, we are interested in pursuing feedback from potential users and working toward the next design with a view of developing a more practical, aesthetically appealing prototype. We also aim to address the challenge of using this device outdoors, which might lead to changes in the basic design of the system, though the philosophy of interaction with a high-level interface will remain unchanged. We are also tempted to investigate how the use of advanced joysticks, such as force feedback joysticks, will contribute towards making the system more user- friendly.

We must note however that the scope of our work is limited in one sense. We address interfaces for legacy systems, computer-controlled wheelchairs and typical human-made environments. Obviously if homes were redesigned to accomodate smart mobility systems and mobility systems could be designed to work in smart homes, some of these issues would be addressed very differently.

24.9 Acknowledgments

The authors would like to acknowledge the grants (US 0083240 and DUE 9979635) provided by the National Science Foundation for this research effort. They would also like to acknowledge Ian Glaser's help in building the system hardware.

24.10 References

Canudas deWit C, Sordalen OJ (1992) Exponential stabilization of mobile robots with nonholonomic constraints. IEEE Transactions on Automatic Control, 37: 1791-1797

Cowan NJ, Koditschek (1999) DE Planar image based visual servoing as a navigation problem. In: Proceedings of the IEEE International Conference on Robotics and Automation, pp 611-617

Eberst C, Anderson M, Christensen HI (2000) Vision based door traversal for autonomous mobile robots. In: Proceedings of the 2000 IEEE/RSJ International Conference on Intelligent Robots and Systems

Faugeras O (1993) Three- Dimensional Computer Vision. MIT Press

Kumar V, Rahman T, Krovi V (1997) Assistive devices for people with motor disabilities. Wiley Encyclopedia for Electrical and Electronic Engineers

Levine S, Koren Y, Borenstein J (1990) Navchair control system for automatic assistive wheelchair navigation. In: Proceedings of the 13th Annual RESNA International Conference, Washington, DC, RESNA Press, pp 193-194

Orpwood RD (1990) Design methodology for aids for the disabled. Journal of Medical Engineering and Technology 14(1): 2-10

Patel S, Jung SH, Ostrowski J, Rao RS, Taylor CJ (2002) Sensor Based Door Navigation for a Nonholonomic Vehicle. Submitted to the IEEE International Conference on Robotics and Automation (ICRA), Washington, DC

Rahman T, Harwin W, Chen S, Mahoney R (1994) Rehabilitation robot control with enhanced sensory feedback. In: Proceedings of the 4th International Conference on Rehabilitation and Robotics, pp 43-48

Simpson R, Poirot D, Baxter MF (1999) Evaluation of the hephaestus smart wheelchair system. In: Proceedings of International Conference on Rehabilitation Robotics, Stanford University, pp 99-105

Taylor CJ (1999) Virtual keyboards. Technical report, Department of Computer and Information Science, University of Pennsylvania

Wagner JJ, Van der Loos HFM, Smaby N, Chang K, Burgar C (1999) Provar assistive robot interface. In: Proceedings of International Conference on Rehabilitation Robotics, Stanford University, pp 250-254

Chapter 25

An Ergonomic One-handed Wheelchair

L.A. Porter and S. Lesley

25.1 Introduction

Some people with hemiplegia (paralysis down one side of the body) are unable to walk, so they need a wheelchair. But the standard manual wheelchair is designed for people with two active hands. If operated with only one hand, the chair tends to veer towards the patient's inactive side with each push of the handrim. Some hospitals teach a technique for coping, in which patients correct their direction of travel by continually 'walking' their active foot on the ground while applying a corrective sideways push. It works, but is slow and undignified, (Kirby *et al.*, 1999). There are also problems with turning (Kitano *et al.*, 1997).

Special one-handed wheelchairs are available: those that incorporate two handrims on one side (dual handrims), and those that use a reciprocating lever. But both types have major design faults.

The dual-handrim drive requires the user to grip both handrims with one hand, and rotate them simultaneously through the same angle at the same angular velocity. Hence, travelling in a straight line is not easy, and is stressful on the hand and wrist. Even worse, when driving around a bend, the handrims have to be rotated at different angular velocities; the left handrim operating the right wheel and the right handrim operating the left wheel! Consequently, tight bends are very difficult to achieve.

The lever mechanism drives only one wheel, and does so via a reversible one-way clutch. Hence, each thrust of the lever tends to make the wheelchair veer away from the intended line, requiring continual adjustment of the steering. Also, the lever load increases significantly when driving around a bend towards the lever side of the chair, which limits the minimum radius of turn on that side. Similarly, the lever brakes only one wheel, which makes the chair veer to that side when braking. Also, an additional mechanism is required to switch the one-way clutch between forward and backward motions.

Electrically-driven wheelchairs are one solution; but they are expensive, and are not permitted in some retirement homes and day-care centres. For these places, and for users who like to take some exercise, a manual wheelchair is preferred. Also, manual wheelchairs are smaller and lighter, and can be folded or dismantled and put in the boot/trunk of a car.

Hence there is still a need for a suitable manual hemiplegic wheelchair, which is safe, ergonomic and easy to learn.

Table 25.1. Functional specification

Demand/ Wish	Weighting	Feature
		OPERATION
		Able to:
D		- Travel in a straight line forwards and backwards
D		- Steer when going forwards
W	3	- Steer when going backwards
W	3	- Turn with a minimum radius of 600 mm
W	3	- Pirouette
D		- Brake in a straight line
D		- Brake progressively
D		- Brake without delay in an emergency
D		Parking brake controllable by both user and attendant
D		Can be pushed by attendant
D		Footrests to clear a kerb
D		Usable indoors and outdoors
W	3	Propulsion, steering and braking to be intuitive
W	2	Usable on unpaved surfaces
W	1	Switchable left and right-sided operation
		ERGONOMICS
D		Suitable for 5th to 95th percentile adults
D		Easy to transfer user in/out of wheelchair
W	3	No change of hand position between propelling and steering
W	3	No change of hand position between propelling and braking
W	3	Maximises use of muscles
W	3	Encourages good posture
W	3	No need to look at the controls
W	3	Does not soil the user's hands or clothing

Table 25.1. (cont.) Functional specification

D/W	Weighting	Feature
		GEOMETRY
D		Fits in car boot/trunk
W	3	Maximum width 660 mm
W	3	Same length as standard manual wheelchair
		SAFETY
D		Safe to use
D		Stable on 16*f* incline
W	3	No finger traps
		STORAGE
W	3	May be folded
		FORCES
W	3	Handrim force less than dual-handrim hemiplegic wheelchair
W	3	Suitable for persons weighing 38 - 115 kg
W	3	Wheelchair weight less than 23 kg
		ENERGY
W	3	Maximises efficiency
W	3	Needs no electric power
W	3	Allows optional input from hemiplegic side
		COSTS
W	2	Maximum sale price £600
W	3	Non-rusting
		PRODUCTION
D		Prototype manufacturable in University workshops
W	3	Suitable for batch production
W	3	Add-on unit to existing models
		QUALITY
D		BS ISO 7176-1:1999, BS 6937:1998, BS 6935-5:1998
		LIFETIME
W	3	Ten years life
		MAINTENANCE
W	3	Maintenance less than once per year

25.2 The Solution

25.2.1 Brainstorming

A functional specification was drawn up, Table 25.1, and used as a prompt for ideas during extensive brainstorming. In addition to the spontaneous production of specification requirements, based on knowledge learned from wheelchair users, attendants and common sense, a more structured approach was also employed. This used a template to ensure that a wide range of relevant fields was included in the process.

The most promising idea was one with a differential gear drive and foot steering, Figure 25.1. It provides straight-line propulsion via a single handrim, and steering via the patient's foot. In addition, the wheelchair may be pirouetted on the spot, again using only one handrim.

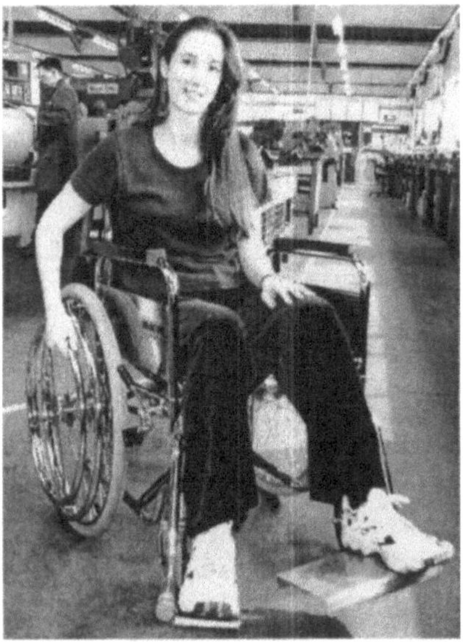

Figure 25.1. The ergonomic one-handed wheelchair

A differential allows a single handrim to propel both drive wheels in such a way that they each receive the same torque. This gives the wheelchair a strong tendency to go in a straight line without continual adjustment of the steering. However, by adding a steering mechanism to one of the two front wheels, the wheelchair can also be steered freely in any direction, because the differential allows the two drive wheels to rotate at different speeds. In stroke-induced hemiplegia, the user has full use of one foot, so it is convenient to use foot steering.

A differential also has another advantage: if the central member is locked with a brake, and a second handrim is attached directly to the drive wheel on the active side of the wheel-chair, then forward rotation of the second handrim causes rearward rotation of the opposite drive wheel. This makes the wheelchair pirouette on the spot - a feature which the authors believe to be unique. Pirouetting produces very compact turns, and is particularly useful in confined spaces.

Superficially, the new wheelchair looks just like the old dual-handrim hemiplegic wheelchair. However, it works very differently: one handrim provides only forward and rearward motion, and the other provides only a pirouetting motion. And because only one handrim is used at any time, there is far less stress on the user's hand and wrist, and the handrims are far more intuitive and easy to use. Also, it has foot steering.

Steering around a bend, left or right, has no effect on the force required to drive the outer handrim.

25.2.2 The Propulsion Mechanism

Figure 25.2 shows a transverse cross-section of the differential. The planet carrier carries three compound planets. By making the gear ratio between the larger planet (27t) and the annulus (54t) the same as the gear ratio between the smaller planet (9t) and the sun (18t), the torque generated in the annulus is the same as the torque generated in the sun. Hence, if the annulus drives the adjacent wheel and the sun drives the opposite wheel, then both wheels receive the same driving torque - equal to half the input torque. This drives the wheelchair in a straight line, using only a single handrim, without the need for any steering. The user can then relax with both feet on a fixed footrest.

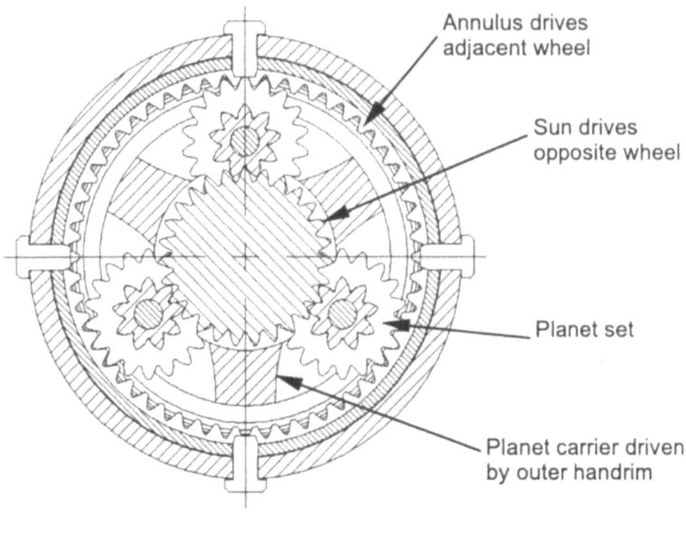

Figure 25.2. Cross-section of the differential (Scale approx. 1.3×)

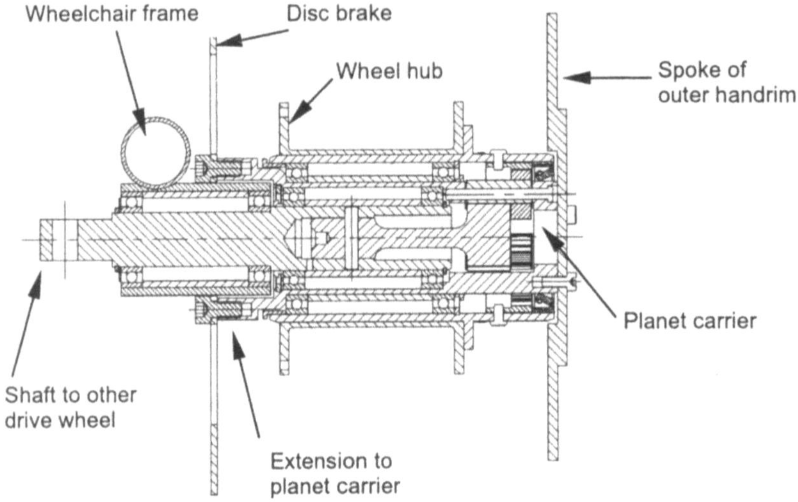

Figure 25.3. Longitudinal section of the differential

Figure 25.3 shows a longitudinal cross-section. The planet carrier passes through the wheel hub and out of the other side. On the other side, a bicycle disc brake is attached to it. When this brake is applied, the planet carrier is prevented from rotating. So, if one driving wheel is rotated forward, then the other driving wheel rotates rearward, causing the wheelchair to pirouette about a point mid-way between the two driving wheels. For convenience, another handrim is attached to the adjacent driving wheel for pirouetting.

To initiate a pirouette, the pirouette lever is moved to lock the disc brake, and the user transfers their hand from the outer (propulsion) handrim to the inner (pirouette) handrim. Their active foot is moved to the fixed footplate to allow the steerable castor to move freely.

The pirouette lever is placed beside the single parking brake. When both levers are operated, both wheels become locked. Hence the pirouette lever also acts as a parking brake.

25.2.3 The Steering Mechanism

Because the propulsion mechanism provided no steering, an independent means of steering was required. Foot steering was chosen because users with hemiplegia still have one active foot, which can provide enough force and control for the purpose.

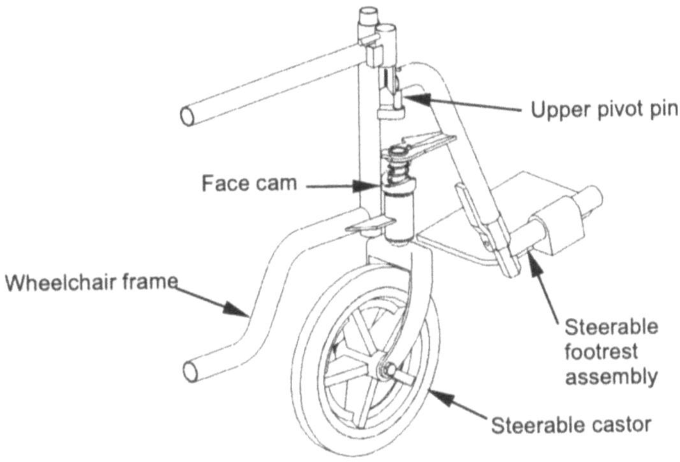

Figure 25.4. Foot-steering mechanism

Foot steering is not required during pirouetting, and is optional when going straight, either forwards of backwards; so the fixed footrest for the inactive foot is made wide enough to allow the user to rest their active foot beside the inactive foot when not steering. Hence the mechanism has to allow the steerable footrest to engage and disengage at various times.

A general view of the foot steering is shown in Figure 25.4. (For clarity, other parts of the wheelchair are not shown.) The steerable footrest assembly can translate along and swivel about a vertical axis through the castor stem and the upper pivot pin. The footrest is normally kept in its upper (disengaged) position by a spring, Figure 25.5.

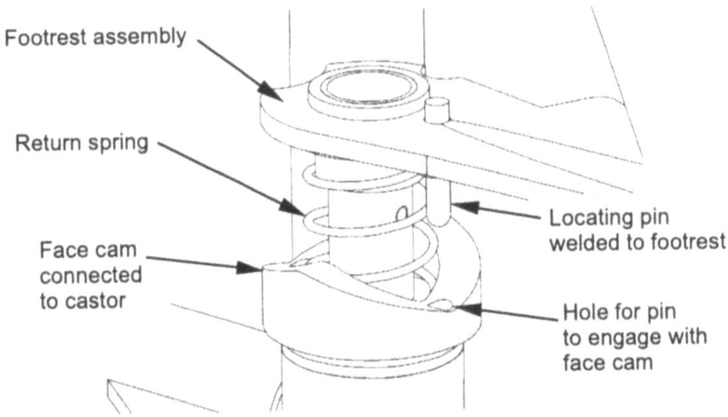

Figure 25.5. Face-cam with footrest disengaged

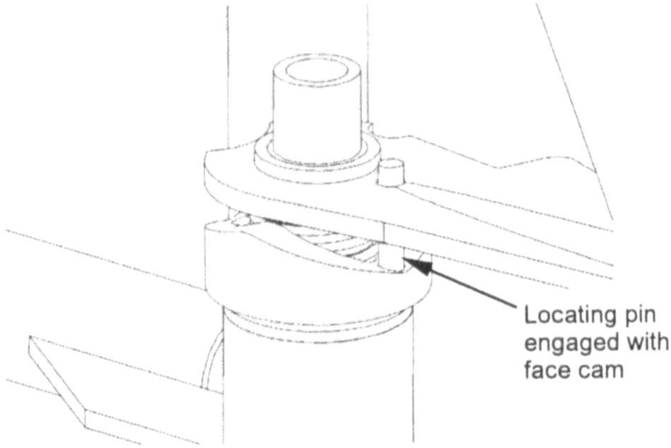

Figure 25.6. Face-cam with footrest engaged

When the user places their foot on the steerable footrest, the weight of the leg compresses the spring and the footrest descends. As the locating pin slides down the flank of the cam, the castor and footrest are moved into alignment, and the locating pin then engages with the hole, Figure 25.6. Swivelling the foot and footplate then causes swivelling of the castor, which steers the wheelchair.

When going backwards, it is easier to steer if the steerable castor trails in the normal way. For this reason, the face cam has two sets of cams and two holes, arranged 180° apart, allowing the steering to engage even after the castor has swivelled through 180°. A minimum turn radius of 600 mm is achievable.

When the foot steering is disengaged, the steerable footrest is locked in a straight-ahead position by the docking pin entering the docking plate, Figure 25.7. The footplate may be detached by lifting it further.

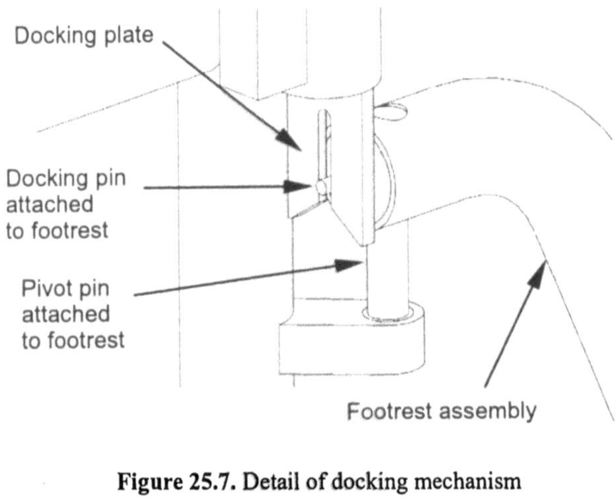

Figure 25.7. Detail of docking mechanism

25.3 Test Results

25.3.1 Clinical Staff Trials

Initial back-to-back trials against a dual-handrim hemiplegic wheelchair were conducted by three clinical staff from Addenbrooke's Disablement Services Centre. Their comments included: "The idea is sound," and "Using only one handrim at a time requires less mental effort, and is therefore an advantage with stroke patients." The staff believed that the new design could offer hemiplegic patients "a viable alternative" to a standard (non-hemiplegic) wheelchair and so extends the range of available options.

However, there were also criticisms: too much force to engage the steering, too much lateral movement of the foot when steering, too much force to initiate a pirouette from the straight-ahead position, too much backlash when parked. These criticisms are valid and will be addressed in the next prototype.

25.3.2. Able-bodied User Trials

Five able-bodied users tested the prototype against a dual-handrim hemiplegic wheelchair over a series of tests. The comparative tests covered a broad range of issues, from "Ease and intuitiveness of use" to "Energy required for use" and "Manoeuvrability." The testers were then asked to complete a questionnaire. All of them preferred the prototype. On average the prototype scored 50% higher than the dual-handrim wheelchair.

25.4 Conclusions

25.4.1 General

The prototype has demonstrated a design of manual hemiplegic wheelchair which far exceeded the existing designs, both in performance (range of motions possible) and usability (ergonomic and intuitive ease of use).

Dual-handrim hemiplegic wheelchairs often remain in hospital cupboards because they do not meet the users' needs. This design provides a means of adapting these unused wheelchairs so that they become fit for use.

25.4.2 Advantages of the New Design

The foot-controlled steering mechanism, together with the differential unit, solve many of the problems suffered by the existing manual hemiplegic wheelchair options:

- more ergonomic, intuitive and easier to learn;
- straight-line travel is easier and does not require continual steering on level ground;
- steering is independent of propulsion;
- propulsion and braking are via hand-rims;
- only one hand-rim is gripped at any time - easier than gripping two;
- braking is applied equally to both drive wheels, with no tendency to veer to the side;
- both parking-brake levers are on the same side of the chair;
- a longer propulsive arc is possible than with dual-handrim hemiplegic wheelchairs;
- pirouetting is possible;
- no ‘gear-shifting’ is needed between forward and reverse travel;
- more compact than reciprocating-lever hemiplegic wheelchairs;
- recycling of redundant dual-handrim hemiplegic wheelchairs may be possible.

25.4.3 Disadvantages of the New Design

- costs more than dual-handrim hemiplegic models;
- unusable by people who do not have one active leg.

25.5 The Next Step

Further development work is needed to overcome the limitations listed in Section 3.1. This may require another prototype. Trials with hemiplegic patients will then be conducted. Also, CE and Medical Devices Agency approvals must be obtained. Separate patent applications have been submitted for the foot steering and the differential. A licensing agreement for manufacture is currently being investigated.

25.6 References

Kirby RL, Ethans KD, Duggan RE, Saunders-Green LA, Lugar JA, Harrison ER (1999) Wheelchair propulsion: descriptive comparison of hemiplegic and two-handed patterns during selected activities. American Journal of Physical Medicine and Rehabilitation

Kitano Y (1997) Necessary turning area for single arm and single leg driven wheel-chair. In: Proceedings of the 12th Japanese Conference of Advancement of Rehabilitation Technology, vol. 12, pp 19-22

Chapter 26

Gathering User Needs in the Development of the POWER-HAND Opening Aid – A Successful Consumer Product for the Wider Market

J. Smith, R. Huxley, M. Topping, S. Alcock and P. Hawkins

26.0 Abstract

How can we improve the chances of success of future products during the development process? This should be one of the foremost questions during the formulation of a project plan and the conceptualisation of a new product. Without commercial initiative from the start, many research projects fail to reap the rewards that are associated with successful implementation of genuine ideas.

The aims of this chapter are to offer an insight into our experiences in the gathering of user needs for the development of a new assistive product, POWER-HAND, a consumer kitchen appliance currently being developed from concept to commercial reality. Developed as part of the PACKAGE project (Provision for improved lifestyles via Access to Consumer pacKAGEs), funded by the European Commission IST programme, the aim of the finished product is to improve access to a wide range of packaging types, for a wide range of users. Throughout the designers have relied upon a close and ongoing relationship with end-users in order to deliver a successful product.

26.1 Introduction

The PACKAGE project began in February 2000 with set deliverables to improve access to consumer packaging. There are two main areas within the project:

- To develop three new technical products that provide access to packaging for a wide range of consumers, POWER-HAND being the basic model. The two further models, MAGIC-HAND and TELE-HAND, offer automated opening and integrate into both care home and the forthcoming SmartHome environments.

- To develop simple modifications to consumer packaging so that they are more easily openable. The packaging industry craves new ideas and the opportunity to increase market share leads to constant innovation – however this innovation commonly leads to problems for many users who have physical and mental impairments. PACKAGE has developed innovative packaging and collaborated with some of the worlds largest manufacturers to facilitate change.

There are few assistive products on the market that are designed for wider use. Many assistive products, however effective, continue to stigmatise users with their bland design a fact often commented on by some of the users in our trials. The retail window for many of these devices remains isolated within the pages of 'Care Catalogues', available exclusively to care homes and centres and often our trial candidates were not aware of the range of devices available.

Our methods of gathering user needs and interpreting the results to form successful products have been well proven over the last 10 years, notably through our work with Handy 1, a robotic aid to independence for the severely disabled.

In order for POWER-HAND to succeed as a useful and sellable product, an effective development strategy was adopted from selecting a variety of potential end-users and product champions to managing the risk of showing the product early in it's development. Through our user-led strategy, POWER-HAND has accelerated from an outline brief to a protected production prototype in 18 months.

26.2 Objectives of the POWER-HAND User Requirements Analysis

The User requirements phase lasted for twelve months. In order to create a user-centred design process, work began prior to the start of the project to identify various disability groups and invitations were sent asking disability group representatives to attend a User Needs Workshop held in the second week of the project.

The main objectives of the user requirements analysis for the POWER-HAND product were to:

- quantify the difficulties which disabled and elderly people encounter with consumer packaging;
- identify disabled and elderly groups and invite them to participate in the project as major players;
- establish the characteristics of the various users;
- hold a two-day workshop to learn about the specific problems of various disability groups with regard to packaging;
- form a User Group Forum (UGF), which will retain a permanent presence in the project as an evaluation group and will attend relevant meetings;
- initiate low tech solutions for opening existing packages;

- provide a basis for the technical and functional specifications for development;
- gather data which will satisfy designers, commercial and market interests.

26.3 Methodology

An important aim of the PACKAGE project is to develop a mainstream product which will be of use to both disabled and able-bodied persons. In order to adopt 'Design for All' principles, all the prototypes that will be developed throughout the project will be developed from a thorough user centred design process with all testing completed with 'real' users who are able to give an expert opinion as to which aspects of the tools are suitable or unsuitable for their disability group. Several POWER-HAND prototype iterations have been produced so far following user feedback during testing. The method of adjusting and developing through the project is much more beneficial than trying to change the final production system.

26.3.1 Product Trials: 3 Phases

On the path to production prototype, alongside the ongoing development work were three main phases.

26.3.1.1 Phase 1: Testing with Partners

POWER-HAND was initially tested briefly with work colleagues and partners. These were selected from areas of influence such as user requirements, quality assurance, sales and marketing. It was important at this stage to select partners who were closely related to the project and whose personal input would benefit development.

- We tested the initial prototype with a group containing between 5 and 8 members and conducted a group discussion and brainstorming session where members were invited to look at the prototype and share their comments. A few simple design errors were fixed in this manner.
- It is important that all foreseen design errors are fixed before user testing.

This method allowed us to alleviate any obvious design flaws, gave us easy and unlimited access to the subjects and enabled us to start work immediately. However, as this group had an involvement and prior knowledge of the project and also did not have any physical disabilities, it was essential to ensure that the product then went out for testing with 'real' users and with a variety of different disability groups.

26.3.1.2 Phase 2: Testing with Users

After fixing initial design errors, the UGF meeting plan became active. UGF candidates were selected based on a target market, known user groups and demographics. Every week, separate UGF meetings were run to gather data – these were in small groups of approximately 4 members with larger group meetings held quarterly. The smaller group meetings enabled us to discover in detail the difficulties people had with specific aspects of the POWER-HAND design, gather video evidence of people trying the system and conduct questionnaire studies. The larger group meetings enabled us to gather the general opinions of a larger number of people (typically 10-15 members) and to conduct brainstorming sessions.

- Through these user trials, Powerhand developed several iterations. It was important that any changes could be implemented quickly to benefit the continued gathering of data.
- Video evidence under user discretion proved to be a great aid. Many design issues were resolved through careful video analysis.

26.3.1.3 Characteristics of the User Group Forum

The main impairments of the disability groups involved in the study are summarised in Table 26.1 below:

Table 26.1. Summarising various characteristics of elderly and disabled groups within the UGF that might hinder package-opening ability.

	Visual Imp**	**Weak -ness**	**Pain**	**Dext-erity Imp****	**Stiffness / Reduced Motion**	**Sensi-tivity Loss**	**Tremor/ Spasm**
Elderly	✓	✓	✓		✓	✓	
Cerebral Palsy		✓		✓			✓
Multiple Sclerosis	✓	✓		✓		✓	✓
Arthritis		✓	✓	✓	✓		
Parkinson's Disease		✓		✓	✓		✓
Stroke		✓*	✓			✓	
Arthro-gryposis		✓			✓		
Osteo-porosis		✓	✓				
Spina Bifida		✓			✓		

* one-sided weakness or paralysis is a common result of stroke.
** Imp = Impairment

26.3.1.4 Protocol for the User Group Forum Meetings

Initial trials focussed on examining opening aids currently available. Four tools were selected that require different opening techniques, squeezing and twisting for example. We decided to concentrate on a small number of typical tools in the initial UGF meeting so that we could identify the positive and negative aspects of each tool and the specific movements required by the users of different disability to use the tool. Suggestions as to how users felt the features of these tools might be improved were also gathered.

Participants were also asked to bring in any devices which they currently used at home. These were examined by the group and comments were given.

The larger group meetings held in September and December followed the same basic protocol expanded to include a larger selection of opening tools in addition to the PACKAGE POWER-HAND prototype tools. During the meetings, lunch was provided and travel expenses were offered to participants.

Members of the User Group Forum were videoed trying to open a selection of bottles and jars with their hands. Thus, the opening could be studied later, to see how the user attempted to open the packaging and what problems, if any, it posed. If they were unable to open the packaging they were asked in the initial meetings to try either a device which they usually used at home, or one of the low tech opening devices currently available.

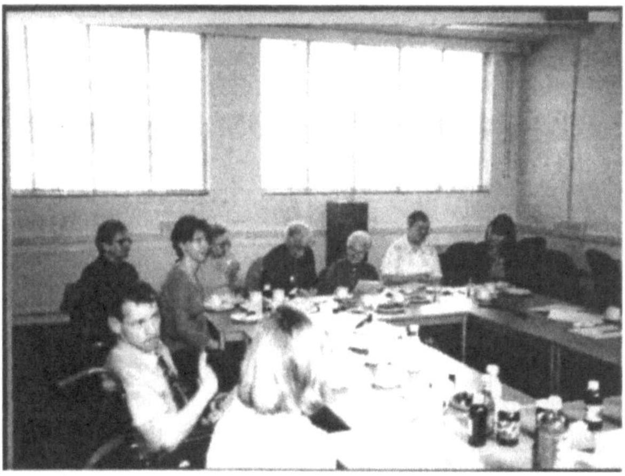

Figure 26.1. The first User Group Forum meeting

Whilst attempting to open the jars, participants were asked to think about how difficult or easy they found the task and how comfortable or uncomfortable it felt.

The final POWER-HAND prototype was presented to subjects individually and a questionnaire study conducted. This gave us the opportunity to conduct an in-depth interview and to ensure that responses were given to all questions. Also, it avoided the bias that could have occurred if the users had tried to use POWER-HAND in front of the rest of the group. After each meeting, the information obtained was presented to the designers who took the views into account during each iteration of POWER-HAND. The relationship between the researchers and the UGF has remained strong throughout the project and we now have a large database of users who would be willing to participate in future

26.3.1.5 Phase 3: Potential Manufacturers

Once a good final prototype design was developed, the design was taken to potential manufacturers identified early in the PACKAGE project

We were able to demonstrate that:

- all applicable European Standards had been met;
- POWER-HAND had achieved commercial product protection at an early point.

Convincing a major brand to agree to the manufacture of Powerhand required the demonstration of commercial value. At this stage, compiled usability data provided design conclusions and validated the decisions taken.

An additional marketing questionnaire conducted with people of all ages provided effective sales potential - surprisingly of the people surveyed, a large percentage of those under 25 years old would buy a product to aid package opening.

A successful meeting was arranged with production and marketing directors to demonstrate the effectiveness of the design and communicate the usability and market results.

26.4 POWER-HAND: Final Design Overview

The design of POWER-HAND incorporated users comments in order to develop a product accessible by a large and varied population. Some examples of the main problems the User Group found with the existing tools and how the development of POWER-HAND has tried to overcome these are listed below.

- The tools often required too much dexterity of the user groups, for example, placing a loop around a bottle top or opening handles in order to place over the top of a tool. The POWER-HAND has been designed to be as simple as possible so that even people with very limited movement in their fingers could benefit from the system.
- The plastic of some tools was too rigid. Many people commented that they would prefer a softer or smoother material, which would not hurt their hands as they held it. POWERHAND tools are made from smooth, rounded materials.
- Many tools required a two handed operation which often meant that it was difficult for people to secure the product during opening. The central holder of the POWER-HAND will allow users to secure their product whether opening by hand or one of the tools provided, also we have intended our tools to be operable by one hand for the majority of users.

- Often tools required a twisting or turning action, which proved painful and impossible for some of the disability groups with conditions such as arthritis.
- Similarly, squeezing actions often proved difficult. The POWER-HAND enables the user to open screw top jars and bottles by simply holding the electric holder and pressing down on the jars. For particularly stubborn jars, the jar pop can be used prior to the electric opener to release the vacuum seal.
- Some of the tools studies worked well but had gnarled or ridged edges which several users stated dug into their hands which were often swollen and painful. Therefore, the POWER-HAND tools have all got smooth edges which should not hurt the user.

These findings were amongst many that were taken into consideration whilst designing the final POWER-HAND prototype.

26.4.1 Final Prototype Design

A final POWER-HAND prototype was developed following the end of the user requirements analysis, incorporating as many desirable features as possible. The User Group Forum stated that the five tools which they would find most useful would be:

- holder;
- jar pop;
- bag slicer;
- ring-pull opener;
- electric jar opener;
- metal bottle top opener.

Thus these tools have been incorporated into the current multi-purpose POWER-HAND prototype and the device is currently undergoing user evaluation in the UK, France and Italy.

POWER-HAND consists of two modular units:

1. Hand-held electrical opener with ergonomic grip – Ergonomic enclosure with a powered rubber cone. Torque tests were conducted on 90 screw top packs to determine the required motor characteristics.
2. Base unit in translucent polyurethane. A central conical bottle holder is surrounded by four detachable manual tools – these tools were identified by users as being the most useful in trials. The base can be washed easily and transported without the tools becoming detached.

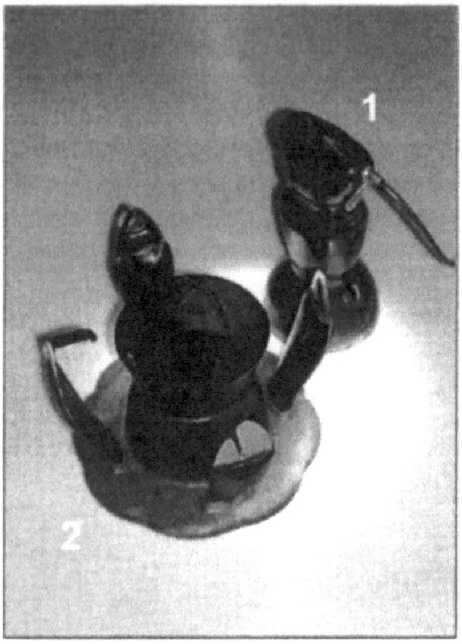

Figure 26.2. POWER-HAND prototype

26.4.2 The POWER-HAND Tools

Figure 26.3 shows the full range of POWER-HAND tools currently under development.

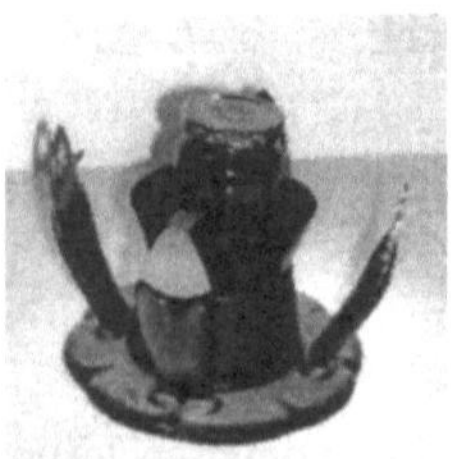

POWER-HAND Holder

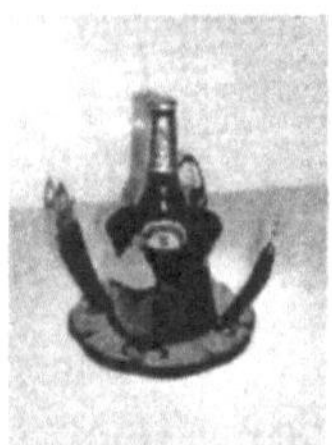

Jar in POWER-HAND holder

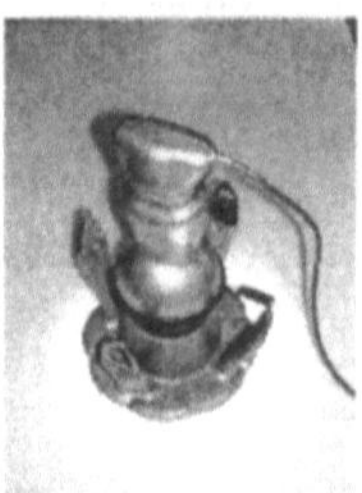

POWER-HAND Electronic Opener

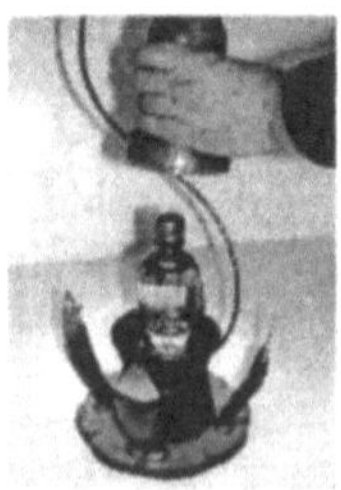

POWER-HAND Electric Opener being lowered over a bottle top

Figure 26.3. The POWER-HAND tools

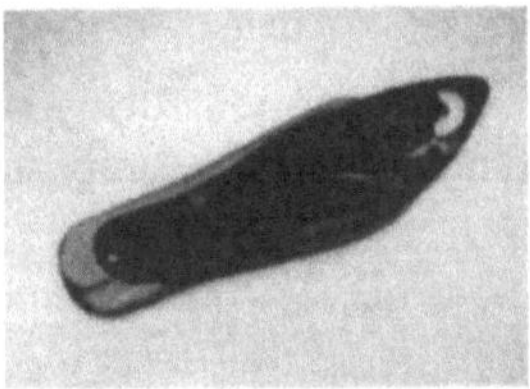

POWER-HAND Jar pop

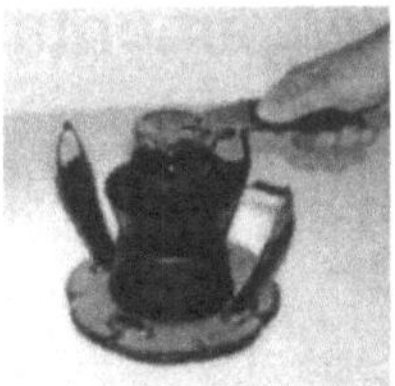

POWER-HAND JAR POP releasing vacuum on jar

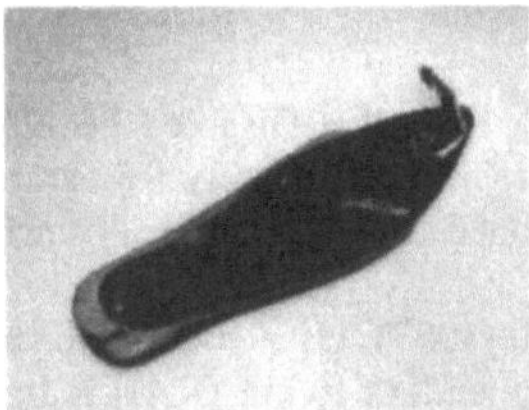

POWER-HAND Ring-pull opener

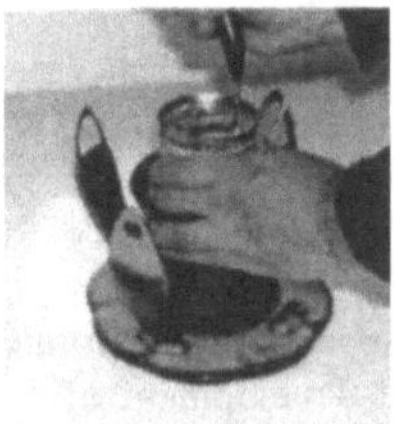

POWER-HAND Ring-pull opener hooked under ring-pull

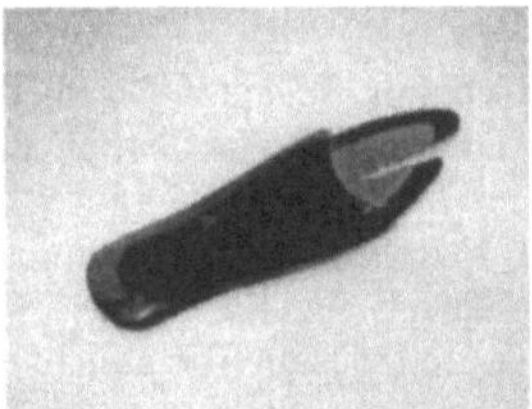

POWER-HAND Bag Slicer

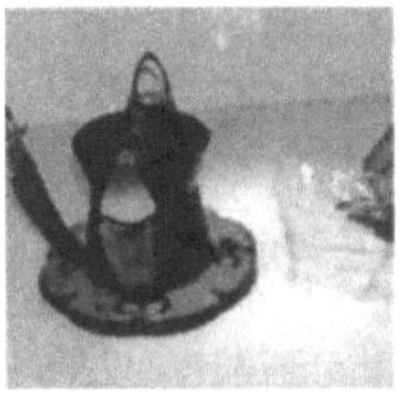

POWER-HAND Bag Slicer in use.

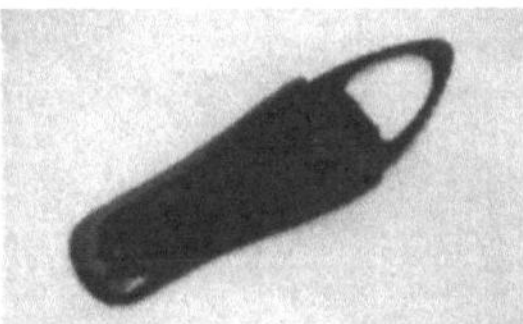

The POWER-HAND Bottle Opener

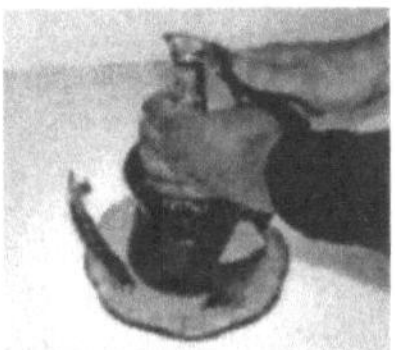

POWER-HAND Bottle Opener hooked under the bottle top.

Figure 26.3. (cont.) The POWER-HAND tools

26.5 Conclusions

Our methods of gathering user needs and interpreting the results to form successful products have been well proven. The key elements of a totally user-driven approach including a variety of able-bodied, elderly and disabled participants has ensured that Design-for-All principles have been adopted and applied. Also, the method of iteration and rapid prototyping has ensured that the design process has evolved throughout the requirements phase, giving users a chance to give real feedback on potential products and concepts. The results of the PACKAGE user requirements analysis are now being analysed and a POWER-HAND prototype is currently being evaluated in the UK, France and Italy.

26.6 Acknowledgements

The project partners are pleased to acknowledge funding from the European commission IST programme framework

26.7 References

Department of Trade and Industry (2000) A Study of the Difficulties that Disabled People have when Using Everyday Consumer Products. Government Consumer Safety Research - Department of Trade and Industry Research commissioned by Consumer Affairs Directorate, HMSO, London

Heck H, Buhler Ch, Hedenborn P, Bolmsjo G, Topping M (1997) User requirements analysis and technical development of a robotic aid to independent living (RAIL). In: Proceedings of 4th European Conference on Engineering and Medicine - Bridging East and West, Warsaw, Poland

Topping MJ (2000) Handy 1, A Robotic Aid To Independence For Severely Disabled People. In: Proceedings of RIMS Annual Conference, The Future of Rehabilitation in Multiple Sclerosis, Venice, p 21

Topping MJ, Smith J (2000) The Development of Handy 1 a Rehabilitation Robotics System. In: Proceedings of 16th IMACS World Congress, Lausanne, Switzerland

Userfit (1996) Userfit: a practical guide handbook on user-centred design for assistive technology. Brussels-Luxembourg, ECSC-EC-EAEC

Chapter 27

Locomotion Assistance for the Blind

R. Farcy and Y. Bellik

27.0 Summary

We have developed a triangulating laser telemeter adapted to the space perception for the blind: the "Teletact." Two parts compose the Teletact. The first part is a laser telemeter, which detects the distances to obstacles, and the second one is an interface, which presents these distances to the blind user. The Teletact was developed originally with a sonorous interface. Due to the long time training required by this interface we have tested some new interfaces based on other modalities (tactile and force feedback). In this chapter, we present all these interfaces and discuss them.

27.1 Introduction

The long cane is the most popular navigational aid for the blind. It is relatively easy to use, light and not expensive. However its reach is very limited and it is only used to scan the ground one metre in front of the walker. Therefore blind people must be in a permanent state of muscular contraction to be able to stop suddenly at every moment. A system of high angular resolution providing information about the surrounding area in a range of a few meters could relieve blind people of some of the actual constraints and stress when walking. Previous works in this field (Blash *et al.*, 1991; Jansson, 1991), have shown the importance of such a system for mobility assistance for the blind.

We have developed a triangulating laser telemeter adapted to the space perception for the blind: the Teletact (Farcy *et al.*, 1997). The Teletact is composed of 2 parts. The first part is a laser telemeter, which detects the distances to obstacles, and the second one is an interface, which presents these distances to the blind user. The Teletact was developed originally with a sonorous interface. Due to the long time training required by this interface we have tested some new interfaces based on other modalities (tactile and force feed-back). In this chapter, we present all these interfaces and discuss them.

27.2 Description of the Teletact

The Teletact is a hand held laser telemeter (Farcy *et al.*, 1997). The distance to the first obstacle encountered by the laser beam is measured with about 1% accuracy in the 10cm – 10 m range. Figure 27.1 gives the basic scheme of the telemeter, and Figure 27.2 shows the original commercial device. The blind person perceives the direction he points thanks to the internal consciousness of the position of its members (proprioception). To identify an obstacle it is necessary to scan the environment. The rate of distance measurements is 40 measurements per second.

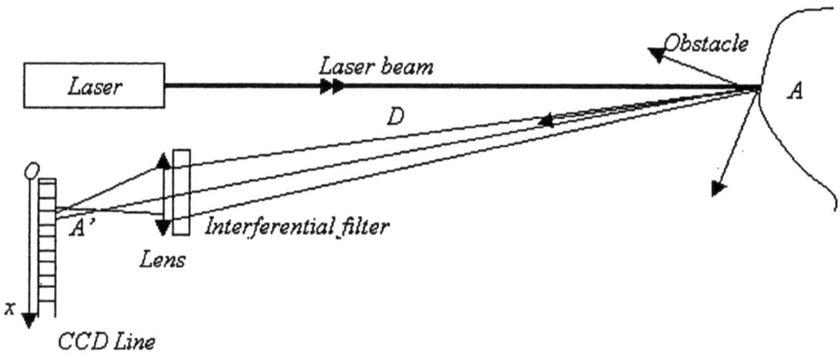

Figure 27.1. Basic principle of the Telemeter

The laser diode emits a collimated one milliwatt 670 nm laser beam. The beam meets the obstacle at a distance D and creates a laser spot A. The image of the laser spot A through the lens on the CCD line is A′. The position of A′ on the line gives the distance D. As we can see on the figure, for $x_{A'}$ great, D is short. The basic principle is very simple, the main difficulty is to achieve immunity to diurnal light (i.e. up to 200klux summer sunny days), that need some optical and electrical additive systems.

27.3 Description of the Interfaces Tested

In this section, we describe the principles of the different tested interfaces: the sonorous interface, the tactile interface and the force-feedback interface. We have exclude electro-tactile interfaces because they are very uncomfortable and their installation is too complex (Kaczmarek *et al.*, 1991; Szeto *et al.*, 1982). In the next section, we will compare and discuss these three interfaces.

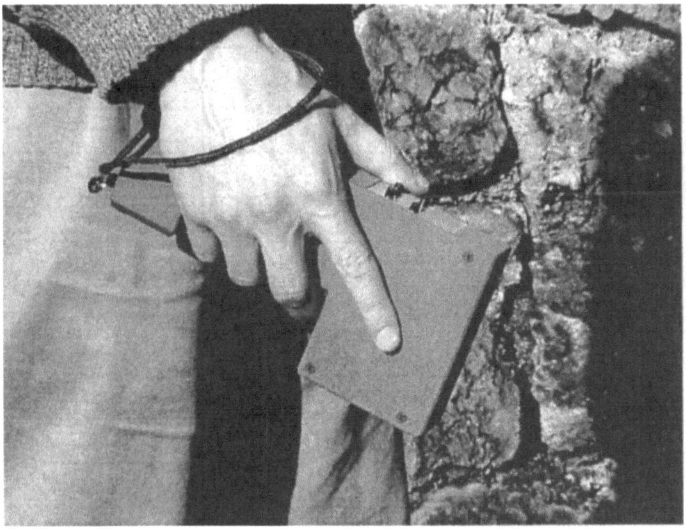

Figure 27.2. Photo of the Teletact

27.3.1 The Sonorous Interface

To communicate to the blind the information of distance, we use 28 different musical notes, which correspond to 28 unequal intervals of distances (intervals are smaller at short distances), the higher the tone, the shorter the distance. The telemeter gives a precision of about 1% on the distance measurement. The number of available musical notes is then the limitation for the precision. We use flute sounds over 4 octaves of the major scale (131Hz, 2.1 kHz). We have finally 28 useful notes. The range 10 cm - 30 m is divided in 28 unequal intervals of distance so as to reduce the width of the intervals at short distances. The correspondence between notes and distances is given in table 27.1. The most important information is not identification of musical notes but the sense and the rate of their variations, in other word the transcription of the profile of the obstacles into a "melody."

Table 27.1. Correspondence between musical notes and distance intervals.

Distance interval (cm)	Musical note	Frequency (Hz)
12 - 16	B	1974
16 - 21	A	1760
21 - 27	G	1567
27 - 34	F	1396
34 - 42	E	1318

Table 27.1. (cont.) Correspondence between musical notes and distance intervals.

Distance interval (cm)	Musical note	Frequency (Hz)
42 - 51	D	1174
51 - 61	C	1046
61 - 72	B	987
72 - 84	A	880
84 - 97	G	783
97 - 111	F	698
111 - 126	E	658
126 - 142	D	587
142 - 160	C	523
160 - 180	B	492
180 - 205	A	440
205 - 235	G	391
235 – 270	F	348
270 - 310	E	329
310 – 360	D	293
360 - 420	C	261
420 – 500	B	246
500 – 600	A	220
600 – 730	G	195
730 – 900	F	174
900 – 1200	E	164
1200 – 2000	D	146
2000 – 3000	C	131

Figure 27.3 represents musical lines corresponding to 2 different profiles. The lower line in white notes concerns the profile of a down stairs in a moving up movement of the wrist. The musical line in black notes represents the reference profile obtained with the same movement of the hand if the floor was remaining horizontal, without stairs. In this example, the white and black colours should not be interpreted as note lengths. We use these 2 colours just to distinguish the 2 profiles The distance intervals corresponding to the different musical notes are chosen so as a flat floor would correspond as best as possible to a temporal regular

musical scale (in the case of a fluid movement of the wrist). In other cases neither the succession of the intervals between the notes, nor the duration of the notes are regular.

We can see in Figure 27.3 that for the down stairs the distance increases more rapidly than for a flat floor and that the profile discontinuities of the stairs are reverberated on the note succession and duration. The identification of the down stairs relative to the flat floor do not result in practice to an analyse note by note of the correspondence between musical note and distance. A flat floor corresponds to a particular melody, and a down stair corresponds to another one. Actually, the perception of space profiles are achieved thanks to melody identification processes developed by the users.

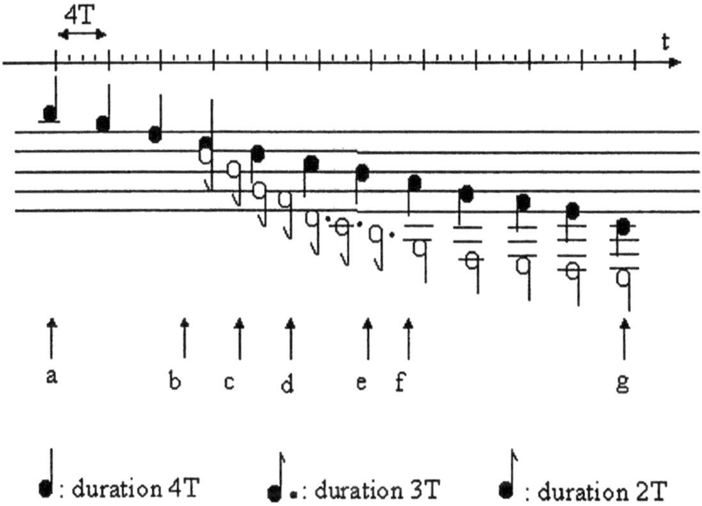

Figure 27.3. Musical lines corresponding to 2 profiles: down stairs and flat floor

27.3.2 The Tactile Interface

To obtain a silent device we replaced the sonorous output by vibrating devices localised under the fingers. We tested the tactile interface under 2 ways: in the first way we used two vibrating devices and in the second way we used eight vibrating devices.

27.3.2.1 Using Two Vibrating Devices

To code the distance we used two effects on the first vibrating device: the vibrating amplitude increases as the distance to the obstacle decreases, at the same time the period of the vibration decreases. So a decrement of the distance to an obstacle is coded by an increment of the amplitude of the vibration and a decrement of the vibrating period. The second vibrating device is used to code the detection of discontinuities on the floor; we use a 50 ms strong burst of vibration.

27.3.2.2 Using Eight Vibrating Devices

Using only 2 devices appears not to be precise enough. We decided then to experiment the use of eight vibrating devices (Figure 27.4). The principle is that each vibrating device corresponds to a particular distance interval. The users can use this interface in two different ways depending on their preferences. The first way consists in putting the index finger on the vibrating devices to feel the vibrations. The second way consists in putting a different finger between each couple of two vibrating devices. This method requires using four fingers.

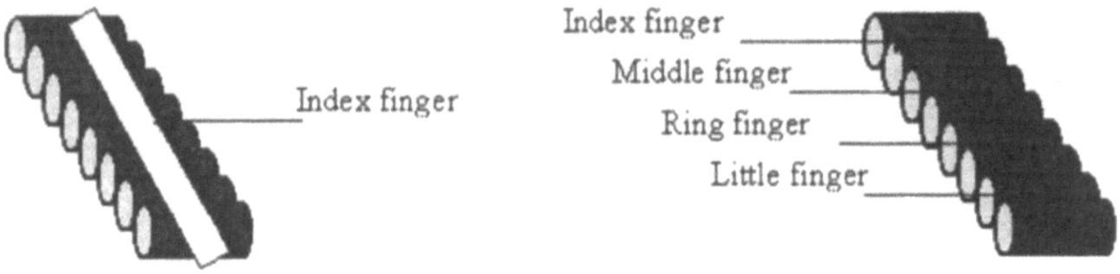

Figure 27.4. The 2 ways of using the 8 vibrating devices interface

27.3.3 The Force Feedback Interface

The principle of the force feedback interface (Figure 27.5) consists in using a linear potentiometer. The cursor of the potentiometer can be used as a mean to adjust the length of a virtual walking stick. When the user moves the cursor forward the length of the virtual walking stick increases. When he moves the cursor backward, the length decreases. When the virtual walking stick reaches an obstacle, the user feels that he cannot increase the length of the stick because the cursor is blocked.

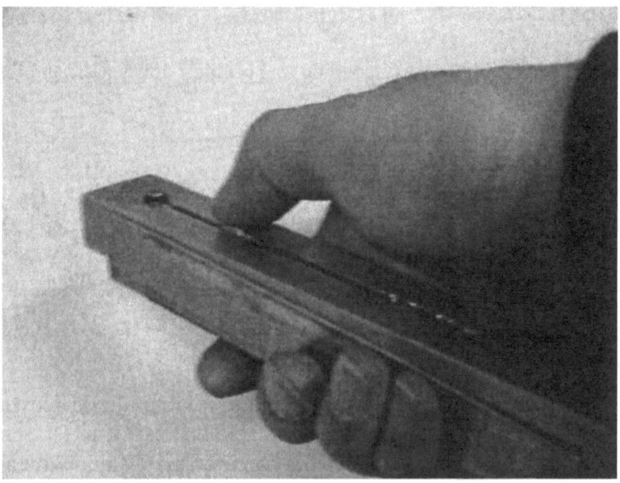

Figure 27.5. The force feedback interface

27.4 Discussion

The sonorous interface has various defects. To make the difference between musical sounds and street sounds is not really a problem. An earphone is used to clearly ear the information. When the ambient sonorous level often fluctuates it is possible to adjust the sonorous level. The real problem is that some people have difficulties to merge rapidly the sonorous information with the proprioceptive one (movement of the wrist) to deduce spatial data. This information merge has to become instinctive after learning, and if the person has to think about it, using the device becomes a too difficult intellectual work.

Using the vibrating interface is easier; the perception is more direct and intuitive. Beginners generally prefer it. People trained to sonorous output say it's less precise but sufficient. The 8 vibrating devices interface seems to be better than the 2 device one and users prefer to use it according to the second way.

The force feedback interface is a promising solution but it still presents some technical problems. The device presents watertightness problems. So, it is not possible to use it under raining weather. Another technical problem is that the motor used with the potentiometer presents some weakness after a long time use.

However we are now sure of different points: in its actual form, using the Teletact needs a good spatial representation, a good proprioception, and an active attitude: to scan to look for obstacles. It is very difficult for blind from birth to use it because of lack in spatial representation. For old persons (although we get some exceptions) it is difficult because of the long learning period. The main advantage of the device is the good anticipation users get and the optimisation of the navigation. For the moment it is a system for typically very active 20-40 year blind persons who have seen before.

The sonorous interface has been evaluated with about 50 persons. The tactile interface is still under evaluation and the results presented here have been deduced from preliminary tests.

Finally, it is important to notice that the long cane is not only an obstacle detector for blind persons but it is also a mean which allows sighted people to recognise blind people. Consequently, our device must be used complementarily with the long cane because it is not an indicator of blindness.

27.5 Conclusion

We have presented a laser profilometer dedicated to the spatial perception for the blind. We have tested the sonorous interface with about 50 blind persons for detection of obstacles, avoiding holes, using the orientation of a wall to find his way... A training course is necessary to use correctly the profilometer. For congenital blindness, the procedure is longer, the three dimensional spatial representation of space and perspective laws have to be learnt (Damashani *et al.*, 1999). It is developed in association with the centre of locomotion of the Association Valentin Haüy (Paris). The tactile and force feedback interfaces are still under experiment, but the tests we have made with 3 blind persons gave us very encouraging results. These interfaces still have large possibilities of improvement. In particular we will try in the future to experiment multimodal interfaces (Bernsen, 1994; Oviatt *et al.*, 2000). Combining touch with sound, for instance by using touch in normal situations and sound in dangerous situations.

27.6 References

Blash BB, Long RG (1991) Use or non-use of electronic travel aids in the united states. In: Proceedings of the 6th International Mobility Conference, Madrid, Spain, pp 49-58

Bernsen NO (1994) Modality theory in support of multimodal Interface design. In: Proceedings of the AAAI Spring Sympoium on Intelligent Multi-Modal Systems, pp 37-44

Damaschini R, Farcy R (1999) A space perception aid for the blind, ODIMAP II, Pavia, Italy

Farcy R, Damaschini R, Milchberg N, Sampaio E, Brenière Y (1997) Laser profilometer as a three-dimensional space perception system for the blind. In: Proceedings of Bios Europe 97, San Remo Italy

Farcy R, Damaschini R (1997) Triangulating laser profilometer as a three dimensional space perception system for the blind. Applied Optics

Jansson G (1991) The functions of present and future electronic travel aids for visually impaired children and adults. In: Proceedings of the 6th International Mobility Conference, Madrid, Spain, pp 59-64

Kaczmarek KA, Webster JG, Bach-y-Rita P, Tompkins WJ (1991) Electrotactile and vibrotactile displays for sensory substitution systems. IEEE Transactions on Biomedical Engineering 38(1)

Oviatt S, Cohen P, Wu LZ, Vergo J, Duncan L, Suhm B, Bers J, Holzman T, Winograd T, Landay J, Larson J, Ferro D (2000) Designing the user interface for multimodal speech and pen-based gesture applications: State-of-the-art systems and future research directions. Human-Computer Interaction 15(4): 263-322

Szeto AYJ, Saunders FA (1982) Electrocutaneous stimulation for sensory communication in rehabilitation engineering. IEEE Transactions on Biomedical Engineering BME-29(4)

Chapter 28

'Keep Taking the Medication': Assistive Technology for Medication Regimes in Care Settings

S. Kember, K. Cheverst, K. Clarke, G. Dewsbury, T. Hemmings, T. Rodden and M. Rouncefield

28.1 Introduction

This chapter presents some of the early design work of the 'Care in the Digital Community' research project - begun under the EPSRC IRC Network project EQUATOR. One objective of the project is to improve the quality of everyday life by building and adapting technologies for a range of user groups and application domains. Consequently, it is very much concerned with developing supporting technologies based on a comprehensive understanding of user needs. Meeting this objective will require us to address fundamental and long-term research challenges in how computing technologies and concepts relate and adapt to a range of everyday domestic environments, including those characterised as 'care' settings. The Digital Care project employs a multidisciplinary research team to facilitate the development of enabling technologies to assist care in the community for particular user groups with different support needs. The general aim is to examine how digital technology can be used to provide various kinds of support to sheltered housing residents and their staff. Although the project anticipates exploring the affordances of a variety of technological configurations, including the use of virtual environments replicating real world situations and the use of handheld and wearable digital technology, the focus of this chapter is on our early work on providing support for the medication regime.

Gaining a comprehensive understanding of needs or a perspicuous view on user requirements in this domain poses a number of interesting methodological challenges. It is not just that many of the important ethical and deployment issues concerning the development, deployment and evaluation of real systems remain unexplored, but that methods for eliciting needs in such a complex setting are relatively under-developed. Moreover, any system of determining needs must reflect the complexity of this multifaceted state (Sheaff, 1996). There are issues concerning the translation of the identified needs into a realistic, practical solution that can enable the person within their daily routine. Domestic environments in general and 'care' settings in particular are very different spaces from working environments and represent a very different set of challenges for those involved in the design of systems. Technology can benefit disabled and older people.

> *The benefits can be measured in terms of the extent to which they may be able to live more independently and, importantly, the extent to which they may be empoered and socially included though availability and use of such technologies.*
>
> (Fisk, 2001)

When technology is incorporated within the home, the people who live with the technology on a day-to-day basis have tended to be overlooked (Tweed and Quigley, 2000). It is also important to recognise that the imposition of technology must be undertaken in such a way that it does not remove choice and control from the user (Fisk, 2001). These people not only include the occupants of the living space but the support workers and others who have regular access to the domestic space. Technology can be incorporated into the person's life, such that they come to depend on it as Lupton and Seymour (2000) suggest:

> *Any human body using any form of technology may be interpreted as in some way adopting prostheses to enhance its capacities. Nearly everyone in contemporary western societies has developed a close dependency on technologies to function in everyday life, such as using spectacles to see clearly or a car to achieve greater mobility. As this suggests, the category of 'disability' is not fixed, but rather is fluid and shifting, a continuum rather than a dichotomy.*

The nature of the home, and the character of everyday home life is evolving and undergoing constant change in definition and is thus required to be responsive to the needs of people throughout their whole lifetime. Any design process requires the designer to consider the home from a proactive and lifetime perspective:

> *The home as a fixed entity is unresponsive and unable to accommodate the new demands placed upon it. The social care/housing sectors act as reactive bodies to situations such as this and provide mechanical aids to enable the individual to reside within the home, but here there are obvious limitations and constraints embedded in this process. The home, it is contended, should be considered as more than just a physical entity.*
>
> (Dewsbury and Edge, 2001)

The Digital Care project has begun to explore some of the methodological options open to those working in the domestic domain, in particular the translation of research into design recommendations and the attempt to elicit or validate 'requirements.' The problem is that research in these contexts is often regarded as not only difficult, but inappropriate and intrusive. The deeply personal nature of many social activities limits just *what* can be investigated, as well as *how* it can be investigated, and reporting the interactional elements in a range of activities and contexts is often difficult. These and other delicate issues represent potentially obdurate problems and methodological responses have taken a number of forms. At present the Digital Care project research method for technology development includes experimenting with combinations of ethnographic study, user-centred design and evaluation and the use of 'cultural probes' with both residents and staff.

Ethnographic studies (Hughes *et al.*, 1993, 1994) claim to provide a 'sensitising' to the 'real world,' 'real time' character and context of everyday life and the facilitation of what Anderson (1994) calls 'the play of possibilities for design.' We are undertaking long term ethnographic, observational studies of the work of the staff as well as more 'lightweight' ethnographic studies with residents. However, the precise nature and value of the ethnographic input into design is controversial since much of our experience comes from ethnographic investigation of the workplace. It may be that we require significant shifts in our investigative techniques as well as in our understanding of design, to consider how technology relates to domestic, specifically 'care' settings and the requirement to support everyday living rather than productivity. One way in which we have attempted to increase the repertoire of available techniques is through the employment and adoption of 'cultural probes.' 'Cultural Probes' (Gaver *et al.*, 1999), originating in the traditions of artist–designers rather than science and engineering, and deployed in a number of innovative design projects (e.g. the Presence project) may prove a way of supplementing ethnographic investigations. We use 'cultural probes' (cameras, diaries, maps, dictaphones, photo-albums, postcards, etc.) in the Digital Care project, as a way of uncovering information from a group that is difficult to research by other means and as a way of prompting responses to users emotional, aesthetic, and social values and habits. The probes furthermore provide an engaging and effective way to open an interesting dialogue with users.

The eclectic approach adopted attempts to meet some of the ethical and moral dilemmas through careful involvement and acknowledgement of users in the design process. One particular technical concern, perhaps a dominant if unusual one, is that of dependability and associated issues of diversity, responsibility and timeliness (see: DIRC). Given the care setting it is imperative that technologies designed for the setting are reliable and dependable. Bjorneby (2000) notes that reliability of the technology is essential. Just as technology can enable it can equally be the cause of disablement and low self-concept. In amongst the technical challenges are other issues concerning the location of the interface, the generalisability of design solutions, the transfer of skills to real world situations, and support for independent living in the community. These challenges highlight some of the moral and ethical components of the design enterprise, in particular the need to carefully think through and balance issues of 'empowerment' and 'dependence.' As Gitlin (1995) argues:

> *The use of technology appears to present dramatic compromises in social activities, role definition, and identity.*

The challenge is to provide support for individuals in the move towards independent living, rather than create new, technological, forms of dependence. This requires a certain ethical awareness and recognition that technology can impinge on individual care pathways and sensitivity towards the social implications of any technological intervention such as that technology is not a static imposition but as Freeberg (1996) suggests:

> *Technology is a medium in which instrumental action co-ordination replaces communicative understanding through interest-biased designs. Simply put,*

sometimes technology is overextended, sometimes it is politically biased, sometimes it is both. Several different critical approaches are needed, depending on the case.

Embodying a philosophy of care into design necessitates considering issues of empowerment and dependence and then thinking how these might usefully become incorporated into design guidelines.

28.2 Hostel and Semi-Independent Living

The setting for the project is a hostel and nearby associated semi-independent living accommodation, for former psychiatric patients. The hostel is the first step for patients leaving the psychiatric wards of local hospitals that are currently being closed down. In the hostel residents are provided with a room and helped to develop independent living skills by a number of staff. Residents can then move on to the other, semi-independent living site of sheltered housing, consisting of a number of flats and bed-sits, prior to moving out to flats in the local area, or, if they need further support, back to the hostel. The overall aim of these facilities is to gradually introduce the patients back into the community and allow them to support themselves. Emphasis is on the learning of daily living routine and skills. As a general principle any technology introduced into the setting should contribute to this goal. A technology that merely completes a task for residents does little in producing independence but merely shifts reliance onto the technology.

28.3 Supporting Medication: Fieldwork

Although our research is at an early stage, a number of issues and requirements have already arisen. Initial introductory and debriefing meetings at the hostel and semi-independent living accommodation and the early ethnographic fieldwork and return of cultural probes indicate some major preoccupations of both residents and care workers. One important concern of both residents and staff focuses on issues surrounding the routine taking of daily medication. Many of the residents are on daily medication regimes and a number of residents have expressed concern about the possible grave consequences of them forgetting to take their medication. Observation and interview confirm the role of the medication regime in the maintenance of normal everyday life and residents emphasised their, often graphic, fears and anxieties over the likely consequences of forgetting their medication.

Medication issues - dosage, delivery of 'medi-pacs,' reminders, re-assuring residents about delivery and so on also feature heavily in the everyday work of the staff. At the hostel medication is kept in a locked drug cabinet, distributed by the staff when required with records kept in a written log. At the semi-independent living site patients must manage their own medication and, as stated, it is a source of continuing anxiety. Although provided with a week's supply of packaged daily doses by the pharmacy - 'medi-pacs' - there is some concern that they may either forget to take their medication or accidentally overdose. Technical devices that may prove useful in these circumstances are various medication reminders that help patients manage their own medication, i.e. when to take it, record acknowledgements of reminders and so on allied with a system to automate the recording of drug information. But the functionality of any technology provided must be carefully considered and sensitively deployed. The devices are intended to act as 'reminders' to residents to take their medication and are not indicators that any medication has been taken and obviously such devices must be dependable as failure of the technology could have potentially disastrous consequences.

Where residents are responsible for taking their own medication, this fact has significant implications for the way in which medication is monitored and tracked. For example, the use of a bar-code scanning approach would place an inappropriate burden on the resident. One possible approach we have considered for the hostel has been to use RFID-based smart labels in order to ascertain whether a resident has taken their medication from the medication store - as used in the 'Magic Medicine Cabinet' system (Dadong, 1999). Another possibility we have explored is building certain reminder and recording features into the 'medi-packs' themselves. While this will not control the medication regime to prevent deliberate overdosing, it may contribute to the prevention of accidental overdosing. Some instances from the early fieldwork - coincidentally occurring on the same day - illustrate this point. In one case the care worker, following a phone call from the resident's doctor was concerned to intercept the delivery of a 'medi-packs' in order to replace one dosage of tablets with another. In another incident there was some concern that an elderly resident was accidentally overdosing as a consequence of the design and delivery system for the 'medi-packs.' As the 'medi-packs' are delivered from the pharmacy at about 6:30pm the resident was required to take only the evening dose for that day, leaving the two earlier doses to be taken the next week. Problems were arising both because the resident, used to emptying each daily dose, was accidentally overdosing by taking all the medication for the delivery day, but also was being left with no morning or afternoon medication for the same day on the following week. Finally, one of the residents deliberately overdosed by taking all the medication in the newly delivered 'medi-pack.' This incident also highlighted other issues to do with medication and the recording of, access to and integration of information as the care worker gave information on the resident and the medication to the ambulance service.

28.4 Requirements

The initial studies have identified a range of requirements regarding the resident's medication and the design of technologies to support the medication regime (Cheverst *et al.*, 2001). In the semi-independent living area residents are expected to manage their own medication and weekly supplies are provided by the pharmacy packaged into individual doses within a plastic container known as a 'medipack' (Figure 28.1). This arrangement causes anxiety and inconvenience for both staff and residents. Residents, who have previously relied on the staff to provide their medication at the correct time, must now remember what to take and when, leading to worries about missed medication, taking pills at the wrong time or even accidental overdoses. This in turn, leads to residents relying on staff to provide reassurance about the medication and in some cases reminders of when and what to take. This kind of reliance is detrimental to the aims of the semi-independent unit and a solution that bridges the two stages was thought to be desirable.

In order to achieve this intermediary stage residents primarily need a system that will reassure them that they are following the correct regimen, whilst leaving the task of managing their medication in their own hands. It is important that the system does not take over the task for them completely as many commercial products attempt to do by fully automating the dispensing of drugs at the correct time. The aim here is not to automate a task and remove a cognitive load, but to encourage self-reliance and allay any fears of getting it wrong. In addition to these requirements it would also be desirable to provide some form of unobtrusive feedback, accessible by the staff for monitoring the residents progress. This function of the system may be also be used to alert the staff to possible problems such as a deliberate overdose.

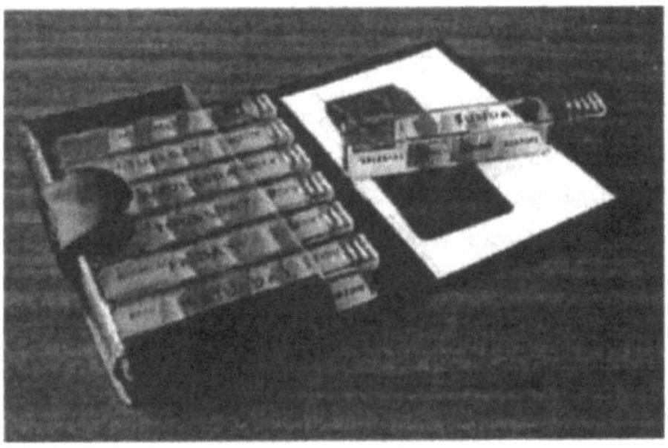

Figure 28.1. A 'medipack'

28.5 Medication manager or 'MediPic'

Initial design proposals looked at augmenting the medipack, but observation showed that residents did not tend to carry the medipack with them and therefore a mobile system was not required. The current system consists of a simple box divided into compartments separating individual doses. This compact form-factor can be easily restocked and delivered to the resident's accommodation and is therefore a positive point to carry over into the new design. The box itself would not be augmented but exist as a replaceable 'cartridge' for a separate housing containing the medication management device. Figure 28.2 illustrates the design for the initial prototype device.

The transparent pill container sits on top of a layer containing a grid of coloured light emitting diodes. Looking from above, each compartment has two lights to indicate which pills can be taken and which not. In this case red and green lights are used, red for stop, green for go as it is a familiar colour combination. However, it should be noted that these colours may pose a problem for some people with colour blindness and can be easily replaced with another combination. Once a pill is taken or has been missed the lights go out indicating that the compartment is no longer 'live,' and should be ignored. An initial prototype (Figure 28.3) has been constructed using this design.

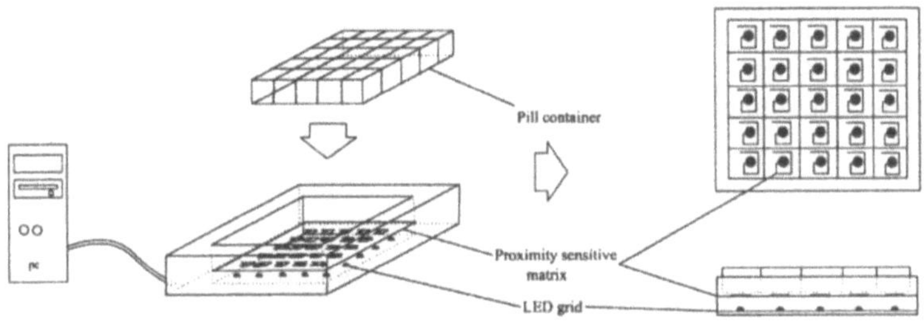

Figure 28.2. Prototype medication manager

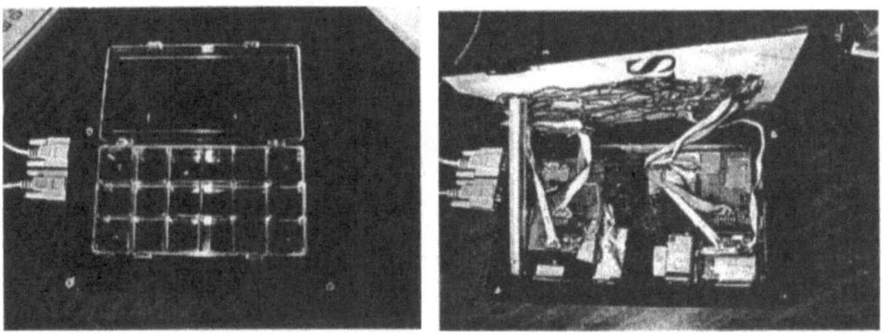

Figure 28.3. Version 1 of the medication manager. Internal view shows two circuits controlling two banks of LEDs

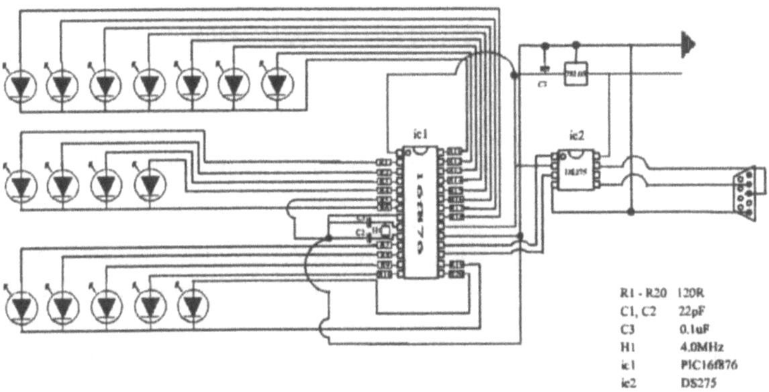

Figure 28.4. Basic circuit for serial light control in the medication manager

Control of the lights is through a simple micro controller circuit (Figure 28.4), which receives commands via a serial connection from a PC. The use of a PC as the controlling system for the medication manager, simplifies development and future prototypes will consist of an entirely embedded system. At the moment software on the controlling PC provides a calendar function controlling the lights directly (Figure 28.5). This design provides residents with visual reminders of when to take medication and provides reassurance that the correct medication is being taken. Omitting the use of audio reminders or other more tangible reminders, forces the resident to actively check on the current state of the lights thus reinforcing the routine.

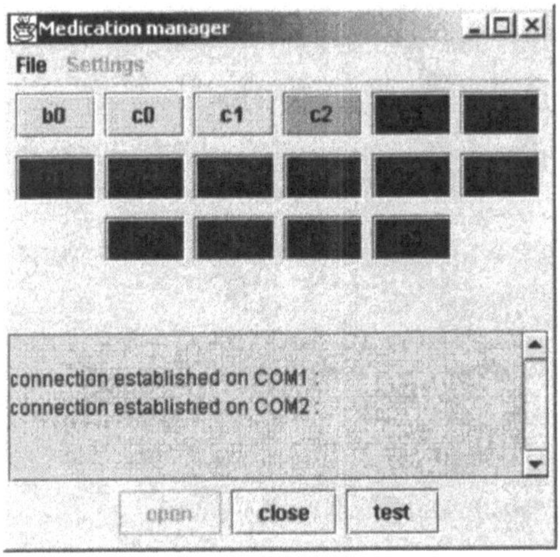

Figure 28.5. Screenshot of medication management software.

28.6 Conclusion: Research Challenges

The next version of the medication manager will be larger to allow the management of a week's supply of medication. This will involve the use of a more complex micro controller with a larger number of bi-directional I/O ports. The PIC16f876 (Microchip, 2001) currently being used, has a simple 35-word instruction set and is relatively easy to program, however, this chip has support for only 16 lights (= 4 days). The initial prototype design also includes support for feedback to the staff, though this has yet to be implemented. The design incorporates a layer of 'charge transfer' touch sensors, which can be activated through the pill container, registering a touch on the bottom surface of the container as a pill is removed. Version 2 of the prototype will incorporate this technology and will allow staff to gather data on a resident's progress in this area. This may also be of help in an emergency situation where a deliberate overdose has occurred. Information on what has been taken will be available and an early warning may be possible.

Further work is also needed to address dependability and feedback issues. It is extremely important the system function in a dependable manner before any thought of field tests is considered. We must remember that this application domain requires high standards of reliability as any failure of the system could affect the residents in an extremely adverse manner. Clearly much of the potential of assistive devices relies upon the successful operation of a range of new technologies as well as the readiness of users to accept and embrace a new technology. Just as we should not allow ourselves to rely upon overly negative stereotyping of these particular users, so too must we avoid the temptation to make exaggerated claims as to their technological adeptness. Instead we make the case that special thought needs to be given to the design of technological artefacts, that takes into account such factors as a different learning curve and a different place for the artefact within the lifestyle of the user.

Over the coming months we will be deploying the chosen solutions within the setting. This deployment process will itself raise a whole series of important and necessary issues for research into assistive technologies. Following deployment a period of evaluation will commence which (in addition to raising further issues) will no doubt lead to refinements in our initial set of requirements and therefore modifications to our adopted approach. In particular we anticipate the emergence of design challenges in matching generic and specific requirements with available technology; in addressing the 'tailorability' of COTS systems and devices; and in ensuring the delivery of genuinely mobile and dependable devices.

At present we envisage a prolonged period of extensive continuous testing to determine the systems performance, before deployment in the setting. In addition a number of design workshops have been scheduled both for user evaluation and feedback and for considering the integration of the medication manager with other devices - such as interactive picture displays or digital family portraits (Mynatt *et al.*, 2001) - that may be incorporated into the resident's home, as well as consideration of training and tailoring issues. The medication manager is thus part of an iterative design process (Clarkson and Keates, 2001), in which problem specification, matching the system to the real world and evaluation should be a continuous process. In this view design issues do not cease with the initial deployment of the device or initial evaluation, with everything occuring after this being given the status of 'maintenance.' Instead deployment is regarded as another opportunity for design considerations to be highlighted, challenged and reassessed.

This chapter has presented our early work on a project investigating the role of computing technologies in supporting a community housing project. The driving aim of the project is to explore the extent to which the requirements of a community care trust can be met by technology whilst staying within the political and ethical boundaries imposed by the given application domain. In devising a medication manager, an assistive technology supporting aspects of everyday life seldom addressed by conventional computers, we are also faced with the research challenge of investigating new aesthetics and new functionality in support of a wider range of personal and social values.The challenge is to understand how best to integrate devices into our surrounding environment and how these may be used as part of everyday life (see: Dewsbury, 2001). We need to ask whether current approaches to design are appropriate in such complex care settings. The preliminary research of the Equator project suggests that new conceptual models, theories and guidelines are needed for explaining and informing the design of these emerging technologies. It also requires a shift in research, towards using and developing theories, practices and techniques that are interdisciplinary.

28.7 Acknowledgements

This work is funded by the UK Engineering and Physical Sciences Research Council, EQUATOR and Dependability (DIRC) Interdisciplinary Research Collaborations. We also thank the Croftlands Charitable Trust for their support.

28.8 References

Anderson R (1994) Representations and Requirements: The value of Ethnography in System Design. Human-Computer Interaction 9: 151-182

Bjørneby S (2000) Signpost: 'Smart Houses': Can they really benefit Older People? 5: 2

Cheverst K, Cobb S, Hemmings T, Kember S, Friday A, Phillips P, Procter R, Rodden T, Rouncefield M (2001) Design With Care. In: Proceedings of Workshop Symposium on Adding the user into the design of the home in the Digital Age, Edinburgh

Clarkson PJ, Keates S (2001) A practical inclusive design approach. In: Proceedings of INCLUDE 2001, London, 72-73.

Wan D (1999) Magic Medicine Cabinet: A Situated Portal for Consumer Healthcare. In: Proceedings of 1st International Symposium on Handheld and Ubiquitous Computing, Karlsruhe, Germany, pp 352-355

Dewsbury G (2001) The Social and Psychological Aspects of Smart Home Technology within the Care Sector. New Technology in Human Services, Forthcoming

Dewsbury G, Edge M (2001) Designing the Home to Meet the Needs of Tomorrow ... Today: Smart technology, health and well-being. Open House International, 26(2), Available at: http://www.smartthinking.ukideas.com/_ OHI.pdf

Feenberg A (1996) Marcuse or Habermas: Two critiques of technology. Enquiry 39, 45-70

Fisk M (2001a) The implications of SMART home technology. In: Peace S and Holland C (eds.) Inclusive housing in an ageing society: Innovative approaches, Policy Press. London, pp101-124

Fisk M (2001b) In-view magazine: Focus on technical issues in housing. May 2001, Northern Ireland Housing Executive, pp30-31

Gaver W, Dunne A, Pacenti E (1999) Design: Cultural probes. In: Interactions: New Visions of Human-Computer Interaction. ACM Press

Gitlin L (1995) Why Older People Accept or Reject Assistive Technology. Generations: Journal of the American Society of Ageing 19, 1

Hughes JA, King V, Rodden T, Andersen H (1994) Moving out from the control room: Ethnography in system design. In: Proceedings of CSCW '94, Chapel Hill, NC

Lupton D, Seymour W (2000) Technology, selfhood and physical disability. Social Science and Medicine, 50: 1851-1862

Microchip (2001) Microchip PIC 16F87X data sheet. Available at: www.microchip.com

Mynatt E, Rowan J, Jacobs A, Craighill S (2001) Digital Family Portraits: Providing Peace of Mind for Extended Family Members. In: Proceedings of Conference on Human factors in computing systems (CHI '01), Seattle, ACM Press, pp 333-340

Phillip H (2001) Charge Transfer Sensing. Quantum Research Group White Paper 2001. Available at: www.qprox.com

Shaeff R (1996) The Need For Healthcare. Routledge, London

The DIRC Project - go to http://www.dirc.org.uk/

The Equator Project - go to http://www.equator.ac.uk/

Tweed C, Quigley G (2000) The design and technological feasibility of home systems for the elderly. The Queens University, Belfast

Chapter 29

"I can't talk now," and Other Design Stories: Four Assistive Technologies for People With and Without Disabilities

G. Pullin

29.1 Overview of Four Projects

This chapter seeks to challenge the division between assistive technology and design in general and argues that boundaries should be blurred: not only should design become more inclusive, but assistive technology should involve industrial and interaction designers in order to better balance emotional and functional needs.

Four of the author's projects from design consultancy and postgraduate art education are considered: The LECKEY WOOSH stander, the SPYFISH underwater video system, the BESPOKE HAND prosthesis and the PHONOPHOBIA mobile phone.

29.1.1 For People With and Without Disabilities

All four projects constitute assistive technologies, but only the LECKEY WOOSH stander and the BESPOKE HAND prosthesis are designed for people with particular disabilities. The SPYFISH underwater video system and the PHONOPHOBIA mobile phone are for people defined other than in terms of their (long-term) abilities.

The value of juxtaposing them is that each has an intimate and emotional interaction with its user. This they have in common with most medical devices, from crutches to robotic aids, which involve not only vital functionality but issues of individual identity, self-esteem and social perceptions.

29.1.2 Commercial and Exploratory Intent

The LECKEY WOOSH stander and the SPYFISH video system are commercial products developed for manufacture, whereas the BESPOKE HAND prosthesis and the PHONOPHOBIA phone are concepts intended to explore new possibilities and provoke new conversations.

Designers sometimes choose to prioritise emotional and qualitative issues in such conceptual projects in order to gain insights, but these insights will be lost if this intent is not communicated and understood.

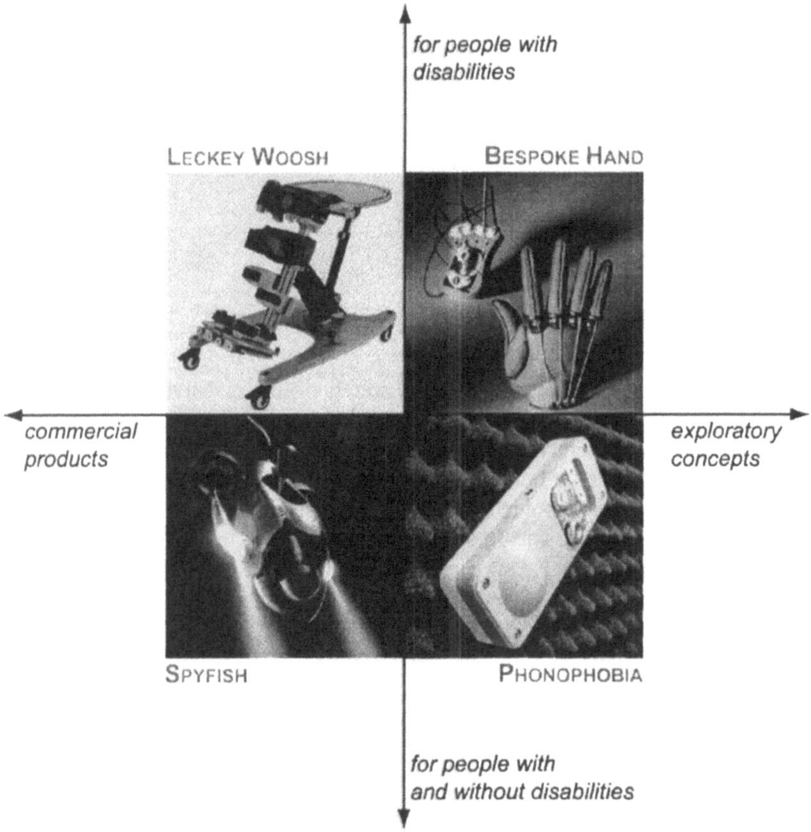

Figure 29.1. Overview of four projects

29.1.3 Four Assistive Technologies

The LECKEY WOOSH stander supports disabled children and allows them to interact with their peers face to face. (LECKEY and WOOSH are trademarks of James Leckey Design Ltd.) The SPYFISH underwater video system creates the experience of diving without getting wet. (SPYFISH is a trademark of H2Eye International Ltd.) The BESPOKE HAND prosthesis explores ways in which amputees might further express themselves through their prosthetic hands. The PHONOPHOBIA mobile phone enables emotional dialogue when a person receives a telephone call and cannot speak aloud.

29.2 LECKEY WOOSH Stander

The LECKEY WOOSH stander is a commercial product and has been in manufacture for five years. It was designed by design consultancy Isis, for and with Leckey.

This supportive furniture for children with severe disabilities provides their therapists with 25 independent adjustments, to fit it to children of different sizes and accommodate different postures. The clinical and technical demands are challenging but appearance and approachability are important too.

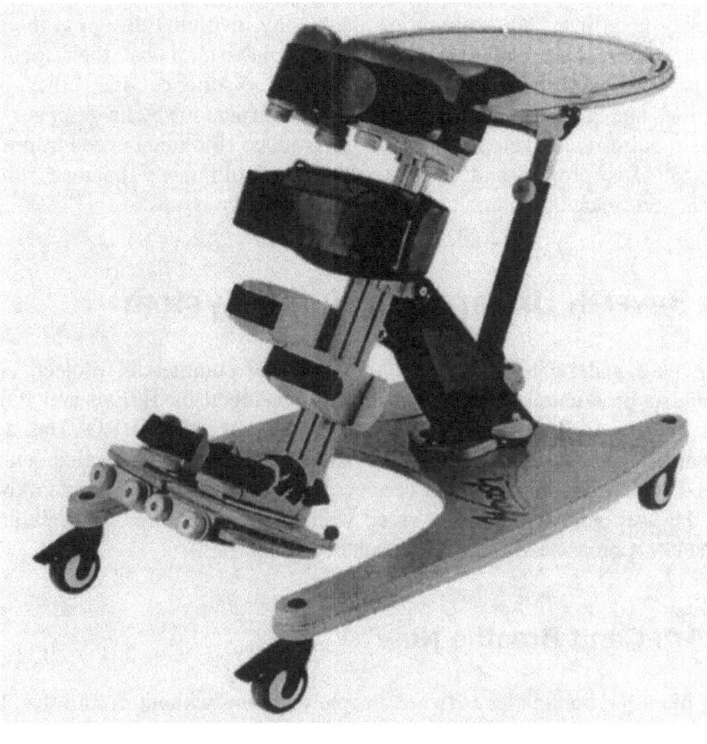

Figure 29.2. LECKEY WOOSH stander

29.2.1 Emotional Support

Supportive furniture plays an emotional role for the children themselves in their developing self-image, for their parents who may still be coming to terms with their child's disabilities, and for other children whose perceptions of any child will include anything unfamiliar.

If such assistive technology can sometimes allow disabled children to attend mainstream schools, then this is defeated if its very presence increases the social isolation of the children amongst their peers.

29.2.2 Design at the Heart

Leckey have involved graphic design and product design consultancies Triplicate and Isis as part of their multidisciplinary team of occupational therapists, physiotherapists, engineers, marketing and manufacturing departments and children and their parents.

> *"[Leckey] wanted to look at cosmetic aspects; not for the sake of it, but primarily to focus on the needs of the user."*
>
> (Evamy, 1997)

Leckey is an inspiring example of a company involving design at the heart of equipment for people with disabilities. They understand that their identity and products both contribute to their customers' experience and other people's perceptions and that good design is often most conspicuous by its absence.

This requires the development team to introduce emotional needs from the very beginning of a project and to be prepared to ultimately balance functional, technical and financial criteria against more qualitative issues.

29.3 SPYFISH Underwater Video System

The SPYFISH underwater video system is another commercial project, currently approaching production. It has been jointly developed by H2Eye and IDEO and reinvents the marine researcher's remotely operated vehicle (ROV) as a leisure experience. The system includes a miniature remote-controlled submarine equipped with video cameras and connected to the surface by a cable. Above the water, the user watches real-time video with overlaid graphics, and interacts with the SPYFISH submarine via a wireless hand control.

29.3.1 "I Can't Breathe Now"

Diving blurs the boundaries between people with and without disabilities, because everyone is disabled when it comes to breathing underwater. We all require assistive technology, be this an aqualung or a SPYFISH video system.

29.3.2 Can't Dive? Won't Dive!

If 'disability' instead means being denied access to existing assistive technology, then the SPYFISH video system could be considered an alternative to scuba-diving equipment. This alternative is equally available to those who can't dive due to a disability, don't know how to dive or don't want to dive, as well as those who can and do dive (and the development team included people from each of these groups). This represents a broad cross-section of users and a large potential market.

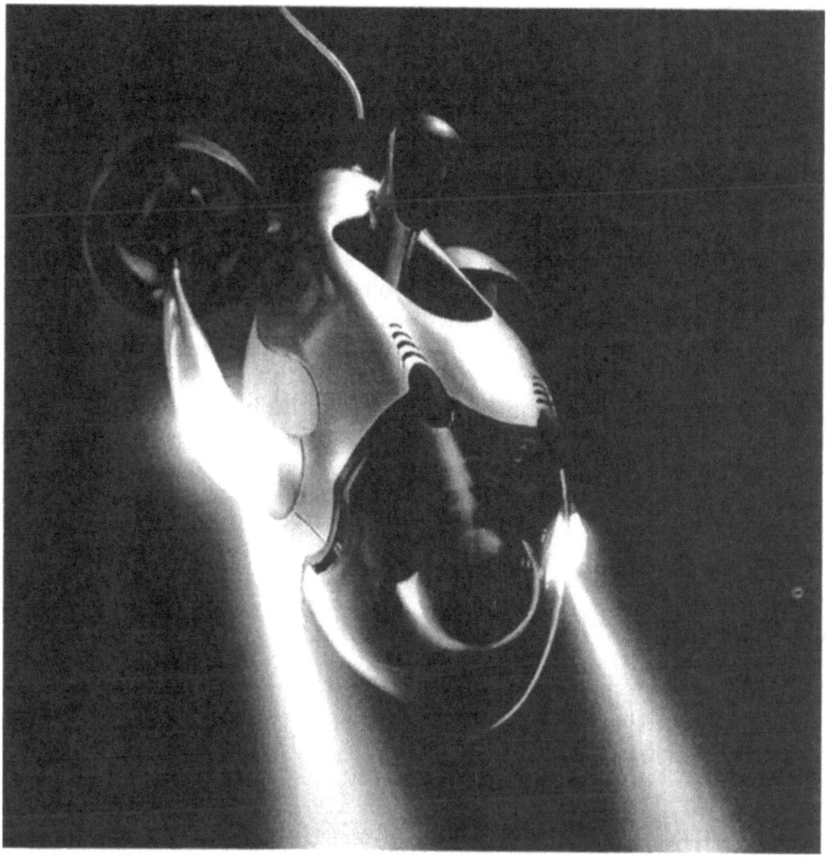

Figure 29.3. SPYFISH underwater video system

29.3.3 Interaction Design

A large multidisciplinary team including human factors experts, engineers and programmers designed the SPYFISH interface to be an iconic, intuitive and immersive experience. However the recently recognised discipline of interaction design more than any other was responsible for defining this experience.

Interaction design has emerged from the art college disciplines of information, graphic and computer-related design. The role of the interaction designer is to balance qualitative and quantitative issues, combining a feel for behaviour, choreography and aesthetics (and sometimes surprise and intrigue) with an understanding of information, navigation and functionality.

Dynamic graphics and sounds are overlaid onto the SPYFISH video to provide additional feedback, but so as to enhance the overall experience of 'swimming' underwater, not detract from it.

29.3.4 Can't Use? Won't Use!

The physical controls for the five degrees of freedom on the SPYFISH submarine are one-handed, so that users always have a hand free to steady themselves on a moving boat. This challenge of simple control of an inherently complex interface shares many issues with rehabilitation robotics, from which some experience was drawn (Hillman *et al.*, 1990).

No-one is dependent on using the SPYFISH system, however. In this sense the design of such a leisure experience might be seen as less critical than that of an assistive technology for daily living, but in other ways this increases the challenge: Since this is a product that no-one strictly *needs* to use, it follows that they have to *want* to use it. Designers are well practised at creating engaging and rewarding user experiences.

This book's themes of "utility, usability and accessibility" are issues in which interaction designers can complement the approaches of human factors experts, computer scientists and software engineers. Beyond these important functional requirements we should be setting our sights on engagement, experience and emotion.

29.4 BESPOKE HAND Prosthesis

The BESPOKE HAND prosthesis was a research project at the Royal College of Art. Whilst not a general rejection of the discretion of existing cosmetic hands or of the functional robustness of existing hooks, it explored an alternative approach.

29.4.1 Whose Hand is it Anyway?

In interviews, some amputees mentioned that their prescribed prosthesis wasn't 'their' hand. For one this is because the standard proportions of his prostheses are not those of his massively broad remaining hand. Another amputee said that although her prosthetic hand is a fairly realistic visual imitation to other people, it is unpleasant to the touch so she doesn't feel comfortable with it herself.

The BESPOKE HAND prosthesis aspires to be 'their' hand not as an accurate replica of an amputee's missing hand (it is an abstraction and made from wood and fabric) but because they have defined it themselves. The user chooses the materials from which their hand is made, on the basis of whatever criteria (aesthetic or tactile, ethnic or cultural) are important to them. Their hand is then made specially for them, to the proportions of their remaining hand. As no two pieces of wood are identical each hand, like each fingerprint, is unique and over time the wood ages gracefully and records its relationship with its wearer.

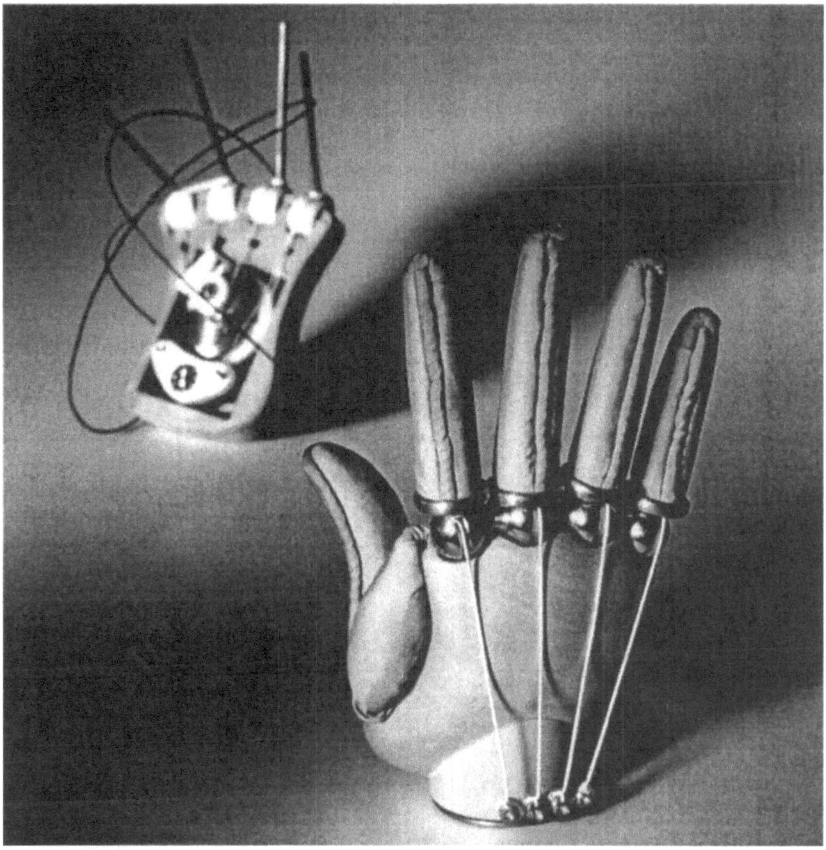

Figure 29.4. BESPOKE HAND prosthesis

29.4.2 "I Can't Point Now"

One amputee spoke of an incident when she was carrying shopping in her good hand and was asked directions in the street. She was embarrassed when she couldn't point but had to gesture with a clenched prosthetic hand. She also finds pressing buttons on lifts and buses difficult.

The BESPOKE HAND prosthesis features an indexing mechanism hidden within its palm. Operation is via a conventional shoulder harness and cable, but the user has access to different gripping actions, an open hand posture and a pointing finger.

Most textbooks focus exclusively on the different types of prehension, the opposition of surfaces of the hand to afford the grasp of objects. Hands are not just tools however, but instruments of expression, gesture and communication. These issues demand a broader definition of functionality.

29.5 PHONOPHOBIA Mobile Phone

The PHONOPHOBIA mobile phone is part of an internal IDEO project creating a series of exploratory alternatives to conventional mobile phone interactions. The target is the anti-social side effects of mobile phone use, so these concepts are designed as much for the people around the user as for the users themselves.

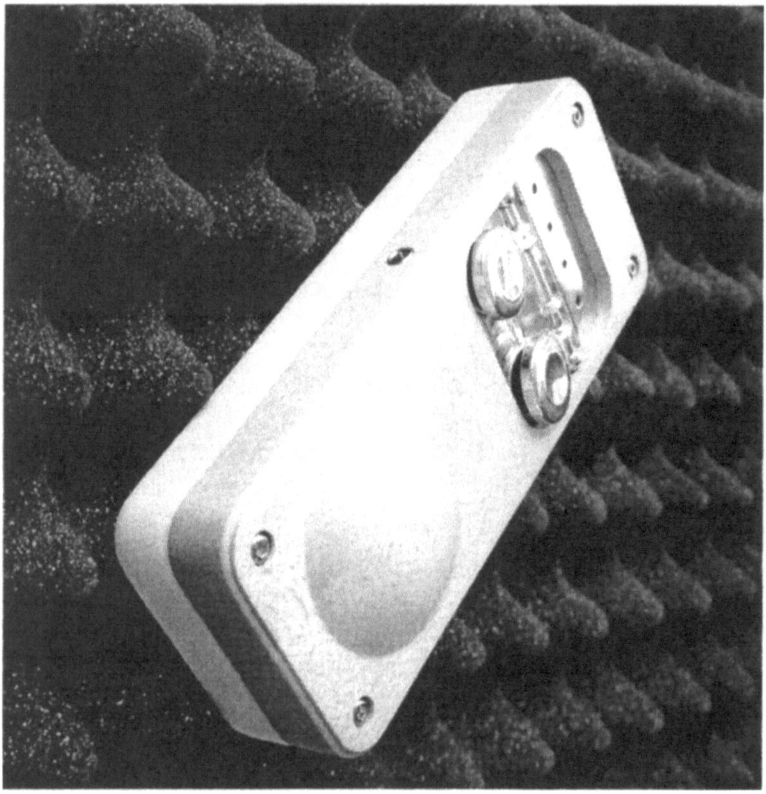

Figure 29.5. PHONOPHOBIA mobile phone

29.5.1 "I Can't Talk Now"

People receiving a telephone call in a public place, for example on a bus, face a dilemma: If they take the call, they invade the privacy of their neighbours whilst losing their own. The socially sensitive user acquires a temporary contextual disability. "I can't talk now" is often all they can say.

In this situation, as in many others, there is an overlap between the contextual needs of 'able-bodied' people and the constant needs of people with a disability, in this case speech impairment. These overlaps can inspire more inclusive design.

29.5.2 It Ain't What You Say, It's The Way That You Say It

PHONOPHOBIA means "fear of talking aloud". The user has manual control of a small number of primitive vocal sounds which only they and their caller can hear. These sounds include interjectives such as "huh" and "eh?" which people use to support and sustain even the most one-sided conversation.

Whilst the interface is restricted to simple vowel sounds, it allows subtle control of their articulation and pitch. The response "yeah" has a dozen different meanings depending on how it is said, ranging from enthusiasm to cynicism, from surprise to neutrality. With practise, all of these can be expressed.

This project re-examines the balance between functionality and expression and seeks to question the absence of prosody in both short messaging service (SMS) telephone communication and existing text to speech (TTS) communication aids.

29.5.3 "I Can't Look Now"

IDEO recently began designing another non-visual interface with a client. This is intended for a mass market of sighted users but aimed at temporary, contextual user needs where 'eyes-free' operation is beneficial or necessary, for example whilst driving a car or walking down the street.

Nonetheless we invited two blind people onto the design team for reasons we hope will prove mutually beneficial: Blind and partially-sighted people are expert users of non-visual interfaces because they rely on them. The depth of their experience is therefore unique and we believe that involving blind users will help us design a better interaction for sighted users.

In addition, our client recognises that if their product is accessible to blind and partially-sighted people then this in itself represents a sizeable and under-served market, so more inclusive (yet not 'universal') design is good business.

29.6 Conclusions

A designer's role is to balance the emotional and functional, the qualitative and quantitative aspects of a product, interaction or environment. Designers sometimes choose to prioritise these qualitative issues in conceptual projects in order to explore new possibilities, but these insights will be lost if this intent is not communicated and understood.

Involving more disabled people, and other experts in disability, in design in general, would help to make any technology more inclusive. Identifying resonance between the implications of particular disabilities and specific contextual ('able-bodied') user needs can help define inclusive yet focussed product specifications. 'Universal Access' might then be advanced through the collective availability of purposeful and well-designed alternatives.

If interaction designers and industrial designers are involved in developing assistive technologies, this will help to create user experiences which are both accessible and pleasurable. Beyond this book's themes of "utility, usability and accessibility", we should be setting our sights on engagement, experience and emotion.

29.7 Background

For the past five years, the author has practised as an interaction designer with IDEO London. Here he leads a multidisciplinary studio of human factors specialists, mechanical and software engineers, model-makers, interaction designers and industrial designers. IDEO is an international design and development consultancy. It is known for its distinctive user-focused design methodologies, including 'user experience prototyping,' and for a culture of innovation (Myerson, 2001). It designs products, services and environments across many different industries with clients ranging from multinational corporations to technology start-ups.

During the late 1980's at the Bath Institute of Medical Engineering (BIME) the author was responsible for the mechanical design of the Bath workstation and wheelchair-mounted robotic manipulators. This work was presented at the first and second Cambridge Workshops on Rehabilitation Robotics. In 1991 he left BIME to study design at the Royal College of Art, exploring prostheses and accessible interfaces for automated teller machines (ATMs). Since then the author has worked as a design consultant and project leader at Isis and IDEO on numerous products, both medical and non-medical.

29.8 References and Other Sources

Evamy M (1997) Able bodies. Design, Spring 1997, pp 20-23

Hillman MR, Pullin GM, Gammie AR, Orpwood RD, Stammers CW (1990) Development of a robot arm and workstation for the disabled. Journal of Biomedical Engineering 12: 199-204

Myerson J (2001) IDEO: Masters of innovation. Laurence King, p 157

Pullin G (1993) Prosthetic hand. MDesRCA thesis, Royal College of Art, DIC thesis, Imperial College, London

Pullin G (1992) The design of a robotic manipulator for disabled users. MPhil thesis, University of Bath

Pullin G (1991) The importance of aesthetics in the design of rehabilitation robotics. In: Proceedings of the International Conference on Rehabilitation Robotics, Atlanta, Georgia, pp 124-133

Pullin G (1986) Keyboard emulator for disabled children. BA report, Department of Engineering Science, Oxford University

Index of Contributors

Adams R. 53
Alcock S. 267
Arnott J.L. 161

Bates R. 75
Beattie W. 161
Bellik Y. 277
Bien Z. 201
Billard A. 179
Brewster S. 97
Brown D.J. 63
Brown S.S. 109

Capobianco A. 131
Carbonell N. 131
Chang P-H. 201
Cheverst K. 285
Clarke K. 285
Clarkson P.J. ... 13, 23, 33
.... 53, 87
Colello M.S. 223
Conn K. 245
Coy J. 3

Dautenhahn K. 179
Dewsbury G. 285

Evans J. 171
Evans N.M. 213

Farcy R. 277
Fergadis G. 151

Gheerawo R.R. 43
Gow D. 193
Gregor P. 171

Han J-S. 201
Hawkins P. 267
Hawley M. 235
Hemmings T. 285
Hillman M.R. 213
Hine N. 161, 171
Huxley R. 267
Hwang F. 87

Inglis E. 171
Istance H.O. 75

Jung S.H. 245

Katupitiya J. 245
Keates S. ... 13, 23, 33, 87
Kember S. 285
Kientz T. 245

Kim D-J. 201
Kumar V. 245
Kyberd P.J. 193

Langdon P. 53, 87
Lannen T.L. 63
Lebbon C.S. 43
Lesley S. 257

Mahoney R.M. 223
Malassiotis S. 151
Morasch H. 119

Newell A.F. 171
Nikolakis G. 151

O'Neill P. 235

Orpwood R.D. 213
Ostrowski J. 245

Park H-S. 201
Patel S. 245
Piéla G. 119
Pieper M. 119
Porter L.A. 257
Poulton A.S. 193
Pullin G. 295

Rao R.S. 245
Reid D. 97
Roast C. 235
Robinson P. 87, 109
Rodden T. 285
Rouncefield M. 285

Sergeant P. 161
Smith J. 267
Standen P.J. 63
Stavrakis M. 151
Stefanov D.H. 201
Szymkowiak A. 171

Taylor C.J. 245
Topping M. 267
Tzovaras D. 151

Wilson B.A. 171

Young R.T.P. 141
Yu W. 97

MIX
Papier aus verantwortungsvollen Quellen
Paper from responsible sources
FSC® C105338

If you have any concerns about our products,
you can contact us on
ProductSafety@springernature.com

In case Publisher is established outside the EU,
the EU authorized representative is:
Springer Nature Customer Service Center GmbH
Europaplatz 3, 69115 Heidelberg, Germany

Printed by Libri Plureos GmbH
in Hamburg, Germany